THE COMPLETE VITAMIN K COUNTER FOR WARFARIN USERS

MORE THAN 5500 BRAND-NAME AND GENERIC FOODS LISTED WITH VITAMIN K CONTENT

DR. H. MAHER

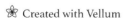 Created with Vellum

CONTENTS

INTRODUCTION

Warfarin is the most frequently used vitamin K antagonist. It is in the anticoagulant class of medication and decreases blood's ability to clot. This helps prevents new clots from forming and stops existing clots from growing larger. However, Warfarin's effectiveness is affected by vitamin K intake. Therefore Warfarin users should be consistent in how much vitamin K they get daily and aim for stable daily vitamin K intakes.

Warfarin (brand names Coumadin and Jantoven) is an anticoagulant (blood thinner) medication. It has been available in the united states since its first approval by the Food and Drug Administration (FDA) in 1954.

Warfarin is used as a valuable medication in the prophylaxis and treatment of deep vein thrombosis (DVT), pulmonary embolism (PE), atrial fibrillation (AF), and myocardial infarction.

Mechanism of Action

Warfarin blocks vitamin K from producing active clotting factors in the liver and consequently reduces the number of vitamin-K-dependent clotting factors in your blood. The anticoagulant effect of Warfarin is due to the inhibition of vitamin K epoxide reductase complex I, an enzyme required for activating the vitamin K available in the body. Your blood will then be less likely to form unwanted clots and inhibits existing clots from growing larger.

What Does Warfarin Treat?

Warfarin is commonly prescribed to:

- Prevent and manage venous thromboembolism (blood clots in the veins) and its related medical conditions, deep vein thrombosis (DVT), and pulmonary embolisms (PE).
- Prevent and treat thromboembolism in patients with atrial fibrillation, which is characterized by an irregular, abnormal heart rhythm.
- Prevent and treat thromboembolic complications in patients who undergo mechanical heart valve replacement.
- Reduce the risk of recurrent myocardial infarction, stroke, systemic embolization after myocardial infarction

It's also prescribed to people with certain health conditions or risks to prevent blood clots from forming in their blood vessels.

What does PT/INR stand for?

PT/INR stands for prothrombin time / international normalized ratio and is a type of calculation based on the results of prothrombin time (PT).

Prothrombin is a vitamin K–dependent plasma protein made by the liver. It is also referred to as factor II, one of about 13 active clotting factors in the blood. Clotting factors work together to help stop bleeding after an injury or cut. The test measures how much time it takes for a clot to form in your blood sample and will determine if Warfarin is working the way it should:

- PT/INR too low: An INR level that is too low indicates that the patient's warfarin dose is too low and his blood is clotting too quickly, putting him at risk for harmful blood clots.
- PT/INR too high: An INR level that is too high indicates that the patient's warfarin dose is too high and his blood is clotting too slowly, putting him at risk of bleeding.

What is vitamin K?

Vitamin K—the generic name given to a group of fat-soluble vitamins with a similar chemical structure—is naturally present in some foods and available as a dietary supplement. The lactic acid bacteria also produce some vitamin K in our intestines.

Vitamin K exists naturally as phylloquinone (vitamin K1), and a group of menaquinone (vitamin K2)—each of these forms has very different contributions to human health. Vitamin K1 (phylloquinone) is the primary dietary source of vitamin K, accounting for roughly 90% of total vitamin K intake. It is found in green leafy vegetables like kale, broccoli, green salads, spinach, olive oil, and soybean oil.

The most important forms of vitamin K2 are MK-4 and MK-7. Both are found in animal products such as meat, dairy, eggs, cheese, yogurt, liver, natto, butter, egg yolks, and fermented soybeans.

Vitamin K alters the body's ability to metabolize Warfarin

For most warfarin-treated patients, vitamin K may change how Warfarin works and cause your prothrombin time (PT) test (or INR test) to change. Vitamin K works against Warfarin and lowers your

INR values. If you eat more vitamin K, it will reduce your INR and alters warfarin effectiveness putting you at risk of dangerous blood clots. If you eat less vitamin K, it will raise your INR, putting you at risk of bleeding.

Thus, you need to keep close control of your daily intake of vitamin K and should **keep the amounts from food and supplements about the same every day.**

How much vitamin K do you need?

The daily amount of vitamin K you need depends on your age and sex. Recommended Dietary Allowances (RDAs) for vitamin k are listed below in micrograms (mcg).

- for 1 to 3 years old males, the RDA is 30 mcg daily
- for 1 to 3 years old females, the RDA is 30 mcg daily
- for 4 to 8 years old, male the RDA is 55 mcg daily
- for 4 to 8 years old, female the RDA is 55 mcg daily
- for 9 to 13 years old, male the RDA is 60 mcg daily
- for 9 to 13 years old, female the RDA is 60 mcg daily
- for 14 to 18 years old males, the RDA is 75 mcg daily
- for 14 to 18 years old females, the RDA is 75 mcg daily
- for 14 to 18 years old pregnant females, the RDA is 75 mcg daily
- for 14 to 18 years old lactating females, the RDA is 75 mcg daily
- for 19+ years old males, the RDA is 120 mcg daily
- for 19+ years old females, the RDA is 90 mcg daily
- for 19+ years old pregnant female, the RDA is 90 mcg daily
- for 19+ years old lactating female, the RDA is 90 mcg daily

How this book is organized?

"The Complete Vitamin K Counter for Warfarin Users" is your indispensable guide to monitoring your Vitamin K intake and keeping your INR within its therapeutic range while taking Warfarin.

Foods are sorted alphabetically within a food category, such as "Vegetables" or "Fruit." This makes it simple to compare the sorts of foods you eat every day and helps you identify which high-Vitamin-K foods you must replace with low-Vitamin-K ones. The food categories used are:

1. Vegetables and Vegetable Products
2. Fruit and Fruit Products
3. Meats
4. Bread & Bakery Products
5. Beans and lentils
6. Finfish and Shellfish Products
7. Grains and Pasta
8. Breakfast Cereals
9. Dairy and Egg Products
10. Beverages
11. Prepared Meals
12. Restaurant Foods
13. Fast Food Items
14. Soups, Pasta and Noodles
15. Nuts and Seeds
16. Spices and Herbs
17. Snack Foods

PART I

THE WARFARIN THERAPY: BASICS

1

UNDERSTANDING BLOOD CLOTS

Blood clotting

Blood clotting, or coagulation, is a critical process by which the body reduces and stops bleeding when you get injured. It occurs each time a blood vessel ruptures and blood starts to flow out. It involves two interrelated stages:

1. primary hemostasis, which consists of the formation of a weak plug
2. secondary hemostasis, which consists of stabilizing the formed weak plug into a blood clot

Primary Hemostasis

Primary hemostasis leads to the initial sealing of the vascular damage by forming a weak plug. It involves four sequences:

1. blood vessel constriction. Vasospasm of the damaged blood vessel is triggered by the injury and induces, in turn, the constriction of the blood vessel by small muscles in its wall,

   which decreases blood flow and results in less blood leaking
   out.

2. platelet adhesion. When a blood vessel is damaged, collagen
   becomes exposed and attracts platelets—the smallest cell
   fragments of blood—to the injury site. Platelet adhesion is
   the mechanism by which platelets bind to nonplatelet
   surfaces.

3. platelet activation is a key process of hemostasis following
   adhesion. It activates platelet by agonists such as adenosine
   diphosphate and collagen fibers present at the sites of injury
   of the blood vessel. During this sequence, the shapes of
   platelets change from plate-like forms to extend long
   filaments.

4. platelet aggregation. In this final sequence. Activated
   platelets aggregate with each other at the site of vascular
   injury.

Second Hemostasis

Secondary hemostasis refers to the sequence of enzymatic reactions
that stabilize the weak platelet plug. It converts fibrinogen, a soluble
protein found in the blood plasma, into an insoluble protein known
as fibrin. Fibrin molecules then merge to form extended fibrin
networks that enmesh platelets, building up a sponging patch that
progressively solidifies and contracts to form the blood clot.

Blood clotting disorder

Your bodies usually break down the formed clot after you have
healed. However, clots sometimes form in veins or arteries without
reason or don't dissolve after vascular damage. Thrombosis occurs
when a blood clot—thrombus—forms within a blood vessel.

Thrombosis is divided into two main types:

- arterial thrombosis occurs when one or more thrombus form, travel in the circulatory system and **blocks an artery**— a vessel that carries blood away from your heart. Arterial blood clots can block blood flow to critical organs like the heart, lungs, or brain, resulting in deadly conditions such as heart attack or stroke.
- venous thromboembolism (VTE, or venous thrombosis,) occurs when one or more blood clots form and **block a vein** —a vessel that carries blood to your heart. VTE is a medical condition that comprises deep vein thrombosis (DVT) and pulmonary embolism (PE). DVT generally occurs in the leg but can also affect other parts of your body. PE happens when a clot travels through the bloodstream to the lungs artery causing blood flow blockage. This blood vessel blockage can be extremely dangerous if the clot is large.

Symptoms of Blood Clotting Disorder

Blood clotting disorders can be life-threatening depending on which part of your body is affected by the blood clot. A blood clot generally does not have any signs until it blocks the blood flow to parts of the body.

If the blood clot blocks the coronary arteries (i.e., a heart attack occurs), the symptoms are:

- chest pain or discomfort
- jaw, neck, or back pain or discomfort
- Shortness of breath
- lightheadedness
- arms pain or discomfort

- shoulders Pain or discomfort
- tiredness
- nausea or vomiting
- shortness of breath
- dizziness

If this blood clot blocks an artery in the brain (i.e., stroke occurs), the symptoms are:

- Sudden and abrupt numbness on one side of the body
- Sudden and abrupt weakness on one side of the body
- Sudden confusion
- Abrupt trouble speaking,
- difficulty understanding speech.
- weakness in the face, arm, or leg
- Sudden trouble of vision in one or both eyes.
- confusion (stroke)
- Sudden loss of balance
- lack of coordination.

If this blood clot blocks an artery in the lung (i.e., pulmonary embolism occurs), the symptoms are:

- chest pain
- difficulty breathing,
- coughing,
- coughing up blood, and irregular heartbeats.
- shortness of breath
- sharp and abrupt chest pains
- rapid or irregular heartbeats
- unexplained cough
- hemoptysis—coughing up blood
- apprehension or anxiety
- sweating
- feeling faint

- tiredness

If this blood clot blocks a vein a the leg (i.e., Deep Vein Thrombosis occurs), the symptoms are:

- leg warm to touch
- swelling
- pain in the leg
- tenderness in the leg
- redness of the skin

How are blood clotting disorders treated?

Once a patient is diagnosed with a blood clot, anticoagulants, are prescribed to reduce the blood's ability to clot. Depending on the type and location of the blood clot, the patient will often be prescribed an anticoagulant for approximately three to six months, but sometimes he will need to take the treatment for the rest of his life.

THE ANTICOAGULANT THERAPY

Vitamin K antagonists—VKAs are the most commonly prescribed anticoagulants and have a favorable benefit-risk ratio. Regular blood tests to measure the INR allow your provider to assess the effectiveness of the treatment and the absence of over or under dosage.

Anticoagulants are drugs that prevent blood clots by increasing the time it takes for blood to clot. They are prescribed to people at high risk of blood clots to lower their risk of severe conditions such as strokes, heart attacks, and pulmonary embolisms. There are four main classes of anticoagulants medications:

- **Vitamin K antagonist (VKA)** works by reducing the availability of vitamin K and, consequently, the blood's ability to clot. Warfarin belongs to the VKA class and is the most widely prescribed anticoagulant in the world.
- **Factor Xa inhibitors** bind to activated factor X (Xa) to

decrease their activity, which leads to less thrombin and, consequently, less clotting.

- **Heparin** is an injectable anticoagulant that inhibits thrombin and factor Xa by activating antithrombin III.
- **Direct Thrombin inhibitors** bind to and inhibit the activity of clotting protein thrombin which prevents blood clot formation.
- **Platelet inhibitors** inhibit platelet function, which helps reduce the formation of clots. Several classes of platelet inhibitor drugs are available such as Aspirin and Clopidogrel.

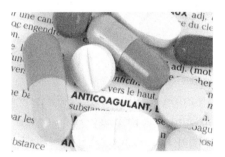

Side effects of anticoagulants

The most common side effect risk with anticoagulant therapy is excessive bleeding. Common side effects include:

- severe bruising
- prolonged nosebleeds
- bleeding gums
- heavy periods in women

Severe side effects include:

- blood in the urine
- blood in stools
- coughing up or vomiting blood

THE WARFARIN THERAPY

Warfarin therapy continues to be essential in preventing arterial and venous thrombosis and the primary and secondary prevention of stroke related to atrial fibrillation. Warfarin therapy requires carefully monitoring to avoid excessive bleeding and to ensure Warfarin is working as intended. Periodic blood testing is required to measure the patient's prothrombin time (PT) and the international normalized ratio (INR).

Warfarin (Coumadin and Jantoven) is an anticoagulant (blood thinner) medication. It has been available in the united states since its first approval by the Food and Drug Administration (FDA) in 1954.

Warfarin is used as a valuable medication in the prophylaxis and treatment of deep vein thrombosis (DVT), pulmonary embolism (PE), atrial fibrillation (AF), and myocardial infarction.

Mechanism of Action

Warfarin is a Vitamin K antagonist which blocks vitamin K from producing active clotting factors in the liver and consequently reduces the number of vitamin-K-dependent clotting factors in your blood. The anticoagulant effect of Warfarin is caused by the inhibition of vitamin K epoxide reductase complex, an enzyme required for activating the vitamin K available in the body. Your blood will then be less likely to form unwanted clots and will inhibit existing clots from growing larger.

What Does Warfarin Treat?

Warfarin is commonly prescribed to:

- prevent and manage venous thromboembolism (blood clots in the veins) and its related medical conditions, deep vein thrombosis (DVT), and pulmonary embolisms (PE).
- prevent and treat thromboembolism in patients suffering from atrial fibrillation
- prevent and treat thromboembolic complications in patients who undergo mechanical heart valve replacement.
- reduce the risk of recurrent myocardial infarction, stroke, systemic embolization after myocardial infarction

It's also prescribed to people with certain health conditions or risks to prevent blood clots from forming in their blood vessels.

What does PT/INR stand for?

PT/INR stands for prothrombin time / international normalized ratio and is a calculation based on prothrombin time (PT) results.

Prothrombin is a vitamin K–dependent plasma protein made by the liver. It is also referred to as factor II, one of about 13 active clotting factors in the blood. Clotting factors work together to help stop bleeding after an injury or cut. The test measures how much time it takes for a clot to form in your blood sample and will determine if Warfarin is working the way it should. The target INR range is between 2 and 3. an INR below or above the range can be dangerous for the patient. The dose of warfarin should be adjusted accordingly to bring the target INR back to 2 to 3.

- PT/INR stays within your therapeutic range: your risk of getting a blood clot or bleeding is small.
- PT/INR is below your therapeutic range: your blood is clotting too quickly, putting you at risk for harmful blood clots.
- PT/INR is above your therapeutic range: your blood is clotting too slowly, putting you at risk of bleeding.

Drug interactions and Warfarin

Warfarin interacts with many prescriptions and nonprescription medicines (over-the-counter or OTC medicines). The interaction may lower the anticoagulant effect of Warfarin or increase the risk of bleeding. A total of 606 prescriptions and OTC medicines are known to interact with Warfarin. Common medications that can interact with Warfarin include aspirin or aspirin-containing products, acetaminophen (Tylenol), or acetaminophen-containing products, many antibiotics, some cold or allergy medicines, and antacids or laxatives.

You can check warfarin interaction at https://www.drugs.com/drug-interactions/warfarin.html

VITAMIN K AND WARFARIN

Vitamin K is an essential micronutrient the liver needs to produce the vitamin K-dependent coagulation factors required for blood to clot correctly. Vitamin K also plays a critical role in calcium metabolism by activating calcium-bound proteins, which guide calcium to bones and prevent its depositions into arteries, organs, and joint spaces. Without enough vitamin K, the regulation of calcium concentration will be severely affected in various tissues.

On the other hand, the purpose of warfarin therapy is to lower the blood's ability to clot but not prevent it from clotting completely. Increasing your vitamin K intake will interfere with the action of warfarin and substantially decrease its effectiveness.

What is vitamin K?

Vitamin K—the generic name given to a group of fat-soluble vitamins with a similar chemical structure—is naturally present in some foods and available as a dietary supplement. The lactic acid bacteria also produce some vitamin K in our intestines.

Vitamin K exists naturally as phylloquinone (vitamin K1), and a group of menaquinone (vitamin K2)—each of these forms has very different contributions to human health. Vitamin K1 (phylloquinone) is the primary dietary source of vitamin K, accounting for roughly 90% of total vitamin K intake. It is found mainly in green leafy vegetables like spinach, kale, broccoli, green salads, olive oil, and soybean oil.

The most important forms of vitamin K2 are MK-4 and MK-7. Both are found in animal products such as meat, dairy, eggs, cheese, yogurt, liver, natto, butter, egg yolks, and fermented soybeans.

Vitamin K alters the body's ability to metabolize Warfarin

For most warfarin-treated patients, vitamin K may change how Warfarin works and cause your prothrombin time (PT) test (or INR test) to change. Vitamin K works against Warfarin and lowers your INR values. If you eat more vitamin K, your INR will decrease, showing an alteration of Warfarin's effectiveness. If you eat less vitamin K, your INR will rise, showing that you are at a higher risk of bleeding.

Because vitamin K is essential for your overall health, you don't need to stop eating foods containing vitamin K. Still, you should make informed and more intelligent food choices by focusing on the vitamin k content of foods and try to **keep the amounts from food and supplements about the same every day.**

For this reason, knowing the vitamin K content in all the foods you prefer and knowing how much you can safely eat while keeping your INR in the therapeutic range is essential.

How much vitamin K do you need?

The daily amount of vitamin K you need depends mainly on your age and sex. Recommended Dietary Allowances (RDAs) for vitamin k are listed below in micrograms (mcg).

- for 19+ years old males, the RDA is 120 mcg daily
- for 19+ years old females, the RDA is 90 mcg daily
- for 19+ years old pregnant female, the RDA is 90 mcg daily
- for 19+ years old lactating female, the RDA is 90 mcg daily

PART II

MEAL PLANNING GUIDELINES

MEAL PLANNING GUIDELINES

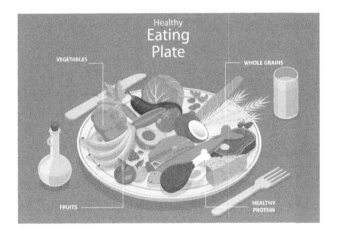

Meal planning allows you to make making informed choices and will work for your personal daily life and tastes. It will ensure that optimal recommendations for a successful Warfarin diet are met. Instead of giving strict recommendations, it gives you options for each food group you can choose.

All foods are assumed to be:

- unprocessed or minimally processed
- in nutrient-dense forms
- lean or low-fat

prepared and cooked with minimal added sugars, salt (sodium), refined carbohydrates, saturated fat, or trans fats.

The total daily calories depend on your personal needs. You have to follow the general guidelines in the next chapters. Recommended amounts of foods in each food group are given to allow you to design your weekly and monthly eating plan.

The five categories of foods are:

- vegetables
- fruits
- grains
- dairy and fortified soy alternatives
- protein foods

General Guidelines

When taking warfarin you must be consistent in how much vitamin K you get daily and aim for stable daily vitamin K intakes. You have to be aware of these guidelines when planning your meals:

1. **aim for a maximum vitamin k (from all sources) in the range of 90-350 mcg per day.**
2. plan regular, balanced meals to avoid high blood sugar levels.
3. **choose healthy cooking methods**, such as broiling, roasting, stir-frying, or grilling.
4. **choose fresh or frozen, unprocessed or canned foods with no added sugar or salt.**

5. **do not eat foods with a vitamin K content greater than 600% DV per serving size.** A recommended DV for adult males equals 120 mcg and for females to 90 mcg.

6. **eat a maximum of 5 servings** (from all sources) **per day of food containing 10%-50% DV of vitamin K.**

7. **eat a maximum of 2½ servings of food** (from all sources) with 50-100% DV of vitamin K.

8. **eat a maximum of 1 serving per day of food** (from all sources) containing 100%-150% DV of vitamin K.

9. **reduce serving sizes for foods with vitamin K content greater than 150% DV** per serving size. If you eat a half-serving size then divide vitamin K content by 2.

10. **choose fresh or frozen, unprocessed**, or canned foods with no added sugar or salt.

11. **exclude trans fats in foods.** Trans fats include margarine, vegetable shortening, French fries, powdered milk, and frozen pizza.

12. **avoid highly processed foods.** Examples of highly processed foods include sugary drinks, flavored potato chips, poultry nuggets and sticks, and fish nuggets.

6

VEGETABLES AND VEGETABLES PRODUCTS

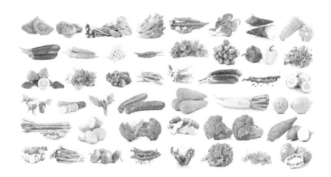

■ **What is the portion size?**

The typical serving sizes for vegetables and vegetable juices are equivalent to:

- 1 cup raw or salad vegetables
- ½ cup cooked vegetables
- ¾ cup (6oz) vegetable juice homemade and unsweetened
- ½ cup of cooked beans, lentils, and peas

▣ How Much a Day?

Total vegetable intake: up to 10 servings

Foods listed here have vitamin k content greater than or equal to 60 mcg per serving size, which corresponds to 50% of the recommended daily value. This simplified list aims to increase your awareness of some foods rich in vitamin K. More comprehensive lists and details about serving sizes are provided in part III (Vitamin K Foods Lists)

▣ Vegetables containing 60%-100% DV of vitamin K: The Simplified List

Examples of foods include:

- **Asparagus Cooked, From Canned (82.9% DV)**; Serving size = 1 cup, 242 g
- **Broccoli Raw (77.1% DV)**; Serving size = 1 cup chopped , 91 g
- **Broccoli, Raab (74.7% DV)**; Serving size = 1 cup chopped , 40 g
- **Cabbage Common, Cooked Boiled, Drained (67.9% DV)**; Serving size = 1/2 cup, shredded, 75 g
- **Cabbage, Creamed (99.3% DV)**; Serving size = 1 cup , 200 g
- **Carrot Dehydrated (66.6% DV)**; Serving size = 1 cup , 74 g
- **Chicory Greens (71.9% DV)**; Serving size = 1 cup, chopped , 29 g
- **Chinese Broccoli, Cooked, From Fresh or Frozen (61.4% DV)**; Serving size = 1 cup, 88 g
- **Chrysanthemum (72.9% DV)**; Serving size = 1 cup, 25 g
- **Endive (96.3% DV)**; Serving size = 1 head, chopped , 50 g
- **Jute Potherb (molokhia), Cooked Boiled (78.3% DV)**; Serving size = 1 cup, 87 g

- Luffa, Cooked With Fat (63.9% DV); Serving size = 1 cup, 183 g
- Pea Salad (96.3% DV); Serving size = 1 cup , 214 g
- Pumpkin Leaves, Cooked Boiled, Drained (63.9% DV); Serving size = 1 cup, 71 g
- Radicchio (85.1% DV); Serving size = 1 cup, shredded , 40 g
- Savoy Cabbage, Cooked Without Fat (86% DV); Serving size = 1 cup, 145 g
- Sour Pickled Cucumber (60.8% DV); Serving size = 1 cup, 155 g
- Sweet Potato Leaves, Raw (88.2% DV); Serving size = 1 cup, chopped, 35 g
- Watercress (70.8% DV); Serving size = 1 cup, chopped , 34 g

■ Vegetables containing 100%-200% DV of vitamin K: The Simplified List

- Beet Greens, Raw (126.7% DV); Serving size = 1 cup, 38 g
- Broccoli Fresh or Frozen, Cooked Without Fat (182.3% DV); Serving size = 1 cup, fresh, cut stalks, 156 g
- Broccoli, Cooked Boiled, Drained (183.4% DV); Serving size = 1 cup, fresh, cut stalks, 156 g
- Brussels Sprouts Cooked, From Fresh or Frozen, Without Fat (180.1% DV); Serving size = 1 cup, 155 g
- Brussels Sprouts, Cooked Boiled, Drained (129% DV); Serving size = 1/2 cup, 80 g
- Brussels Sprouts, From Fresh or Frozen, Creamed (148.6% DV); Serving size = 1 cup, 228 g
- Brussels Sprouts, Raw (129.8% DV); Serving size = 1 cup, 88 g
- Cabbage Mustard (123.3% DV); Serving size = 1 cup, 128 g
- Cabbage Salad Or Coleslaw, Made With Various Dressing (average value) (141% DV); Serving size = 1 cup, 219 g

- Chrysanthemum Garland, Cooked Boiled, Drained (118.9% DV); Serving size = 1 cup, 100 g
- Collards (131.2% DV); Serving size = 1 cup, chopped, 36 g
- Escarole, Creamed (183.8% DV); Serving size = 1 cup, 200 g
- Fennel Bulb, Cooked Without Fat (174.3% DV); Serving size = 1 fennel bulb, 211 g
- Green Cabbage, Cooked Without Fat (135% DV); Serving size = 1 cup, 150 g
- Mustard Greens (120.2% DV); Serving size = 1 cup, chopped, 56 g
- New Zealand Spinach (157.3% DV); Serving size = 1 cup, chopped, 56 g
- Poke Greens, Cooked Without Fat (138.6% DV); Serving size = 1 cup, 155 g
- Spinach (120.8% DV); Serving size = 1 cup, 30 g
- Spring Onions (172.5% DV); Serving size = 1 cup, chopped, 100 g
- Turnip Greens (115.1% DV); Serving size = 1 cup, chopped, 55 g
- Turnip Greens With Roots, Cooked, From Canned, Cooked With Fat (187.8% DV); Serving size = 1 cup, 168 g

---

■ Vegetables containing 200%-600% DV of vitamin K: The Simplified List

- Amaranth Leaves, Raw (266% DV); Serving size = 1 cup, 28 g
- Beet Greens, Cooked Boiled, Drained (580.8% DV); Serving size = 1 cup, 144 g
- Beet Greens, Cooked, Without Fat (576.8% DV); Serving size = 1 cup, 144 g
- Broccoli, Raab, Cooked, Without Fat (360.6% DV); Serving size = 1 cup, 170 g

- Chamnamul, Cooked, Without Fat (492.7% DV); Serving size = 1 cup, 146 g
- Chard Swiss, Cooked Boiled, Drained (477.3% DV); Serving size = 1 cup, chopped, 175 g
- Collards Canned, Cooked Without Fat (542% DV); Serving size = 1 cup, canned, 162 g
- Cress, Fresh, Frozen Or Canned, Cooked Without Fat (428.2% DV); Serving size = 1 cup, 135 g
- Dandelion Greens, Cooked Boiled, Drained (314% DV); Serving size = 1 cup, chopped, 105 g
- Escarole, Cooked, Without Fat (227.8% DV); Serving size = 1 cup, 130 g
- Kale (422.1% DV); Serving size = 1 cup, chopped, 130 g
- Onions Green Fresh or Frozen, Cooked Without Fat (393.7% DV); Serving size = 1 cup, chopped, 219 g
- Spinach, Cooked Boiled, Drained (390.8% DV); Serving size = 1/2 cup, 95 g
- Swiss Chard (249% DV); Serving size = 1 cup, 36 g
- Watercress, Cooked, Without Fat (283.7% DV); Serving size = 1 cup, 137 g

FRUITS AND FRUITS PRODUCTS

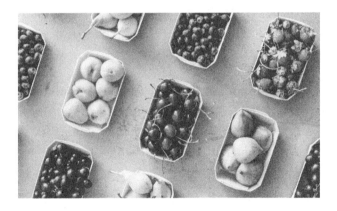

The majority of fruit and vegetables are nutrient-dense, low-calorie, and packed full of essential nutrients such as vitamins, minerals, and fiber.

▦ What is the portion size?

The typical serving sizes for fruits and fruits juices are equivalent to:

- 1 medium piece

- 1 cup (6 oz) of sliced fruits
- ¾ cup (6 oz) of fruit juice

How Much a Day?

2 to 4 servings per day

■ Fruits containing > 50% DV of vitamin K: The Simplified List

- **Fruit Salad, Including Citrus Fruits (53.6% DV)**; Serving size = 1 cup, 188 g
- **Kiwifruit (60.4% DV)**; Serving size = 1 cup, sliced, 180 g
- **Plums Dried (53.9% DV)**; Serving size = 1 cup, pitted, 248 g

---

The fruit food group comprises whole fruits and fruit products (100% fruit juice). Whole fruits can be eaten in various forms, such as cut, cubed, sliced, or diced. At least 60% of the recommended amount of total fruit should come from whole fruit rather than 100% juice. Juices should be without added sugars or food additives.

Strategies to increase total fruit intake include

1. often consuming fruits
2. adding fruits to breakfast.
3. choosing more whole fruits as snacks
4. choosing and carrying fruit with you to eat later
5. creating adequate pairings with your favorite foods

■ Fruits: The Simplified List

- **apples** (all fresh, frozen, dried fruits or 100% fruit juices)
- **Asian pears** (all fresh, frozen, dried fruits or 100% fruit juices)
- **bananas** (all fresh, frozen, dried fruits or 100% fruit juices)
- **blackberries** (all fresh, frozen, dried fruits or 100% fruit juices)
- **blueberries** (all fresh, frozen, dried fruits or 100% fruit juices)
- **currants** (all fresh, frozen, dried fruits or 100% fruit juices)
- **huckleberries** (all fresh, frozen, dried fruits or 100% fruit juices)
- **kiwifruit** (all fresh, frozen, dried fruits or 100% fruit juices)
- **mulberries** (all fresh, frozen, dried fruits or 100% fruit juices)
- **raspberries** (all fresh, frozen, dried fruits or 100% fruit juices)
- **strawberries** (all fresh, frozen, dried fruits or 100% fruit juices)
- **calamondin** (all fresh, frozen, dried fruits or 100% fruit juices)
- **grapefruit** (all fresh, frozen, dried fruits or 100% fruit juices)
- **lemons** (all fresh, frozen, dried fruits or 100% fruit juices)
- **limes** (all fresh, frozen, dried fruits or 100% fruit juices)
- **oranges** (all fresh, frozen, dried fruits or 100% fruit juices)
- **pomelos** (all fresh, frozen, dried fruits or 100% fruit juices)
- **cherries** (all fresh, frozen, dried fruits or 100% fruit juices)
- **dates** (all fresh, frozen, dried fruits or 100% fruit juices)
- **figs** (all fresh, frozen, dried fruits or 100% fruit juices)
- **grapes** (all fresh, frozen, dried fruits or 100% fruit juices)
- **guava** (all fresh, frozen, dried fruits or 100% fruit juices)
- **lychee** (all fresh, frozen, dried fruits or 100% fruit juices)
- **mangoes** (all fresh, frozen, dried fruits or 100% fruit juices)
- **nectarines** (all fresh, frozen, dried fruits or 100% fruit juices)

- **peaches** (all fresh, frozen, dried fruits or 100% fruit juices)
- **pears** (all fresh, frozen, dried fruits or 100% fruit juices)
- **plums** (all fresh, frozen, dried fruits or 100% fruit juices)
- **pomegranates** (all fresh, frozen, dried fruits or 100% fruit juices)
- **rhubarb** (all fresh, frozen, dried fruits or 100% fruit juices)
- **sapote** (all fresh, frozen, dried fruits or 100% fruit juices)
- **soursop** (all fresh, frozen, dried fruits or 100% fruit juices)

8

GRAINS

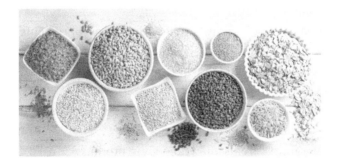

▣ What is the portion size?

The typical serving sizes for cereals and grains are equivalent to:

- ⅓ cup breakfast cereal or muesli
- ½ cup of cooked cereal, or other cooked grain
- ⅓ cup of cooked rice (white rice excluded), and other small grains
- ½ cup of cold cereal

How Much a Day?

Up to 3 servings per day.

■ **Whole grains: The Simplified List**

- **barley** (all whole-grain products or used as ingredients)
- **brown rice** (all whole-grain products or used as ingredients)
- **buckwheat** (all whole-grain products or used as ingredients)
- **bulgur** (all whole-grain products or used as ingredients)
- **millet** (all whole-grain products or used as ingredients)
- **oats (Avena sativa L.)** (all whole-grain products or used as ingredients)
- **quinoa** (all whole-grain products or used as ingredients)
- **dark rye** (all whole-grain products or used as ingredients)
- **whole-wheat bread** (all whole-grain products or used as ingredients)
- **whole-wheat chapati** (all whole-grain products or used as ingredients)
- **whole-grain cereals** (all whole-grain products or used as ingredients)
- **wild rice** (all whole-grain products or used as ingredients)

DAIRY AND FORTIFIED SOY ALTERNATIVES

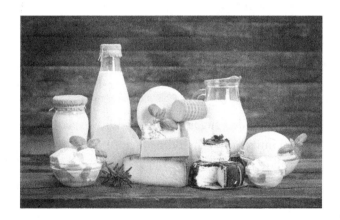

■ What is the portion size?

The typical serving sizes for dairy products are equivalent to:

- 1 cup of milk, soy beverage, or yogurt
- ⅓ cup of cottage cheese
- 1 oz of cheese

People with celiac disease or lactose intolerance should consume dairy alternatives

How Much a Day?

Up to 3 servings per day

◼ **Dairy and Fortified Soy Alternatives: The Simplified List**

- **buttermilk** (all fluid, evaporated milk, or dry including lactose-free and lactose-reduced products)
- **soy beverages** (all fluid, evaporated milk, or dry including lactose-free and lactose-reduced products)
- **soy milk** (all fluid, evaporated milk, or dry including lactose-free and lactose-reduced products)
- **yogurt** (without added sugar and food additives) (all fluid, evaporated milk, or dry including lactose-free and lactose-reduced products)
- **kefir** (without added sugar and food additives) (all fluid, evaporated milk, or dry including lactose-free and lactose-reduced products)
- **frozen yogurt** (without added sugar and food additives) (all fluid, evaporated milk, or dry including lactose-free and lactose-reduced products)
- **cheeses** (all fluid, evaporated milk, or dry including lactose-free and lactose-reduced products)

PROTEIN FOODS

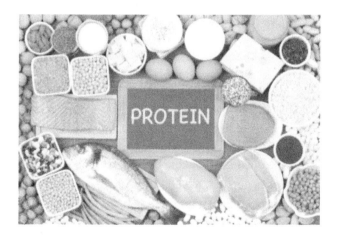

Eating a daily adequate amount of protein is very important for your health. Unlike carbohydrates and fat, your body does not store protein, and you need to eat enough to stay healthy. Animal-based foods are excellent protein sources because they offer a complete composition of essential amino acids with higher bioavailability and digestibility (>90%). Therefore, the main principle to observe here when designing your meal program is to keep a weekly proteins intake equivalent to:

- 30 servings of animal proteins (mainly lean white meat and eggs)
- 10 servings of seafood
- 5 servings of nuts and seeds

■ Meats containing > 50% DV of vitamin K: The Simplified List

- **Beef, Liver Braised (65.2% DV)**; Serving size = 3 oz, 85 g
- **Bockwurst Pork Veal, Raw (53.3% DV)**; Serving size = 1 sausage, 91 g
- **Ham, Or Pork Salad (67.2% DV)**; Serving size = 1 cup, 182 g
- **Veal, Cordon Bleu (53.6% DV)**; Serving size = 1 roll, 229 g

■ Meats, Poultry, Eggs, Seafoods: what is the portion size?

The typical serving sizes for the "meats, poultry, eggs", "seafood", and "nuts, seeds, soy Products" groups are equivalent to:

- 3 to 4 ounces of cooked, baked, or broiled beef
- 3 to 4 ounces of cooked, baked, or broiled veal
- 3 to 4 ounces of cooked, baked, or broiled poultry
- 3 to 4 ounces of cooked or canned fish
- 3 to 4 ounces of seafood
- 2 medium eggs
- ⅓ cup of nuts (5 large or 10 small nuts)
- 2 tablespoons of nut butter
- 2 tablespoons of nut spread

■ Meats, Poultry, Eggs: The simplified List

Meats (lean or low-fats) include:

- beef, goat, lamb, and pork (fat red meats must be limited due to their pro-inflammatory effects). You have to choose lean meats preferably grass-fed beef, lamb, or bison
- game meat (e.g., bison, moose, elk, deer)

Poultry (lean or low-fats) includes

- chicken
- turkey
- cornish hens
- duck
- game birds (e.g., ostrich, pheasant, and quail)
- goose.

Eggs include

- chicken eggs
- turkey eggs
- duck eggs and other birds' eggs

■ **Seafood: The simplified List**

Seafood include

- salmon
- sardine
- anchovy
- black sea bass
- catfish
- clams
- cod

- crab
- crawfish
- flounder
- haddock
- hake
- herring
- lobster
- mullet
- oyster
- perch
- pollock
- scallop
- shrimp
- sole
- squid
- tilapia
- freshwater trout
- tuna

Nuts, Seeds, Soy Products: The simplified List

Nuts (and nut butter) include

- almonds
- pecans
- Brazil nuts
- pistachios
- hazelnuts
- macadamias
- pine nuts
- walnuts
- cashew nuts

Seeds (and seed butter) include:

- pumpkin seeds
- psyllium seeds
- chia seeds.
- flax seeds
- sunflower seeds
- sesame seeds
- poppy seeds

PART III

THE VITAMIN K COUNTER

ABBREVIATIONS

- dia diameter
- fl oz fluid ounce
- g gram
- kcal kilocalorie (commonly known as calories)
- IU International Units
- lb pound
- mcg microgram
- mg milligram
- ml milliliter
- NS not Specified
- oz ounce
- pkg package
- RE retinol equivalent
- sq square
- tbsp tablespoon
- tsp teaspoon
- Tr trace
- tsp teaspoon

BAKED PRODUCTS

Air Filled Fritter—Or Fried Puff Without Syrup Puerto Rican Style ☞ Vitamin K = 13.5 mcg; Serving size: 1 turnover, 57 g

Apple Strudel ☞ Vitamin K = 0.8 mcg; Serving size: 1 oz, 28.4 g

Arepa Dominicana ☞ Vitamin K = 3.8 mcg; Serving size: 1 piece, 115 g

Bagel—(Oat Bran) ☞ Vitamin K = 0.1 mcg; Serving size: 1 mini bagel (2-1/2 inch dia), 26 g

Bagel—Multigrain ☞ Vitamin K = 0.5 mcg; Serving size: 1 piece bagel, 81 g

Bagel—Multigrain ☞ Vitamin K = 0.4 mcg; Serving size: 1 miniature, 26 g

Bagel—Multigrain With Raisins ☞ Vitamin K = 0.4 mcg; Serving size: 1 miniature, 26 g

Bagel—Oat Bran ☞ Vitamin K = 0.4 mcg; Serving size: 1 miniature, 26 g

Bagel—Pumpernickel ☞ Vitamin K = 0.4 mcg; Serving size: 1 miniature, 26 g

Bagel—Wheat ☞ Vitamin K = 1.5 mcg; Serving size: 1 bagel, 98 g

Bagel—Wheat Bran ☞ Vitamin K = 0.4 mcg; Serving size: 1 miniature, 26 g

Bagel—Wheat With Raisins ☞ Vitamin K = 0.4 mcg; Serving size: 1 miniature, 26 g

Bagel—Whole Grain White ☞ Vitamin K = 0.2 mcg; Serving size: 1/2 piece bagel 1 serving, 43 g

Bagel—Whole Grain White ☞ Vitamin K = 0.4 mcg; Serving size: 1 miniature, 26 g

Bagel—Whole Wheat ☞ Vitamin K = 0.4 mcg; Serving size: 1 miniature, 26 g

Bagel—Whole Wheat With Raisins ☞ Vitamin K = 0.4 mcg; Serving size: 1 miniature, 26 g

Bagels ☞ Vitamin K = 0.2 mcg; Serving size: 1 bagel, 99 g

Baklava ☞ Vitamin K = 2.7 mcg; Serving size: 1 piece (2" x 2" x 1-1/2"), 78 g

Basbousa ☞ Vitamin K = 3.4 mcg; Serving size: 1 piece (about 3 x 2-1/2"), 82 g

Biscuit Cheese ☞ Vitamin K = 1.2 mcg; Serving size: 1 biscuit (2" dia), 30 g

Biscuit Cinnamon-Raisin ☞ Vitamin K = 4.5 mcg; Serving size: 1 biscuit (3" dia), 64 g

Biscuit Dough Fried ☞ Vitamin K = 3.1 mcg; Serving size: 1 piece, 43 g

Biscuit Whole Wheat ☞ Vitamin K = 0.9 mcg; Serving size: 1 small (1-1/2" dia), 14 g

Biscuit—Plain Or Buttermilk Frozen Baked ☞ Vitamin K = 1.2 mcg; Serving size: 1 oz, 28.4 g

Biscuit—Plain Or Buttermilk Refrigerated Dough Higher Fat ☛ Vitamin K = 3.6 mcg; Serving size: 1 biscuit, 58 g

Biscuit—Plain Or Buttermilk Refrigerated Dough Higher Fat Baked ☛ Vitamin K = 4.8 mcg; Serving size: 1 biscuit, 51 g

Biscuits—Plain Or Buttermilk Dry Mix ☛ Vitamin K = 7.8 mcg; Serving size: 1 cup, purchased, 120 g

Biscuits—Plain Or Buttermilk Refrigerated Dough Lower Fat ☛ Vitamin K = 1.1 mcg; Serving size: 1 serving 1 biscuit, 58 g

Biscuits—Plain Or Buttermilk Refrigerated Dough Lower Fat Baked ☛ Vitamin K = 0.6 mcg; Serving size: 1 oz, 28.4 g

Blueberry Pie ☛ Vitamin K = 3 mcg; Serving size: 1 oz, 28.4 g

Bread— Chapati Or Roti Whole Wheat—Commercially Prepared, Frozen ☛ Vitamin K = 1.4 mcg; Serving size: 1 piece, 43 g

Bread— Paratha Whole Wheat—Commercially Prepared, Frozen ☛ Vitamin K = 2.7 mcg; Serving size: 1 piece, 79 g

Bread—Barley Toasted ☛ Vitamin K = 1.2 mcg; Serving size: 1 small slice, 22 g

Bread—Boston Brown Canned ☛ Vitamin K = 0.7 mcg; Serving size: 1 oz, 28.4 g

Bread—Caressed Puerto Rican Style ☛ Vitamin K = 0.4 mcg; Serving size: 1 slice, 25 g

Bread—Caressed Toasted Puerto Rican Style ☛ Vitamin K = 0.4 mcg; Serving size: 1 slice, 23 g

Bread—Cheese ☛ Vitamin K = 15.6 mcg; Serving size: 1 slice, 48 g

Bread—Cheese Toasted ☛ Vitamin K = 7.8 mcg; Serving size: 1 small slice, 22 g

Bread—Cinnamon ☛ Vitamin K = 2.7 mcg; Serving size: 1 slice 1 serving, 28 g

Bread—CornBread—Dry Mix Enriched (With Corn Muffin Mix) ☛ Vitamin K = 1.4 mcg; Serving size: 1 oz, 28.4 g

Bread—CornBread—Dry Mix Prepared With 2% Milk 80% Margarine And Eggs ☛ Vitamin K = 1.9 mcg; Serving size: 1 muffin, 51 g

Bread—Crumbs Dry Grated Plain ☛ Vitamin K = 1.9 mcg; Serving size: 1 oz, 28.4 g

Bread—Crumbs Dry Grated Seasoned ☛ Vitamin K = 13.1 mcg; Serving size: 1 oz, 28.4 g

Bread—Cuban Toasted ☛ Vitamin K = 0.1 mcg; Serving size: 1 small slice, 9 g

Bread—Dough Fried ☛ Vitamin K = 2.4 mcg; Serving size: 1 slice or roll, 26 g

Bread—Egg ☛ Vitamin K = 0.3 mcg; Serving size: 1 oz, 28.4 g

Bread—Egg Challah Toasted ☛ Vitamin K = 0.2 mcg; Serving size: 1 small slice, 18 g

Bread—Egg Toasted ☛ Vitamin K = 0.3 mcg; Serving size: 1 oz, 28.4 g

Bread—French Or Vienna Toasted (With Sourdough) ☛ Vitamin K = 0.1 mcg; Serving size: 1 oz, 28.4 g

Bread—French Or Vienna Whole Wheat ☛ Vitamin K = 0.3 mcg; Serving size: 1 slice 1 serving, 48 g

Bread—Fruit ☛ Vitamin K = 5.7 mcg; Serving size: 1 slice, 41 g

Bread—Gluten-Free Toasted ☛ Vitamin K = 0.1 mcg; Serving size: 1 small slice, 22 g

Bread—Gluten-Free White Made With Rice Flour Corn Starch And/or Tapioca ☛ Vitamin K = 0.1 mcg; Serving size: 1 slice, 35 g

Bread—Italian ☛ Vitamin K = 0.9 mcg; Serving size: 1 oz, 28.4 g

Bread—Italian Grecian Armenian ☞ Vitamin K = 0.3 mcg; Serving size: 1 small slice, 24 g

Bread—Italian Grecian Armenian Toasted ☞ Vitamin K = 0.3 mcg; Serving size: 1 small slice, 22 g

Bread—Lard Puerto Rican Style ☞ Vitamin K = 0.1 mcg; Serving size: 1 slice, 25 g

Bread—Multi-Grain (With Whole-Grain) ☞ Vitamin K = 0.4 mcg; Serving size: 1 oz, 28.4 g

Bread—Naan Whole Wheat—Commercially Prepared, Refrigerated ☞ Vitamin K = 3.5 mcg; Serving size: 1 piece, 106 g

Bread—Native Water Puerto Rican Style ☞ Vitamin K = 0.3 mcg; Serving size: 1 slice, 25 g

Bread—Native Water Toasted Puerto Rican Style ☞ Vitamin K = 0.3 mcg; Serving size: 1 slice, 23 g

Bread—Nut ☞ Vitamin K = 7.5 mcg; Serving size: 1 slice, 49 g

Bread—Oat Bran ☞ Vitamin K = 0.3 mcg; Serving size: 1 oz, 28.4 g

Bread—Oat Bran Toasted ☞ Vitamin K = 0.4 mcg; Serving size: 1 oz, 28.4 g

Bread—Oatmeal ☞ Vitamin K = 0.4 mcg; Serving size: 1 oz, 28.4 g

Bread—Oatmeal Toasted ☞ Vitamin K = 0.5 mcg; Serving size: 1 oz, 28.4 g

Bread—Onion ☞ Vitamin K = 0.2 mcg; Serving size: 1 small slice, 24 g

Bread—Onion Toasted ☞ Vitamin K = 0.2 mcg; Serving size: 1 small slice, 18 g

Bread—Pan Dulce Sweet Yeast Bread ☞ Vitamin K = 1 mcg; Serving size: 1 slice (average weight of 1 slice), 63 g

Bread—Potato ☞ Vitamin K = 2.2 mcg; Serving size: 1 slice, 32 g

Bread—Potato Toasted ☛ Vitamin K = 1.8 mcg; Serving size: 1 small slice, 24 g

Bread—Protein (With Gluten) ☛ Vitamin K = 0.4 mcg; Serving size: 1 oz, 28.4 g

Bread—Protein (With Gluten) Toasted ☛ Vitamin K = 0.4 mcg; Serving size: 1 oz, 28.4 g

Bread—Pumpernickel ☛ Vitamin K = 0.2 mcg; Serving size: 1 oz, 28.4 g

Bread—Pumpkin ☛ Vitamin K = 10 mcg; Serving size: 1 slice, 60 g

Bread—Puri Wheat ☛ Vitamin K = 10.2 mcg; Serving size: 1 puri, 36 g

Bread—Raisin Enriched ☛ Vitamin K = 0.5 mcg; Serving size: 1 oz, 28.4 g

Bread—Raisin Enriched Toasted ☛ Vitamin K = 0.5 mcg; Serving size: 1 oz, 28.4 g

Bread—Reduced-Calorie Oat Bran ☛ Vitamin K = 0.5 mcg; Serving size: 1 oz, 28.4 g

Bread—Reduced-Calorie Oat Bran Toasted ☛ Vitamin K = 0.6 mcg; Serving size: 1 oz, 28.4 g

Bread—Reduced-Calorie Rye ☛ Vitamin K = 0.2 mcg; Serving size: 1 oz, 28.4 g

Bread—Reduced-Calorie Wheat ☛ Vitamin K = 0.1 mcg; Serving size: 1 oz, 28.4 g

Bread—Reduced-Calorie White ☛ Vitamin K = 0.2 mcg; Serving size: 1 oz, 28.4 g

Bread—Rice Bran ☛ Vitamin K = 0.3 mcg; Serving size: 1 oz, 28.4 g

Bread—Rice Bran Toasted ☛ Vitamin K = 0.3 mcg; Serving size: 1 oz, 28.4 g

Bread—Roll Mexican Bollilo ☞ Vitamin K = 10.7 mcg; Serving size: 1 piece, 98 g

Bread—Rye Toasted ☞ Vitamin K = 0.4 mcg; Serving size: 1 oz, 28.4 g

Bread—Salvadoran Sweet Cheese (Quesadilla Salvadorena) ☞ Vitamin K = 6.2 mcg; Serving size: 1 serving, 55 g

Bread—Spanish Coffee ☞ Vitamin K = 3.8 mcg; Serving size: 1 piece, 85 g

Bread—Sprouted Wheat Toasted ☞ Vitamin K = 0.3 mcg; Serving size: 1 slice, 24 g

Bread—Sticks Plain ☞ Vitamin K = 1 mcg; Serving size: 1 cup, small pieces, 46 g

Bread—Stuffing Bread—Dry Mix ☞ Vitamin K = 0.3 mcg; Serving size: 1 oz, 28.4 g

Bread—Stuffing Bread—Dry Mix Prepared ☞ Vitamin K = 3.7 mcg; Serving size: 1 oz, 28.4 g

Bread—Stuffing CornBread—Dry Mix Prepared ☞ Vitamin K = 2.5 mcg; Serving size: 1 oz, 28.4 g

Bread—Sweet Potato Toasted ☞ Vitamin K = 0.3 mcg; Serving size: 1 small slice, 22 g

Bread—Vegetable ☞ Vitamin K = 1.8 mcg; Serving size: 1 slice, 44 g

Bread—Vegetable Toasted ☞ Vitamin K = 1.8 mcg; Serving size: 1 slice, 40 g

Bread—Wheat Sprouted ☞ Vitamin K = 0.4 mcg; Serving size: 1 slice 1 serving, 38 g

Bread—Wheat Sprouted Toasted ☞ Vitamin K = 0.5 mcg; Serving size: 1 slice 1 serving, 38 g

Bread—Wheat Toasted ☞ Vitamin K = 1.6 mcg; Serving size: 1 oz, 28.4 g

Bread—White Made From Home Recipe Or Purchased At A Bakery ☞ Vitamin K = 0.3 mcg; Serving size: 1 small slice, 33 g

Bread—White Made From Home Recipe Or Purchased At A Bakery Toasted ☞ Vitamin K = 0.3 mcg; Serving size: 1 small slice, 30 g

Bread—White Wheat ☞ Vitamin K = 2.2 mcg; Serving size: 1 slice, 28 g

Bread—White With Whole Wheat Swirl ☞ Vitamin K = 1 mcg; Serving size: 1 small slice, 24 g

Bread—White With Whole Wheat Swirl Toasted ☞ Vitamin K = 1.4 mcg; Serving size: 1 small slice, 22 g

Bread—White—Commercially Prepared, Low Sodium No Salt ☞ Vitamin K = 0.9 mcg; Serving size: 1 oz, 28.4 g

Bread—Whole Wheat Made From Home Recipe Or Purchased At Bakery ☞ Vitamin K = 0.6 mcg; Serving size: 1 small slice, 33 g

Bread—Whole Wheat Made From Home Recipe Or Purchased At Bakery Toasted ☞ Vitamin K = 0.6 mcg; Serving size: 1 small slice, 30 g

Bread—Whole Wheat Toasted ☞ Vitamin K = 1.9 mcg; Serving size: 1 small slice, 22 g

Bread—Whole-Wheat—Prepared From Recipe Toasted ☞ Vitamin K = 3 mcg; Serving size: 1 oz, 28.4 g

Bread—Whole-Wheat—Prepared From Recipe, ☞ Vitamin K = 2.7 mcg; Serving size: 1 oz, 28.4 g

Bread—Zucchini ☞ Vitamin K = 5.6 mcg; Serving size: 1 slice, 40 g

Breadsticks Soft From Fast Food / Restaurant ☞ Vitamin K = 4.8 mcg; Serving size: 1 small stick, 26 g

Breadsticks Soft From Frozen ☞ Vitamin K = 2.9 mcg; Serving size: 1 small stick, 26 g

Breadsticks Soft With Parmesan Cheese From Fast Food / Restaurant ☛ Vitamin K = 5 mcg; Serving size: 1 small stick, 28 g

Breakfast Tart—Reduced Fat ☛ Vitamin K = 0.2 mcg; Serving size: 1 tart, 52 g

Brioche ☛ Vitamin K = 1.8 mcg; Serving size: 1 piece, 77 g

Butter Croissants ☛ Vitamin K = 0.5 mcg; Serving size: 1 oz, 28.4 g

Cake—Angelfood Dry Mix Prepared ☛ Vitamin K = 0.1 mcg; Serving size: 1 piece (1/12 of 10 inch dia), 50 g

Cake—Batter—RawChocolate ☛ Vitamin K = 1.5 mcg; Serving size: 1 tablespoon, 14 g

Cake—Batter—RawNot Chocolate ☛ Vitamin K = 1.6 mcg; Serving size: 1 tablespoon, 15 g

Cake—Boston Cream Pie—Commercially Prepared, ☛ Vitamin K = 0.9 mcg; Serving size: 1 oz, 28.4 g

Cake—Cherry Fudge With Chocolate Frosting ☛ Vitamin K = 0.7 mcg; Serving size: 1 oz, 28.4 g

Cake—Cream Without Icing Or Topping ☛ Vitamin K = 60.2 mcg; Serving size: 1 cake (8" dia), 510 g

Cake—Dobos Torte ☛ Vitamin K = 122.2 mcg; Serving size: 1 cake (8-1/2" dia), 1472 g

Cake—FruitCake—Commercially Prepared ☛ Vitamin K = 0.4 mcg; Serving size: 1 oz, 28.4 g

Cake—GingerBread—Dry Mix ☛ Vitamin K = 1.8 mcg; Serving size: 1 oz, 28.4 g

Cake—Ice Cream And Cake—Roll Chocolate ☛ Vitamin K = 57.8 mcg; Serving size: 1 ice cream roll (12 oz), 340 g

Cake—Ice Cream And Cake—Roll Not Chocolate ☛ Vitamin K = 14.3 mcg; Serving size: 1 ice cream roll (12 oz), 340 g

Cake—Jelly Roll ☛ Vitamin K = 51.6 mcg; Serving size: 1 jelly roll, 506 g

Cake—Or CupCake—Applesauce With Icing Or Filling ☛ Vitamin K = 10.4 mcg; Serving size: 1 regular cupcake, 75 g

Cake—Or CupCake—Banana With Icing Or Filling ☛ Vitamin K = 10.5 mcg; Serving size: 1 regular cupcake, 75 g

Cake—Or CupCake—Banana Without Icing Or Filling ☛ Vitamin K = 10.6 mcg; Serving size: 1 regular cupcake, 50 g

Cake—Or CupCake—Carrot With Icing Or Filling ☛ Vitamin K = 12.2 mcg; Serving size: 1 regular cupcake, 75 g

Cake—Or CupCake—Carrot Without Icing Or Filling ☛ Vitamin K = 12.3 mcg; Serving size: 1 regular cupcake, 50 g

Cake—Or CupCake—Chocolate Devil's Food Or Fudge Without Icing Or Filling ☛ Vitamin K = 5.9 mcg; Serving size: 1 regular cupcake, 50 g

Cake—Or CupCake—German Chocolate With Icing Or Filling ☛ Vitamin K = 20 mcg; Serving size: 1 regular cupcake, 75 g

Cake—Or CupCake—Gingerbread ☛ Vitamin K = 2.2 mcg; Serving size: 1 regular cupcake, 50 g

Cake—Or CupCake—Lemon With Icing Or Filling ☛ Vitamin K = 7 mcg; Serving size: 1 regular cupcake, 75 g

Cake—Or CupCake—Lemon Without Icing Or Filling ☛ Vitamin K = 5.9 mcg; Serving size: 1 regular cupcake, 50 g

Cake—Or CupCake—Marble With Icing Or Filling ☛ Vitamin K = 13.4 mcg; Serving size: 1 regular cupcake, 75 g

Cake—Or CupCake—Marble Without Icing Or Filling ☛ Vitamin K = 5.9 mcg; Serving size: 1 regular cupcake, 50 g

Cake—Or CupCake—Nut With Icing Or Filling ☛ Vitamin K = 6

mcg; Serving size: 1 regular cupcake, 75 g

Cake—Or CupCake—Nut Without Icing Or Filling ☞ Vitamin K = 6 mcg; Serving size: 1 regular cupcake, 50 g

Cake—Or CupCake—Oatmeal ☞ Vitamin K = 4.4 mcg; Serving size: 1 regular cupcake, 50 g

Cake—Or CupCake—Peanut Butter ☞ Vitamin K = 3.6 mcg; Serving size: 1 regular cupcake, 50 g

Cake—Or CupCake—Pumpkin With Icing Or Filling ☞ Vitamin K = 12.5 mcg; Serving size: 1 regular cupcake, 75 g

Cake—Or CupCake—Pumpkin Without Icing Or Filling ☞ Vitamin K = 12.4 mcg; Serving size: 1 regular cupcake, 50 g

Cake—Or CupCake—Raisin-Nut ☞ Vitamin K = 5.4 mcg; Serving size: 1 regular cupcake, 50 g

Cake—Or CupCake—Spice With Icing Or Filling ☞ Vitamin K = 10.4 mcg; Serving size: 1 regular cupcake, 75 g

Cake—Or CupCake—Spice Without Icing Or Filling ☞ Vitamin K = 10.3 mcg; Serving size: 1 regular cupcake, 50 g

Cake—Or CupCake—White Without Icing Or Filling ☞ Vitamin K = 5.5 mcg; Serving size: 1 regular cupcake, 50 g

Cake—Or CupCake—Yellow Without Icing Or Filling ☞ Vitamin K = 5.9 mcg; Serving size: 1 regular cupcake, 50 g

Cake—Pound Chocolate ☞ Vitamin K = 23.6 mcg; Serving size: 1 loaf, 909 g

Cake—Pound Puerto Rican Style ☞ Vitamin K = 2.2 mcg; Serving size: 1 slice (3-1/2" x 3-1/2" x 1"), 90 g

Cake—Pound With Icing Or Filling ☞ Vitamin K = 72.5 mcg; Serving size: 1 loaf (9-1/4" x 5-1/4" x 3-1/8"), 1228 g

Cake—Pound—Commercially Prepared, Butter (With Fresh And Frozen) ☞ Vitamin K = 1 mcg; Serving size: 1/6 loaf 1/6 of the loaf, 61 g

Cake—Pudding-Type Chocolate Dry Mix ☞ Vitamin K = 0.6 mcg; Serving size: 1 oz, 28.4 g

Cake—Pudding-Type White Enriched Dry Mix ☞ Vitamin K = 1.2 mcg; Serving size: 1 oz, 28.4 g

Cake—Pudding-Type Yellow Dry Mix ☞ Vitamin K = 0.7 mcg; Serving size: 1 oz, 28.4 g

Cake—Ravani ☞ Vitamin K = 39.5 mcg; Serving size: 1 cake, 564 g

Cake—ShortCake—Biscuit Type With Fruit ☞ Vitamin K = 1.1 mcg; Serving size: 1 biscuit (2" dia) with fruit, 65 g

Cake—ShortCake—Biscuit Type With Whipped Cream And Fruit ☞ Vitamin K = 1.3 mcg; Serving size: 1 biscuit (2" diameter) with fruit and whipped cream, 74 g

Cake—ShortCake—Sponge Type With Fruit ☞ Vitamin K = 0.8 mcg; Serving size: 1 cake (3" dia) with fruit, 102 g

Cake—ShortCake—Sponge Type With Whipped Cream And Fruit ☞ Vitamin K = 1.1 mcg; Serving size: 1 cake (3" dia) with fruit and whipped cream, 118 g

Cake—ShortCake—With Whipped Topping And Fruit Diet ☞ Vitamin K = 1.1 mcg; Serving size: 1 individual cake, 94 g

Cake—Snack Cakes Creme-Filled Chocolate With Frosting ☞ Vitamin K = 3 mcg; Serving size: 1 oz, 28.4 g

Cake—Snack Cakes Creme-Filled Chocolate With Frosting Low-Fat With Added Fiber ☞ Vitamin K = 2 mcg; Serving size: 1 cake 1 serving, 27 g

Cake—Snack Cakes Creme-Filled Sponge ☞ Vitamin K = 2.8 mcg; Serving size: 1 oz, 28.4 g

Cake—Snack Cakes Not Chocolate With Icing Or Filling Low-Fat With Added Fiber ☛ Vitamin K = 1.7 mcg; Serving size: 1 cake 1 serving, 27 g

Cake—Sponge Chocolate ☛ Vitamin K = 0.8 mcg; Serving size: 1 tube cake (10" dia, 4" high), 790 g

Cake—Sponge With Icing Or Filling ☛ Vitamin K = 57.7 mcg; Serving size: 1 tube cake (10-1/2" dia, 4-1/4" high), 1109 g

Cake—Sponge—Commercially Prepared, ☛ Vitamin K = 0.1 mcg; Serving size: 1 oz, 28.4 g

Cake—Torte ☛ Vitamin K = 82.1 mcg; Serving size: 1 torte, 912 g

Cake—Tres Leche ☛ Vitamin K = 10.1 mcg; Serving size: 1 cake, 1448 g

Cake—White—Prepared From Recipe, Without Frosting ☛ Vitamin K = 3.8 mcg; Serving size: 1 piece (1/12 of 9 inch dia), 74 g

Cake—Yellow Enriched Dry Mix ☛ Vitamin K = 1.2 mcg; Serving size: 1 serving, 43 g

Calzone With Cheese Meatless ☛ Vitamin K = 29.7 mcg; Serving size: 1 calzone or stromboli, 424 g

Calzone With Meat And Cheese ☛ Vitamin K = 31.4 mcg; Serving size: 1 calzone or stromboli, 424 g

Casabe Cassava Bread ☛ Vitamin K = 3.6 mcg; Serving size: 1 piece (6" dia), 100 g

Cheese Croissants ☛ Vitamin K = 3.1 mcg; Serving size: 1 oz, 28.4 g

Cheese Pastry—Puffs ☛ Vitamin K = 0.8 mcg; Serving size: 1 puff or cheese straw (5" long), 6 g

CheeseCake—Commercially Prepared ☛ Vitamin K = 1.2 mcg; Serving size: 1 oz, 28.4 g

Chocolate Cake—With Frosting ☛ Vitamin K = 39.9 mcg; Serving size: 1 piece (1/12 of a cake), 138 g

Chocolate Coated Graham Crackers ☛ Vitamin K = 1.7 mcg; Serving size: 3 pieces, 27 g

Chocolate Coated Marshmallows ☛ Vitamin K = 2 mcg; Serving size: 1 oz, 28.4 g

Churros ☛ Vitamin K = 3.9 mcg; Serving size: 1 churro, 26 g

Cinnamon Buns Frosted (With Honey Buns) ☛ Vitamin K = 9.9 mcg; Serving size: 1 bun, 65 g

Cinnamon Raisin Bagels ☛ Vitamin K = 0.2 mcg; Serving size: 1 mini bagel (2-1/2 inch dia), 26 g

Cobbler—Apple ☛ Vitamin K = 6.5 mcg; Serving size: 1 cup, 217 g

Cobbler—Apricot ☛ Vitamin K = 9.5 mcg; Serving size: 1 cup, 217 g

Cobbler—Berry ☛ Vitamin K = 29.3 mcg; Serving size: 1 cup, 217 g

Cobbler—Cherry ☛ Vitamin K = 8.7 mcg; Serving size: 1 cup, 217 g

Cobbler—Peach ☛ Vitamin K = 8.7 mcg; Serving size: 1 cup, 217 g

Cobbler—Pear ☛ Vitamin K = 11.3 mcg; Serving size: 1 cup, 217 g

Cobbler—Pineapple ☛ Vitamin K = 5.2 mcg; Serving size: 1 cup, 217 g

Cobbler—Plum ☛ Vitamin K = 14.1 mcg; Serving size: 1 cup, 217 g

Cobbler—Rhubarb ☛ Vitamin K = 42.3 mcg; Serving size: 1 cup, 217 g

Coffee Cake—Crumb Or Quick-Bread—Type ☛ Vitamin K = 9.7 mcg; Serving size: 1 cake (9" square), 692 g

Coffee Cake—Crumb Or Quick-Bread—Type Cheese-Filled ☛ Vitamin K = 7.4 mcg; Serving size: 1 cake (8" square), 568 g

Coffee Cake—Crumb Or Quick-Bread—Type With Fruit ☛ Vitamin K = 7.9 mcg; Serving size: 1 cake (9" square), 785 g

CoffeeCake—Cinnamon With Crumb Topping Dry Mix Prepared ☛ Vitamin K = 1 mcg; Serving size: 1 oz, 28.4 g

Cookies—Batter Or Dough Raw ☞ Vitamin K = 60.3 mcg; Serving size: 1 cup, 250 g

Cookies—Biscotti ☞ Vitamin K = 2.4 mcg; Serving size: 1 cookie, 32 g

Cookies—Brownie With Icing Or Filling ☞ Vitamin K = 1.3 mcg; Serving size: 1 small, 40 g

Cookies—Butter Or Sugar With Fruit And/or Nuts ☞ Vitamin K = 0.1 mcg; Serving size: 1 miniature/bite size, 5 g

Cookies—Butter Or Sugar With Icing Or Filling Other Than Chocolate ☞ Vitamin K = 0.6 mcg; Serving size: 1 miniature/bite size, 7 g

Cookies—Chocolate Chip Made From Home Recipe Or Purchased At A Bakery ☞ Vitamin K = 0.1 mcg; Serving size: 1 miniature/bite size, 5 g

Cookies—Graham Cracker With Chocolate And Marshmallow ☞ Vitamin K = 1.4 mcg; Serving size: 1 suddenly s'mores cookie, 19 g

Cookies—Oatmeal With Chocolate Chips ☞ Vitamin K = 0.4 mcg; Serving size: 1 miniature/bite size, 5 g

Cookies—Peanut Butter With Chocolate ☞ Vitamin K = 0.2 mcg; Serving size: 1 miniature/bite size, 5 g

Cookies—ShortBread—With Icing Or Filling ☞ Vitamin K = 0.8 mcg; Serving size: 1 miniature/bite size, 7 g

Cookies—Animal Crackers—(With Arrowroot Tea Biscuits) ☞ Vitamin K – 1.7 mcg; Serving size: 1 oz, 28.4 g

Cookies—Animal With Frosting Or Icing ☞ Vitamin K = 1.9 mcg; Serving size: 8 cookies 1 serving, 31 g

Cookies—Brownies—Commercially Prepared, ☞ Vitamin K = 1.8 mcg; Serving size: 1 oz, 28.4 g

Cookies—Brownies—Commercially Prepared, Reduced Fat With

Added Fiber ☛ Vitamin K = 2.9 mcg; Serving size: 1 brownie 1 serving, 36 g

Cookies—Butter Or Sugar With Chocolate Icing Or Filling ☛ Vitamin K = 2 mcg; Serving size: 3 cookies, 31 g

Cookies—Butter—Commercially Prepared, Enriched ☛ Vitamin K = 0.5 mcg; Serving size: 1 oz, 28.4 g

Cookies—Chocolate Chip Sandwich With Creme Filling ☛ Vitamin K = 1.4 mcg; Serving size: 1 cookie, 34 g

Cookies—Chocolate Chip—Commercially Prepared, Regular Higher Fat Enriched ☛ Vitamin K = 4.3 mcg; Serving size: 1 cookie, 12.9 g

Cookies—Chocolate Chip—Commercially Prepared, Regular Lower Fat ☛ Vitamin K = 1.4 mcg; Serving size: 1 serving 3 cookies, 34 g

Cookies—Chocolate Chip—Commercially Prepared, Soft-Type ☛ Vitamin K = 0.3 mcg; Serving size: 1 cookie, 14.2 g

Cookies—Chocolate Chip—Commercially Prepared, Special Dietary ☛ Vitamin K = 1.1 mcg; Serving size: 1 oz, 28.4 g

Cookies—Chocolate Cream Covered Biscuit Sticks ☛ Vitamin K = 0.7 mcg; Serving size: 1 serving, 40 g

Cookies—Chocolate Made With Rice Cereal ☛ Vitamin K = 2.5 mcg; Serving size: 1 cookie, 62 g

Cookies—Chocolate Sandwich With Creme Filling Reduced Fat ☛ Vitamin K = 5.4 mcg; Serving size: 1 serving, 34 g

Cookies—Chocolate Sandwich With Creme Filling Regular ☛ Vitamin K = 9.9 mcg; Serving size: 3 cookie, 36 g

Cookies—Chocolate Sandwich With Creme Filling Regular Chocolate-Coated ☛ Vitamin K = 3.2 mcg; Serving size: 1 oz, 28.4 g

Cookies—Chocolate Sandwich With Creme Filling Special Dietary ☛ Vitamin K = 1.5 mcg; Serving size: 1 oz, 28.4 g

Cookies—Chocolate Sandwich With Extra Creme Filling ☛ Vitamin K = 1.8 mcg; Serving size: 1 oz, 28.4 g

Cookies—Chocolate Wafers ☛ Vitamin K = 0.7 mcg; Serving size: 1 oz, 28.4 g

Cookies—Chocolate With Icing Or Coating ☛ Vitamin K = 2.2 mcg; Serving size: 4 cookies, 32 g

Cookies—Coconut Macaroon ☛ Vitamin K = 0.4 mcg; Serving size: 2 cookie 1 serving, 36 g

Cookies—Gluten-Free Chocolate Sandwich With Creme Filling ☛ Vitamin K = 11.3 mcg; Serving size: 3 cookies, 44 g

Cookies—Graham Crackers—Plain Or Honey Lowfat ☛ Vitamin K = 0.9 mcg; Serving size: 1 serving, 35 g

Cookies—Marie Biscuit ☛ Vitamin K = 1.1 mcg; Serving size: 5 cookie, 28 g

Cookies—Marshmallow With Rice Cereal And Chocolate Chips ☛ Vitamin K = 1.5 mcg; Serving size: 1 bar, 22 g

Cookies—Oatmeal Reduced Fat ☛ Vitamin K = 2.8 mcg; Serving size: 1 cookie, 25 g

Cookies—Oatmeal Sandwich With Creme Filling ☛ Vitamin K = 2.1 mcg; Serving size: 1 cookie 1 serving, 38 g

Cookies—Oatmeal—Commercially Prepared, Special Dietary ☛ Vitamin K = 2 mcg; Serving size: 1 oz, 28.4 g

Cookies—Peanut Butter Sandwich Regular ☛ Vitamin K = 1.1 mcg; Serving size: 1 oz, 28.4 g

Cookies—Peanut Butter—Commercially Prepared, Regular ☛ Vitamin K = 1.2 mcg; Serving size: 1 oz, 28.4 g

Cookies—Peanut Butter—Commercially Prepared, Sugar Free ☛ Vitamin K = 10.1 mcg; Serving size: 1 serving 3 cookies, 29 g

Cookies—Raisin Soft-Type ☛ Vitamin K = 1.1 mcg; Serving size: 1 oz, 28.4 g

Cookies—ShortBread—Commercially Prepared Plain ☛ Vitamin K = 3.1 mcg; Serving size: 1 oz, 28.4 g

Cookies—ShortBread—Reduced Fat ☛ Vitamin K = 0.4 mcg; Serving size: 1 cookie, 11.8 g

Cookies—Sugar Refrigerated Dough ☛ Vitamin K = 2.9 mcg; Serving size: 1 serving, 33 g

Cookies—Sugar Refrigerated Dough Baked ☛ Vitamin K = 2.8 mcg; Serving size: 1 oz, 28.4 g

Cookies—Sugar Wafer Chocolate-Covered ☛ Vitamin K = 2 mcg; Serving size: 3 cookie, 29 g

Cookies—Sugar Wafer With Creme Filling Sugar Free ☛ Vitamin K = 0.7 mcg; Serving size: 1 oz, 28.4 g

Cookies—Sugar Wafers With Creme Filling Regular ☛ Vitamin K = 0.8 mcg; Serving size: 3 cookies, 36 g

Cookies—Sugar—Commercially Prepared, Regular (With Vanilla) ☛ Vitamin K = 2.4 mcg; Serving size: 1 oz, 28.4 g

Cookies—Vanilla Sandwich With Creme Filling ☛ Vitamin K = 1.4 mcg; Serving size: 1 oz, 28.4 g

Cookies—Vanilla Sandwich With Creme Filling Reduced Fat ☛ Vitamin K = 1.2 mcg; Serving size: 1 serving cookie, 48 g

Cookies—Vanilla Wafers Higher Fat ☛ Vitamin K = 8.7 mcg; Serving size: 8 wafers, 30 g

Cookies—Vanilla Wafers Lower Fat ☛ Vitamin K = 1.7 mcg; Serving size: 1 oz, 28.4 g

Cookies—Vanilla With Caramel Coconut And Chocolate Coating ☛ Vitamin K = 1.5 mcg; Serving size: 2 cookies, 29 g

Cookies—With Peanut Butter Filling Chocolate-Coated ☛ Vitamin K = 1.2 mcg; Serving size: 2 cookies, 25 g

Corn Muffins ☛ Vitamin K = 0.7 mcg; Serving size: 1 oz, 28.4 g

Corn Pone Baked ☛ Vitamin K = 6.8 mcg; Serving size: 1 pone (8" dia x 3/4"), 377 g

Corn Pone Fried ☛ Vitamin K = 2.9 mcg; Serving size: 1 piece, 61 g

CornBread—Made From Home Recipe ☛ Vitamin K = 0.9 mcg; Serving size: 1 surface inch, 11 g

CornBread—Muffin Stick Round Made From Home Recipe ☛ Vitamin K = 6.1 mcg; Serving size: 1 small, 66 g

Cornmeal Dumpling ☛ Vitamin K = 6 mcg; Serving size: 1 cup, cooked, 240 g

Cornmeal Fritter—Puerto Rican Style ☛ Vitamin K = 5 mcg; Serving size: 1 fritter (2-1/2" x 2-1/2" x 1/4"), 40 g

Cornmeal Stick Puerto Rican Style ☛ Vitamin K = 3.8 mcg; Serving size: 1 stick (3" x 3/4"), 20 g

Cracker Meal ☛ Vitamin K = 0.1 mcg; Serving size: 1 oz, 28.4 g

Crackers—Cheese Low Sodium ☛ Vitamin K = 1.6 mcg; Serving size: 1/2 oz, 14.2 g

Crackers—Cheese Reduced Fat ☛ Vitamin K = 1.1 mcg; Serving size: 1 serving, 30 g

Crackers—Cheese Regular ☛ Vitamin K = 1.3 mcg; Serving size: 1/2 oz, 14.2 g

Crackers—Cheese Sandwich-Type With Cheese Filling ☛ Vitamin K = 8 mcg; Serving size: 6 cracker 1 cracker = 6.5g, 39 g

Crackers—Cheese Sandwich-Type With Peanut Butter Filling ☛ Vitamin K = 1.7 mcg; Serving size: 1/2 oz, 14.2 g

Crackers—Cheese Whole Grain ☛ Vitamin K = 1.2 mcg; Serving size: 1 serving 55 pieces, 31 g

Crackers—Cream Gamesa Sabrosas ☛ Vitamin K = 5.5 mcg; Serving size: 11 crackers, 31 g

Crackers—Flavored Fish-Shaped ☛ Vitamin K = 1.4 mcg; Serving size: 10 goldfish, 5.2 g

Crackers—Gluten-Free Multi-Seeded And Multigrain ☛ Vitamin K = 0.8 mcg; Serving size: 3 crackers, 6.1 g

Crackers—Milk ☛ Vitamin K = 0.5 mcg; Serving size: 1/2 oz, 14.2 g

Crackers—Multigrain ☛ Vitamin K = 5 mcg; Serving size: 4 crackers, 14 g

Crackers—Rye Wafers Plain ☛ Vitamin K = 0.8 mcg; Serving size: 1/2 oz, 14.2 g

Crackers—Saltines (With Oyster Soda Soup) ☛ Vitamin K = 3.8 mcg; Serving size: 5 crackers, 14.9 g

Crackers—Saltines Fat-Free Low-Sodium ☛ Vitamin K = 0.7 mcg; Serving size: 3 saltines, 15 g

Crackers—Saltines Low Salt (With Oyster Soda Soup) ☛ Vitamin K = 2.2 mcg; Serving size: 1/2 oz, 14.2 g

Crackers—Saltines Whole Wheat (With Multi-Grain) ☛ Vitamin K = 2.6 mcg; Serving size: 1 serving, 14 g

Crackers—Sandwich-Type Peanut Butter Filled Reduced Fat ☛ Vitamin K = 1.1 mcg; Serving size: 1 package, 36 g

Crackers—Standard Snack-Type Regular ☛ Vitamin K = 11.1 mcg; Serving size: 5 crackers, 16 g

Crackers—Standard Snack-Type Regular Low Salt ☛ Vitamin K = 0.9 mcg; Serving size: 1/2 oz, 14.2 g

Crackers—Standard Snack-Type Sandwich With Cheese Filling ☛ Vitamin K = 1.2 mcg; Serving size: 1/2 oz, 14.2 g

Crackers—Standard Snack-Type Sandwich With Peanut Butter Filling ☛ Vitamin K = 1.3 mcg; Serving size: 1/2 oz, 14.2 g

Crackers—Standard Snack-Type With Whole Wheat ☛ Vitamin K = 2.1 mcg; Serving size: 5 crackers 1 serving, 15 g

Crackers—Toast Thins Low Sodium ☛ Vitamin K = 8.6 mcg; Serving size: 1 serving, 31 g

Crackers—Water Biscuits ☛ Vitamin K = 0.3 mcg; Serving size: 4 cracker 1 serving, 14 g

Crackers—Wheat Low Salt ☛ Vitamin K = 1.4 mcg; Serving size: 1/2 oz, 14.2 g

Crackers—Wheat Reduced Fat ☛ Vitamin K = 7.2 mcg; Serving size: 1 serving, 29 g

Crackers—Wheat Regular ☛ Vitamin K = 4.8 mcg; Serving size: 16 crackers 1 serving, 34 g

Crackers—Whole Grain Sandwich-Type With Peanut Butter Filling ☛ Vitamin K = 1.9 mcg; Serving size: 6 cracker 1 serving, 43 g

Crackers—Whole-Wheat ☛ Vitamin K = 7.6 mcg; Serving size: 1 serving, 28 g

Crackers—Whole-Wheat Low Salt ☛ Vitamin K = 1.2 mcg; Serving size: 1/2 oz, 14.2 g

Crackers—Whole-Wheat Reduced Fat ☛ Vitamin K = 3.6 mcg; Serving size: 1 serving, 29 g

Cream Puff Shell—Prepared From Recipe, ☛ Vitamin K = 7 mcg; Serving size: 1 oz, 28.4 g

Crisp Apple Apple Dessert ☛ Vitamin K = 8.9 mcg; Serving size: 1 cup, 246 g

Crisp Blueberry ☞ Vitamin K = 58.3 mcg; Serving size: 1 cup, 246 g

Crisp Cherry ☞ Vitamin K = 23.1 mcg; Serving size: 1 cup, 246 g

Crisp Peach ☞ Vitamin K = 23.1 mcg; Serving size: 1 cup, 246 g

Crisp Rhubarb ☞ Vitamin K = 53.1 mcg; Serving size: 1 cup, 246 g

Croutons Seasoned ☞ Vitamin K = 1.1 mcg; Serving size: 1/2 oz, 14.2 g

Crumpet ☞ Vitamin K = 0.2 mcg; Serving size: 1 small (2-1/2" dia), 20 g

Crumpet Toasted ☞ Vitamin K = 0.2 mcg; Serving size: 1 small (2-1/2" dia), 18 g

Danish Pastry—Cheese ☞ Vitamin K = 2 mcg; Serving size: 1 oz, 28.4 g

Danish Pastry—Cinnamon Enriched ☞ Vitamin K = 2.7 mcg; Serving size: 1 oz, 28.4 g

Danish Pastry—Fruit Enriched (With Apple Cinnamon Raisin Lemon Raspberry Strawberry) ☞ Vitamin K = 1.5 mcg; Serving size: 1 oz, 28.4 g

Dessert Pizza ☞ Vitamin K = 13.6 mcg; Serving size: 1 piece, 108 g

Doughnuts—Cake-Type Chocolate Sugared Or Glazed ☞ Vitamin K = 2.8 mcg; Serving size: 1 oz, 28.4 g

Doughnuts—Cake-Type Plain (With Unsugared Old-Fashioned) ☞ Vitamin K = 3.9 mcg; Serving size: 1 donut, 40 g

Doughnuts—Cake-Type Plain Chocolate-Coated Or Frosted ☞ Vitamin K = 2.2 mcg; Serving size: 1 oz, 28.4 g

Doughnuts—Cake—Type Chocolate Covered Dipped In Peanuts ☞ Vitamin K = 4.4 mcg; Serving size: 1 doughnut (3-1/4" dia), 53 g

Doughnuts—Chocolate Cream-Filled ☞ Vitamin K = 5.9 mcg; Serving size: 1 doughnut, 65 g

Doughnuts—Chocolate Raised Or Yeast ☛ Vitamin K = 5.6 mcg; Serving size: 1 doughnut, 50 g

Doughnuts—Chocolate Raised Or Yeast With Chocolate Icing ☛ Vitamin K = 6.7 mcg; Serving size: 1 doughnut (3" dia), 71 g

Doughnuts—Custard-Filled With Icing ☛ Vitamin K = 4.8 mcg; Serving size: 1 doughnut, 70 g

Doughnuts—French Crullers Glazed ☛ Vitamin K = 2.3 mcg; Serving size: 1 oz, 28.4 g

Doughnuts—Raised Or Yeast Chocolate Covered ☛ Vitamin K = 6.8 mcg; Serving size: 1 doughnut (3" dia), 71 g

Doughnuts—Yeast-Leavened Glazed Enriched (With Honey Buns) ☛ Vitamin K = 3.3 mcg; Serving size: 1 oz, 28.4 g

Doughnuts—Yeast-Leavened With Creme Filling ☛ Vitamin K = 2.4 mcg; Serving size: 1 oz, 28.4 g

Doughnuts—Yeast-Leavened With Jelly Filling ☛ Vitamin K = 2 mcg; Serving size: 1 oz, 28.4 g

Dumpling Plain ☛ Vitamin K = 0.3 mcg; Serving size: 1 small, 18 g

Dutch Apple Pie ☛ Vitamin K = 21.5 mcg; Serving size: 1/8 pie 1 pie (1/8 of 9 inch pie), 131 g

Empanada Mexican Turnover Pumpkin ☛ Vitamin K = 14.7 mcg; Serving size: 1 cup, 132 g

Empanada Mexican Turnover Fruit-Filled ☛ Vitamin K = 9.9 mcg; Serving size: 1 cup, 142 g

English Muffins ☛ Vitamin K = 0.2 mcg; Serving size: 1 oz, 28.4 g

English Muffins—Plain Enriched With Ca Prop (With Sourdough) ☛ Vitamin K = 0.3 mcg; Serving size: 1 oz, 28.4 g

English Muffins—Plain Toasted Enriched With Calcium Propionate (With Sourdough) ☛ Vitamin K = 0.4 mcg; Serving size: 1 oz, 28.4 g

English Muffins—Raisin-Cinnamon (With Apple-Cinnamon) ☛ Vitamin K = 0.7 mcg; Serving size: 1 oz, 28.4 g

English Muffins—Raisin-Cinnamon Toasted (With Apple-Cinnamon) ☛ Vitamin K = 0.7 mcg; Serving size: 1 oz, 28.4 g

English Muffins—Whole Grain White ☛ Vitamin K = 1.3 mcg; Serving size: 1 muffin 1 serving, 57 g

English Muffins—Whole-Wheat ☛ Vitamin K = 0.3 mcg; Serving size: 1 oz, 28.4 g

Fig Bars ☛ Vitamin K = 1.6 mcg; Serving size: 1 oz, 28.4 g

Focaccia Italian FlatBread—Plain ☛ Vitamin K = 3.2 mcg; Serving size: 1 piece, 57 g

Forunte Cookies ☛ Vitamin K = 0.3 mcg; Serving size: 1 oz, 28.4 g

French Bread ☛ Vitamin K = 0.2 mcg; Serving size: 1 oz, 28.4 g

Fritter—Apple ☛ Vitamin K = 2 mcg; Serving size: 1 fritter (2-1/2" long x 1-5/8" wide), 17 g

Fritter—Banana ☛ Vitamin K = 3.9 mcg; Serving size: 1 fritter (2" long), 34 g

Fritter—Berry ☛ Vitamin K = 5.2 mcg; Serving size: 1 fritter (1-1/4" dia), 24 g

Funnel Cake—With Sugar ☛ Vitamin K = 14.2 mcg; Serving size: 1 cake (6" dia), 90 g

Funnel Cake—With Sugar And Fruit ☛ Vitamin K = 21.6 mcg; Serving size: 1 cake (6" dia), 135 g

Garlic Bread—From Fast Food / Restaurant ☛ Vitamin K = 10.9 mcg; Serving size: 1 small slice, 37 g

Garlic Bread—Frozen ☛ Vitamin K = 12.7 mcg; Serving size: 1 slice presliced, 43 g

Garlic Bread ☛ Vitamin K = 11.5 mcg; Serving size: 1 small slice, 39 g

Garlic Bread—With Melted Cheese From Fast Food / Restaurant ☛ Vitamin K = 10.5 mcg; Serving size: 1 small slice, 44 g

Garlic Bread—With Melted Cheese From Frozen ☛ Vitamin K = 11.4 mcg; Serving size: 1 small slice, 44 g

Garlic Bread—With Parmesan Cheese From Fast Food / Restaurant ☛ Vitamin K = 11.3 mcg; Serving size: 1 small slice, 39 g

Garlic Bread—With Parmesan Cheese From Frozen ☛ Vitamin K = 11.3 mcg; Serving size: 1 small slice, 39 g

Gingersnaps ☛ Vitamin K = 0.7 mcg; Serving size: 1 oz, 28.4 g

Hush Puppies—Prepared From Recipe, ☛ Vitamin K = 6.7 mcg; Serving size: 1 oz, 28.4 g

Ice Cream Cones Cake—Or Wafer-Type ☛ Vitamin K = 0.5 mcg; Serving size: 1 oz, 28.4 g

Ice Cream Cones Sugar Rolled-Type ☛ Vitamin K = 0.4 mcg; Serving size: 1 oz, 28.4 g

Injera Ethiopian Bread ☛ Vitamin K = 1.2 mcg; Serving size: 1 cup, pieces, 68 g

Johnnycake ☛ Vitamin K = 1.2 mcg; Serving size: 1 piece, 49 g

Ladyfingers ☛ Vitamin K = 0.1 mcg; Serving size: 1 oz, 28.4 g

Melba Toast ☛ Vitamin K = 0.1 mcg; Serving size: 1/2 oz, 14.2 g

Molasses Cookies ☛ Vitamin K = 1.6 mcg; Serving size: 1 oz, 28.4 g

Muffin Blueberry—Commercially Made, Low-Fat ☛ Vitamin K = 4 mcg; Serving size: 1 muffin small, 71 g

Muffin English Cheese ☛ Vitamin K = 0.8 mcg; Serving size: 1 muffin, 58 g

Muffin English Oat Bran With Raisins ☞ Vitamin K = 1 mcg; Serving size: 1 muffin, 58 g

Muffin English Wheat Bran With Raisins ☞ Vitamin K = 0.6 mcg; Serving size: 1 muffin, 58 g

Muffin English Whole Wheat With Raisins ☞ Vitamin K = 0.6 mcg; Serving size: 1 muffin, 58 g

Muffin English With Fruit Other Than Raisins ☞ Vitamin K = 2 mcg; Serving size: 1 muffin, 58 g

Muffin English With Raisins ☞ Vitamin K = 0.8 mcg; Serving size: 1 muffin, 58 g

Muffin—Whole Grain ☞ Vitamin K = 4.5 mcg; Serving size: 1 miniature, 25 g

Muffins Blueberry Toaster-Type ☞ Vitamin K = 5.5 mcg; Serving size: 1 oz, 28.4 g

Muffins Blueberry Toaster-Type Toasted ☞ Vitamin K = 5.9 mcg; Serving size: 1 oz, 28.4 g

Muffins Blueberry—Commercially Prepared, (With Mini-Muffins) ☞ Vitamin K = 11.1 mcg; Serving size: 1 oz, 28.4 g

Muffins Oat Bran ☞ Vitamin K = 3.7 mcg; Serving size: 1 oz, 28.4 g

Muffins Wheat Bran Toaster-Type With Raisins Toasted ☞ Vitamin K = 4.9 mcg; Serving size: 1 oz, 28.4 g

Multi-Grain Toast ☞ Vitamin K = 0.4 mcg; Serving size: 1 oz, 28.4 g

Naan Indian Flatbread ☞ Vitamin K = 1.6 mcg; Serving size: 1 piece (1/4 of 10" dia), 44 g

Nabisco Nabisco Ritz Crackers ☞ Vitamin K = 1.7 mcg; Serving size: 1 cracker, 3.3 g

Oatmeal Cookies ☞ Vitamin K = 2.3 mcg; Serving size: 1 oz, 28.4 g

Pan Dulce With Raisins And Icing ☛ Vitamin K = 2.5 mcg; Serving size: 1 roll, 93 g

Pancakes—Buckwheat Dry Mix Incomplete ☛ Vitamin K = 0.9 mcg; Serving size: 1 oz, 28.4 g

Pancakes—Gluten-Free Frozen—Ready-To-Heat ☛ Vitamin K = 2.1 mcg; Serving size: 1 pancake, 48 g

Pancakes—Plain Dry Mix Incomplete (With Buttermilk) ☛ Vitamin K = 0.2 mcg; Serving size: 1 oz, 28.4 g

Pancakes—Plain Frozen—Ready-To-Heat (With Buttermilk) ☛ Vitamin K = 1.8 mcg; Serving size: 1 oz, 28.4 g

Pancakes—Plain Frozen—Ready-To-Heat Microwave (With Buttermilk) ☛ Vitamin K = 2.1 mcg; Serving size: 1 oz, 28.4 g

Pancakes—Plain Reduced Fat ☛ Vitamin K = 2 mcg; Serving size: 1 serving 3 pancakes, 105 g

Pancakes—Whole Wheat Dry Mix Incomplete ☛ Vitamin K = 0.4 mcg; Serving size: 1/4 cup mix 1 serving, 38 g

Pannetone ☛ Vitamin K = 0.2 mcg; Serving size: 1 slice, 27 g

Pastry—Cheese-Filled ☛ Vitamin K = 3.8 mcg; Serving size: 1 pastry, 28 g

Pastry—Cookies—Type Fried ☛ Vitamin K = 8.7 mcg; Serving size: 1 pastry, 46 g

Pastry—Fruit-Filled ☛ Vitamin K = 13.7 mcg; Serving size: 1 pastry, 78 g

Pastry—Italian With Cheese ☛ Vitamin K = 0.9 mcg; Serving size: 1 pastry, 85 g

Pastry—Made With Bean Or Lotus Seed Paste Filling Baked ☛ Vitamin K = 2.7 mcg; Serving size: 1 small square moon cake, 51 g

Pastry—Made With Bean Paste And Salted Egg Yolk Filling Baked ☞ Vitamin K = 9.2 mcg; Serving size: 1 large square moon cake, 204 g

Pastry—Pastelitos De Guava (Guava Pastries) ☞ Vitamin K = 10.8 mcg; Serving size: 1 piece, 86 g

Pastry—Puff Custard Or Cream Filled Iced Or Not Iced ☞ Vitamin K = 5.6 mcg; Serving size: 1 cream horn, 57 g

Pepperidge Farm Goldfish Baked Snack Crackers—Original ☞ Vitamin K = 1.4 mcg; Serving size: 10 goldfish, 5.2 g

Phyllo Dough ☞ Vitamin K = 0.7 mcg; Serving size: 1 oz, 28.4 g

Pie Crust—Cookie-Type Chocolate Ready Crust ☞ Vitamin K = 33.1 mcg; Serving size: 1 crust, 182 g

Pie Crust—Cookie-Type Graham Cracker Ready Crust ☞ Vitamin K = 6.2 mcg; Serving size: 1 oz, 28.4 g

Pie Crust—Cookie-Type—Prepared From Recipe, Graham Cracker Chilled ☞ Vitamin K = 7.3 mcg; Serving size: 1 piece (1/8 of 9 inch crust), 30 g

Pie Crust—Cookie-Type—Prepared From Recipe, Vanilla Wafer Chilled ☞ Vitamin K = 43.9 mcg; Serving size: 1 cup, 129 g

Pie Crust—Deep Dish Frozen Baked Made With Enriched Flour ☞ Vitamin K = 33.7 mcg; Serving size: 1 pie crust (average weight), 202 g

Pie Crust—Deep Dish Frozen Unbaked Made With Enriched Flour ☞ Vitamin K = 33.8 mcg; Serving size: 1 pie crust (average weight), 225 g

Pie Crust—Refrigerated Regular Baked ☞ Vitamin K = 0.8 mcg; Serving size: 1 pie crust, 198 g

Pie Crust—Standard-Type Frozen Ready-To-Bake Enriched ☞ Vitamin K = 1 mcg; Serving size: 1 piece (1/8 of 9 inch crust), 18 g

Pie Crust—Standard-Type Frozen Ready-To-Bake Enriched Baked ☞

Vitamin K = 12 mcg; Serving size: 1 pie crust (average weight of 1 baked crust), 154 g

Pie Crust—Standard-Type—Prepared From Recipe, Baked ☞ Vitamin K = 3.4 mcg; Serving size: 1 piece (1/8 of 9 inch crust), 23 g

Pie Crust—Standard-Type—Prepared From Recipe, Unbaked ☞ Vitamin K = 3.2 mcg; Serving size: 1 piece (1/8 of 9 inch crust), 24 g

Pie Pudding—Chocolate With Chocolate Coating Individual Size ☞ Vitamin K = 6 mcg; Serving size: 1 individual pie, 142 g

Pie Pudding—Flavors Other Than Chocolate Individual Size Or Tart ☞ Vitamin K = 5.3 mcg; Serving size: 1 small tart, 117 g

Pie Pudding—Flavors Other Than Chocolate With Chocolate Coating Individual Size ☞ Vitamin K = 6 mcg; Serving size: 1 individual pie, 142 g

Pie—Apple Diet ☞ Vitamin K = 1.6 mcg; Serving size: 1 individual serving, 85 g

Pie—Apple—Commercially Prepared, Enriched Flour ☞ Vitamin K = 1 mcg; Serving size: 1 oz, 28.4 g

Pie—Banana Cream Individual Size Or Tart ☞ Vitamin K = 5.9 mcg; Serving size: 1 tart, 117 g

Pie—Banana Cream—Prepared From Recipe, ☞ Vitamin K = 1.8 mcg; Serving size: 1 oz, 28.4 g

Pie—Berry Not Blackberry Blueberry Boysenberry Huckleberry Raspberry Or Strawberry Individual Size Or Tart ☞ Vitamin K = 12.9 mcg; Serving size: 1 tart, 117 g

Pie—Blackberry Individual Size Or Tart ☞ Vitamin K = 19.9 mcg; Serving size: 1 tart, 117 g

Pie—Blueberry Individual Size Or Tart ☞ Vitamin K = 19.8 mcg; Serving size: 1 tart, 117 g

Pie—Cherry—Commercially Prepared, ☛ Vitamin K = 2.2 mcg; Serving size: 1 oz, 28.4 g

Pie—Chocolate Cream Individual Size Or Tart ☛ Vitamin K = 6.8 mcg; Serving size: 1 tart, 117 g

Pie—Chocolate Creme—Commercially Prepared, ☛ Vitamin K = 11.4 mcg; Serving size: 1 serving .167 pie, 120 g

Pie—Chocolate-Marshmallow ☛ Vitamin K = 100.7 mcg; Serving size: 1 pie (8" dia), 819 g

Pie—Coconut Cream Individual Size Or Tart ☛ Vitamin K = 5.5 mcg; Serving size: 1 tart, 117 g

Pie—Coconut Creme—Commercially Prepared, ☛ Vitamin K = 1.5 mcg; Serving size: 1 oz, 28.4 g

Pie—Custard Individual Size Or Tart ☛ Vitamin K = 2 mcg; Serving size: 1 tart, 117 g

Pie—Egg Custard—Commercially Prepared, ☛ Vitamin K = 0.9 mcg; Serving size: 1 oz, 28.4 g

Pie—Fried Pies Fruit ☛ Vitamin K = 1.2 mcg; Serving size: 1 oz, 28.4 g

Pie—Lemon Cream Individual Size Or Tart ☛ Vitamin K = 9.1 mcg; Serving size: 1 tart, 117 g

Pie—Lemon Meringue—Commercially Prepared, ☛ Vitamin K = 0.6 mcg; Serving size: 1 oz, 28.4 g

Pie—Lemon Not Cream Or Meringue Individual Size Or Tart ☛ Vitamin K = 10.8 mcg; Serving size: 1 tart, 117 g

Pie—Mince Individual Size Or Tart ☛ Vitamin K = 9 mcg; Serving size: 1 tart, 117 g

Pie—Mince—Prepared From Recipe, ☛ Vitamin K = 1.5 mcg; Serving size: 1 oz, 28.4 g

Pie—Peach ☛ Vitamin K = 0.9 mcg; Serving size: 1 oz, 28.4 g

Pie—Peach Individual Size Or Tart ☛ Vitamin K = 10.1 mcg; Serving size: 1 tart, 117 g

Pie—Pear Individual Size Or Tart ☛ Vitamin K = 10.8 mcg; Serving size: 1 tart, 117 g

Pie—Pecan—Commercially Prepared, ☛ Vitamin K = 4.4 mcg; Serving size: 1 oz, 28.4 g

Pie—Pumpkin—Commercially Prepared, ☛ Vitamin K = 3.7 mcg; Serving size: 1 oz, 28.4 g

Pie—Raisin Individual Size Or Tart ☛ Vitamin K = 8.9 mcg; Serving size: 1 tart, 117 g

Pie—Rhubarb Individual Size Or Tart ☛ Vitamin K = 22.8 mcg; Serving size: 1 tart, 117 g

Pie—Strawberry Cream Individual Size Or Tart ☛ Vitamin K = 6.3 mcg; Serving size: 1 tart, 117 g

Pie—Strawberry Individual Size Or Tart ☛ Vitamin K = 9 mcg; Serving size: 1 tart, 117 g

Pie—Vanilla Cream—Prepared From Recipe, ☛ Vitamin K = 1.9 mcg; Serving size: 1 oz, 28.4 g

Pita Bread ☛ Vitamin K = 0.1 mcg; Serving size: 1 pita, large (6-1/2 inch dia), 60 g

Pizza—Cheese Gluten-Free Thick Crust ☛ Vitamin K = 6.5 mcg; Serving size: 1 piece, 132 g

Pizza—Cheese Gluten-Free Thin Crust ☛ Vitamin K = 7.3 mcg; Serving size: 1 piece, 119 g

Pizza—Cheese Whole Wheat Thick Crust ☛ Vitamin K = 7.3 mcg; Serving size: 1 piece, 132 g

Pizza—Cheese Whole Wheat Thin Crust ☛ Vitamin K = 7.9 mcg; Serving size: 1 piece, 119 g

Pizza—Cheese With Fruit Medium Crust ☛ Vitamin K = 8.1 mcg; Serving size: 1 piece, 137 g

Pizza—Cheese With Fruit Thick Crust ☛ Vitamin K = 13.4 mcg; Serving size: 1 piece, 150 g

Pizza—Cheese With Fruit Thin Crust ☛ Vitamin K = 8.4 mcg; Serving size: 1 piece, 104 g

Pizza—Cheese With Vegetables From Frozen Thick Crust ☛ Vitamin K = 10.4 mcg; Serving size: 1 piece, 143 g

Pizza—Cheese With Vegetables From Frozen Thin Crust ☛ Vitamin K = 7 mcg; Serving size: 1 piece, 109 g

Pizza—Cheese With Vegetables From Restaurant Or Fast Food Medium Crust ☛ Vitamin K = 8.6 mcg; Serving size: 1 piece, 133 g

Pizza—Cheese With Vegetables From Restaurant Or Fast Food Thick Crust ☛ Vitamin K = 14.2 mcg; Serving size: 1 piece, 149 g

Pizza—Cheese With Vegetables From Restaurant Or Fast Food Thin Crust ☛ Vitamin K = 9.1 mcg; Serving size: 1 piece, 100 g

Pizza—Extra Cheese Thick Crust ☛ Vitamin K = 13.5 mcg; Serving size: 1 piece, 141 g

Pizza—Extra Cheese Thin Crust ☛ Vitamin K = 8.5 mcg; Serving size: 1 piece, 92 g

Pizza—No Cheese Thick Crust ☛ Vitamin K = 11.9 mcg; Serving size: 1 piece, 124 g

Pizza—No Cheese Thin Crust ☛ Vitamin K = 7.4 mcg; Serving size: 1 piece, 75 g

Pizza—Rolls ☛ Vitamin K = 5.7 mcg; Serving size: 1 cup, 119 g

Pizza—With Beans And Vegetables Thick Crust ☛ Vitamin K = 14.7 mcg; Serving size: 1 piece, 173 g

Pizza—With Beans And Vegetables Thin Crust ☞ Vitamin K = 9.9 mcg; Serving size: 1 piece, 129 g

Pizza—With Cheese And Extra Vegetables Medium Crust ☞ Vitamin K = 9 mcg; Serving size: 1 piece, 152 g

Pizza—With Cheese And Extra Vegetables Thick Crust ☞ Vitamin K = 14 mcg; Serving size: 1 piece, 155 g

Pizza—With Cheese And Extra Vegetables Thin Crust ☞ Vitamin K = 9.4 mcg; Serving size: 1 piece, 120 g

Pizza—With Extra Meat And Extra Vegetables Medium Crust ☞ Vitamin K = 8.9 mcg; Serving size: 1 piece, 159 g

Pizza—With Extra Meat And Extra Vegetables Thick Crust ☞ Vitamin K = 14.2 mcg; Serving size: 1 piece, 173 g

Pizza—With Extra Meat And Extra Vegetables Thin Crust ☞ Vitamin K = 9.4 mcg; Serving size: 1 piece, 129 g

Pizza—With Extra Meat Medium Crust ☞ Vitamin K = 8.9 mcg; Serving size: 1 piece, 150 g

Pizza—With Extra Meat Thick Crust ☞ Vitamin K = 14.1 mcg; Serving size: 1 piece, 166 g

Pizza—With Extra Meat Thin Crust ☞ Vitamin K = 9.4 mcg; Serving size: 1 piece, 120 g

Pizza—With Meat And Fruit Medium Crust ☞ Vitamin K = 8.1 mcg; Serving size: 1 piece, 150 g

Pizza—With Meat And Fruit Thick Crust ☞ Vitamin K = 13.2 mcg; Serving size: 1 piece, 157 g

Pizza—With Meat And Fruit Thin Crust ☞ Vitamin K = 8.5 mcg; Serving size: 1 piece, 115 g

Pizza—With Meat And Vegetables From Restaurant Or Fast Food Thick Crust ☞ Vitamin K = 13.9 mcg; Serving size: 1 piece, 149 g

Pizza—With Meat And Vegetables From Restaurant Or Fast Food Thin Crust ☛ Vitamin K = 9.4 mcg; Serving size: 1 piece, 113 g

Pizza—With Meat Gluten-Free Thick Crust ☛ Vitamin K = 6.7 mcg; Serving size: 1 piece, 139 g

Pizza—With Meat Gluten-Free Thin Crust ☛ Vitamin K = 7.2 mcg; Serving size: 1 piece, 124 g

Pizza—With Meat Other Than Pepperoni From Frozen Medium Crust ☛ Vitamin K = 5.8 mcg; Serving size: 1 piece, 102 g

Pizza—With Meat Other Than Pepperoni From Frozen Thick Crust ☛ Vitamin K = 10.5 mcg; Serving size: 1 piece, 144 g

Pizza—With Meat Other Than Pepperoni From Frozen Thin Crust ☛ Vitamin K = 4 mcg; Serving size: 1 piece, 97 g

Pizza—With Meat Other Than Pepperoni From School Lunch Medium Crust ☛ Vitamin K = 6.3 mcg; Serving size: 1 piece, 147 g

Pizza—With Meat Other Than Pepperoni Stuffed Crust ☛ Vitamin K = 12.8 mcg; Serving size: 1 piece, 164 g

Pizza—With Meat Whole Wheat Thick Crust ☛ Vitamin K = 7.4 mcg; Serving size: 1 piece, 139 g

Pizza—With Meat Whole Wheat Thin Crust ☛ Vitamin K = 7.7 mcg; Serving size: 1 piece, 124 g

Pizza—With Pepperoni From Frozen Medium Crust ☛ Vitamin K = 6 mcg; Serving size: 1 piece, 102 g

Pizza—With Pepperoni From Frozen Thick Crust ☛ Vitamin K = 10.7 mcg; Serving size: 1 piece, 144 g

Pizza—With Pepperoni From Frozen Thin Crust ☛ Vitamin K = 4.2 mcg; Serving size: 1 piece, 97 g

Pizza—With Pepperoni From School Lunch Medium Crust ☛ Vitamin K = 11.8 mcg; Serving size: 1 piece, 147 g

Pizza—With Pepperoni Stuffed Crust ☛ Vitamin K = 13.3 mcg; Serving size: 1 piece, 164 g

Plain Graham Crackers ☛ Vitamin K = 4.1 mcg; Serving size: 1 oz, 28.4 g

Popover ☛ Vitamin K = 0.2 mcg; Serving size: 1 popover, 31 g

Puff Pastry ☛ Vitamin K = 4.6 mcg; Serving size: 1 oz, 28.4 g

Puff Pastry—Frozen Ready-To-Bake Baked ☛ Vitamin K = 4.6 mcg; Serving size: 1 oz, 28.4 g

Roll Cheese ☛ Vitamin K = 4.2 mcg; Serving size: 1 roll, 41 g

Roll Sweet Frosted ☛ Vitamin K = 3 mcg; Serving size: 1 small, 54 g

Roll Sweet With Fruit Frosted ☛ Vitamin K = 3.1 mcg; Serving size: 1 small, 54 g

Rolls—Dinner Egg ☛ Vitamin K = 0.6 mcg; Serving size: 1 oz, 28.4 g

Rolls—Dinner Oat Bran ☛ Vitamin K = 0.3 mcg; Serving size: 1 oz, 28.4 g

Rolls—Dinner Plain—Commercially Prepared, (With Brown-And-Serve) ☛ Vitamin K = 3 mcg; Serving size: 1 roll (1 oz), 28 g

Rolls—Dinner Rye ☛ Vitamin K = 1.3 mcg; Serving size: 1 large (3-1/2 inch to 4 inch dia), 43 g

Rolls—Dinner Sweet ☛ Vitamin K = 0.2 mcg; Serving size: 1 roll, 30 g

Rolls—Dinner Wheat ☛ Vitamin K = 0.8 mcg; Serving size: 1 roll (1 oz), 28 g

Rolls—Dinner Whole-Wheat ☛ Vitamin K = 0.6 mcg; Serving size: 1 roll (1 oz), 28 g

Rolls—French ☛ Vitamin K = 0.5 mcg; Serving size: 1 oz, 28.4 g

Rolls—Gluten-Free White Made With Rice Flour Rice Starch And Corn Starch ☛ Vitamin K = 0.1 mcg; Serving size: 1 roll, 78 g

Rolls—Hamburger Or Hot Dog Wheat/cracked Wheat ☛ Vitamin K = 3.5 mcg; Serving size: 1 roll, 51 g

Rolls—Hamburger Or Hot Dog Whole Wheat ☛ Vitamin K = 2.5 mcg; Serving size: 1 roll, 56 g

Rolls—Hamburger Or Hotdog Mixed-Grain ☛ Vitamin K = 0.9 mcg; Serving size: 1 oz, 28.4 g

Rolls—Hamburger Or Hotdog Plain ☛ Vitamin K = 2.1 mcg; Serving size: 1 roll 1 serving, 44 g

Rolls—Hamburger Whole Grain White Calcium-Fortified ☛ Vitamin K = 2.2 mcg; Serving size: 1 piece roll, 43 g

Rolls—Hard (With Kaiser) ☛ Vitamin K = 0.2 mcg; Serving size: 1 oz, 28.4 g

Rolls—Pumpernickel ☛ Vitamin K = 0.5 mcg; Serving size: 1 medium (2-1/2 inch dia), 36 g

Rye Bread ☛ Vitamin K = 0.3 mcg; Serving size: 1 oz, 28.4 g

Rye Crispbread ☛ Vitamin K = 0.9 mcg; Serving size: 1/2 oz, 14.2 g

Scone ☛ Vitamin K = 4.2 mcg; Serving size: 1 scone, 42 g

Scone With Fruit ☛ Vitamin K = 4 mcg; Serving size: 1 scone, 42 g

Sopaipilla With Syrup Or Honey ☛ Vitamin K = 1 mcg; Serving size: 1 sopaipilla (1 1/2" x 1 1/2"), 12 g

Sopaipilla Without Syrup Or Honey ☛ Vitamin K = 1.1 mcg; Serving size: 1 sopaipilla (1 1/2" x 1 1/2"), 10 g

Spoonbread ☛ Vitamin K = 6.7 mcg; Serving size: 1 cup, 187 g

Strudel—Berry ☛ Vitamin K = 11.7 mcg; Serving size: 1 piece, 64 g

Strudel—Cheese ☛ Vitamin K = 3.5 mcg; Serving size: 1 piece, 64 g

Strudel—Cheese And Fruit ☛ Vitamin K = 2.4 mcg; Serving size: 1 piece, 64 g

Strudel—Cherry ☞ Vitamin K = 4.2 mcg; Serving size: 1 piece, 64 g

Strudel—Peach ☞ Vitamin K = 4.6 mcg; Serving size: 1 piece, 64 g

Strudel—Pineapple ☞ Vitamin K = 4 mcg; Serving size: 1 piece, 64 g

Sweet Bread—Dough Filled With Bean Paste Meatless—Steamed ☞ Vitamin K = 3.6 mcg; Serving size: 1 manapua, 103 g

Sweet Rolls—Cinnamon—Commercially Prepared, With Raisins ☞ Vitamin K = 1.2 mcg; Serving size: 1 oz, 28.4 g

Taco Shells Baked ☞ Vitamin K = 1.1 mcg; Serving size: 1 shell, 12.9 g

Tamale Sweet ☞ Vitamin K = 2.2 mcg; Serving size: 1 tamale, 34 g

Tamale Sweet With Fruit ☞ Vitamin K = 2.3 mcg; Serving size: 1 tamale, 49 g

Tiramisu ☞ Vitamin K = 3 mcg; Serving size: 1 piece, 174 g

Toasted Bagels ☞ Vitamin K = 0.2 mcg; Serving size: 1 mini bagel (2-1/2 inch dia), 24 g

Toasted Cinnamon Raisin Bagels ☞ Vitamin K = 0.2 mcg; Serving size: 1 mini bagel (2-1/2 inch dia), 24 g

Toasted White Bread ☞ Vitamin K = 1 mcg; Serving size: 1 oz, 28.4 g

Toasted Whole Wheat Bread ☞ Vitamin K = 2.6 mcg; Serving size: 1 oz, 28.4 g

Toaster Pastries Fruit (With Apple Blueberry Cherry Strawberry) ☞ Vitamin K = 4.4 mcg; Serving size: 1 oz, 28.4 g

Toaster Pastries Fruit Frosted (Include Apples Blueberry Cherry Strawberry) ☞ Vitamin K = 10.3 mcg; Serving size: 1 piece, 53 g

Toaster Pastries Fruit Toasted (Include Apple Blueberry Cherry Strawberry) ☞ Vitamin K = 3.4 mcg; Serving size: 1 pastry, 51 g

Topping From Cheese Pizza ☞ Vitamin K = 3.5 mcg; Serving size: topping from 1 piece, 40 g

Topping From Meat And Vegetable Pizza ☞ Vitamin K = 4.2 mcg; Serving size: topping from 1 piece, 51 g

Topping From Meat Pizza ☞ Vitamin K = 3.1 mcg; Serving size: topping from 1 piece, 41 g

Topping From Vegetable Pizza ☞ Vitamin K = 5.2 mcg; Serving size: topping from 1 piece, 49 g

Tortillas—Ready-To-Bake Or -Fry Flour Refrigerated ☞ Vitamin K = 3.5 mcg; Serving size: 1 tortilla, 48 g

Tortillas—Ready-To-Bake Or -Fry Flour Shelf Stable ☞ Vitamin K = 2.1 mcg; Serving size: 1 tortilla, 49 g

Tortillas—Ready-To-Bake Or -Fry Whole Wheat ☞ Vitamin K = 1.8 mcg; Serving size: 1 tortilla 1 serving, 41 g

Turnover Guava ☞ Vitamin K = 8.1 mcg; Serving size: 1 turnover, 78 g

Turnover Or Dumpling Apple ☞ Vitamin K = 8.1 mcg; Serving size: 1 turnover, 82 g

Turnover Or Dumpling Berry ☞ Vitamin K = 13.3 mcg; Serving size: 1 turnover, 78 g

Turnover Or Dumpling Cherry ☞ Vitamin K = 7 mcg; Serving size: 1 turnover, 78 g

Turnover Or Dumpling Lemon ☞ Vitamin K = 6.5 mcg; Serving size: 1 turnover, 78 g

Turnover Or Dumpling Peach ☞ Vitamin K = 7.6 mcg; Serving size: 1 turnover, 78 g

Turnover Pumpkin ☞ Vitamin K = 9.4 mcg; Serving size: 1 turnover, 78 g

Vans Gluten-Free Totally Original Waffles ☞ Vitamin K = 3.4 mcg; Serving size: 1 waffle, 47 g

Waffles—Buttermilk Frozen—Ready-To-Heat ☞ Vitamin K = 4.1 mcg; Serving size: 1 waffle, square, 39 g

Waffles—Buttermilk Frozen—Ready-To-Heat Microwaved ☞ Vitamin K = 3.8 mcg; Serving size: 1 waffle, 35 g

Waffles—Buttermilk Frozen—Ready-To-Heat Toasted ☞ Vitamin K = 3.5 mcg; Serving size: 1 oz, 28 g

Waffles—Chocolate Chip Frozen—Ready-To-Heat ☞ Vitamin K = 6.5 mcg; Serving size: 2 waffles, 70 g

Waffles—Gluten-Free Frozen—Ready-To-Heat ☞ Vitamin K = 5 mcg; Serving size: 1 waffle, 45 g

Waffles—Plain Frozen Ready -To-Heat Toasted ☞ Vitamin K = 1.9 mcg; Serving size: 1 oz, 28.4 g

Waffles—Plain Frozen—Ready-To-Heat ☞ Vitamin K = 2.2 mcg; Serving size: 1 oz, 28.4 g

Waffles—Plain Frozen—Ready-To-Heat Microwave ☞ Vitamin K = 2.6 mcg; Serving size: 1 waffle, round (4 inchdia), 32 g

Waffles—Whole Wheat Lowfat Frozen—Ready-To-Heat ☞ Vitamin K = 2.3 mcg; Serving size: 1 serving 2 waffles, 70 g

Wheat Bread ☞ Vitamin K = 1.4 mcg; Serving size: 1 oz, 28.4 g

Wheat Flour Fritter—Without Syrup ☞ Vitamin K = 6.9 mcg; Serving size: 1 fritter, 22 g

White Bread ☞ Vitamin K = 0.1 mcg; Serving size: 1 slice, 29 g

White Cake—With Coconut Frosting ☞ Vitamin K = 1.2 mcg; Serving size: 1 oz, 28.4 g

White Pizza—Cheese Thick Crust ☞ Vitamin K = 5.5 mcg; Serving size: 1 piece, 141 g

White Pizza—Cheese Thin Crust ☞ Vitamin K = 4.1 mcg; Serving size: 1 piece, 92 g

White Pizza—Cheese With Meat And Vegetables Thick Crust ☞ Vitamin K = 6.2 mcg; Serving size: 1 piece, 155 g

White Pizza—Cheese With Meat And Vegetables Thin Crust ☞ Vitamin K = 5.4 mcg; Serving size: 1 piece, 118 g

White Pizza—Cheese With Meat Thick Crust ☞ Vitamin K = 6 mcg; Serving size: 1 piece, 154 g

White Pizza—Cheese With Meat Thin Crust ☞ Vitamin K = 4.5 mcg; Serving size: 1 piece, 100 g

White Pizza—Cheese With Vegetables Thick Crust ☞ Vitamin K = 6 mcg; Serving size: 1 piece, 155 g

White Pizza—Cheese With Vegetables Thin Crust ☞ Vitamin K = 4.7 mcg; Serving size: 1 piece, 106 g

Whole Wheat Bread ☞ Vitamin K = 2.5 mcg; Serving size: 1 slice, 32 g

Whole Wheat Pita ☞ Vitamin K = 0.9 mcg; Serving size: 1 pita, large (6-1/2 inch dia), 64 g

Yam Buns; Puerto Rican Style ☞ Vitamin K = 34.9 mcg; Serving size: 1 cup, 153 g

Yellow Cake—With Chocolate Frosting ☞ Vitamin K = 36.1 mcg; Serving size: 1 piece (1/12 of a cake), 144 g

Yellow Cake—With Vanilla Frosting ☞ Vitamin K = 4.6 mcg; Serving size: 1 serving, 67 g

13

BEANS AND LENTILS

Bacon Meatless ☞ Vitamin K = 0 mcg; Serving size: 1 cup, 144 g

Beans—Baked Canned No Salt Added ☞ Vitamin K = 2 mcg; Serving size: 1 cup, 253 g

Beans—Baked Canned With Franks ☞ Vitamin K = 2.6 mcg; Serving size: 1 cup, 259 g

Beans—Baked Canned With Pork And Sweet Sauce ☞ Vitamin K = 1 mcg; Serving size: 1 cup, 249 g

Beans—Black Mature Seeds Raw ☞ Vitamin K = 10.9 mcg; Serving size: 1 cup, 194 g

Beans—Black Mature Seeds—Cooked Boiled ((With Salt)) ☞ Vitamin K = 5.7 mcg; Serving size: 1 cup, 172 g

Beans—Black Turtle Mature Seeds Canned ☞ Vitamin K = 5.5 mcg; Serving size: 1 cup, 240 g

Beans—Black Turtle Mature Seeds Raw ☞ Vitamin K = 10.3 mcg; Serving size: 1 cup, 184 g

Beans—Black Turtle Mature Seeds—Cooked Boiled ((With Salt)) ☞ Vitamin K = 6.1 mcg; Serving size: 1 cup, 185 g

Beans—Chili Barbecue Ranch Style—Cooked ☞ Vitamin K = 1 mcg; Serving size: 1 cup, 253 g

Beans—Dry—Cooked With Ground Beef ☞ Vitamin K = 26.1 mcg; Serving size: 1 cup, 266 g

Beans—Dry—Cooked With Pork ☞ Vitamin K = 16.9 mcg; Serving size: 1 cup, 178 g

Beans—Great Northern Mature Seeds Canned ☞ Vitamin K = 7.9 mcg; Serving size: 1 cup, 262 g

Beans—Great Northern Mature Seeds Raw ☞ Vitamin K = 11 mcg; Serving size: 1 cup, 183 g

Beans—Kidney All Types Mature Seeds Raw ☞ Vitamin K = 35 mcg; Serving size: 1 cup, 184 g

Beans—Kidney All Types Mature Seeds—Cooked Boiled ((With Salt)) ☞ Vitamin K = 5.8 mcg; Serving size: 1 cup, 177 g

Beans—Kidney Red Mature Seeds Canned Drained Solids Rinsed In Tap Water ☞ Vitamin K = 9 mcg; Serving size: 1 cup cup rinsed solids, 158 g

Beans—Kidney Red Mature Seeds Raw ☞ Vitamin K = 10.3 mcg; Serving size: 1 cup, 184 g

Beans—Kidney Red Mature Seeds—Cooked Boiled ((With Salt)) ☞ Vitamin K = 14.9 mcg; Serving size: 1 cup, 177 g

Beans—Navy Mature Seeds Raw ☞ Vitamin K = 5.2 mcg; Serving size: 1 cup, 208 g

Beans—Navy Mature Seeds—Cooked Boiled ((With Salt)) ☞ Vitamin K = 1.1 mcg; Serving size: 1 cup, 182 g

Beans—Pink Mature Seeds Raw ☞ Vitamin K = 12 mcg; Serving size: 1 cup, 210 g

Beans—Pink Mature Seeds—Cooked Boiled ((With Salt)) ☞ Vitamin K = 6.3 mcg; Serving size: 1 cup, 169 g

Beans—Pink Mature Seeds—Cooked Boiled ((Without Salt)) ☞ Vitamin K = 6.3 mcg; Serving size: 1 cup, 169 g

Beans—Pinto Mature Seeds Canned Solids And Liquids ☞ Vitamin K = 5 mcg; Serving size: 1 cup, 240 g

Beans—Pinto Mature Seeds Raw ☞ Vitamin K = 10.8 mcg; Serving size: 1 cup, 193 g

Beans—Pinto Mature Seeds—Cooked Boiled ((With Salt)) ☞ Vitamin K = 6 mcg; Serving size: 1 cup, 171 g

Beans—White Mature Seeds Canned ☞ Vitamin K = 7.6 mcg; Serving size: 1 cup, 262 g

Beans—White Mature Seeds Raw ☞ Vitamin K = 11.3 mcg; Serving size: 1 cup, 202 g

Beans—White Mature Seeds—Cooked Boiled ((With Salt)) ☞ Vitamin K = 6.3 mcg; Serving size: 1 cup, 179 g

Beans—Yellow Mature Seeds—Cooked Boiled ((With Salt)) ☞ Vitamin K = 6.2 mcg; Serving size: 1 cup, 177 g

Beans—Yellow Mature Seeds—Cooked Boiled ((Without Salt)) ☞ Vitamin K = 6.2 mcg; Serving size: 1 cup, 177 g

Black Bean Salad ☞ Vitamin K = 27.3 mcg; Serving size: 1 cup, 231 g

Black Beans ☞ Vitamin K = 5.7 mcg; Serving size: 1 cup, 172 g

Black Beans—Cuban Style ☞ Vitamin K = 11.9 mcg; Serving size: 1 cup, 270 g

Black Brown Or Bayo Beans—Canned Drained —Cooked without Fat ☞ Vitamin K = 6.1 mcg; Serving size: 1 cup, 180 g

Black Brown Or Bayo Beans—Canned Drained Made With Animal Fat Or Meat Drippings ☛ Vitamin K = 5.8 mcg; Serving size: 1 cup, 180 g

Black Brown Or Bayo Beans—Canned Drained Made With Margarine ☛ Vitamin K = 19.1 mcg; Serving size: 1 cup, 180 g

Black Brown Or Bayo Beans—Canned Drained Made With Oil ☛ Vitamin K = 20.5 mcg; Serving size: 1 cup, 180 g

Black Brown Or Bayo Beans—Dry—Cooked—Cooked without Fat ☛ Vitamin K = 5.9 mcg; Serving size: 1 cup, 180 g

Black Brown Or Bayo Beans—Dry—Cooked Made With Animal Fat Or Meat Drippings ☛ Vitamin K = 5.6 mcg; Serving size: 1 cup, 180 g

Black Brown Or Bayo Beans—Dry—Cooked Made With Margarine ☛ Vitamin K = 18.9 mcg; Serving size: 1 cup, 180 g

Black Brown Or Bayo Beans—Dry—Cooked Made With Oil ☛ Vitamin K = 20.9 mcg; Serving size: 1 cup, 180 g

Black Turtle Beans ☛ Vitamin K = 6.1 mcg; Serving size: 1 cup, 185 g

Black-Eyed Peas—(Cowpeas) ☛ Vitamin K = 2.9 mcg; Serving size: 1 cup, 171 g

Boiled SoyBeans—(Edamame) ☛ Vitamin K = 33 mcg; Serving size: 1 cup, 172 g

Broad Beans—(Fava) ☛ Vitamin K = 4.9 mcg; Serving size: 1 cup, 170 g

BroadBeans—(Fava Beans) Mature Seeds Raw ☛ Vitamin K = 13.5 mcg; Serving size: 1 cup, 150 g

BroadBeans—(Fava Beans) Mature Seeds—Cooked Boiled ((With Salt)) ☛ Vitamin K = 4.9 mcg; Serving size: 1 cup, 170 g

Carob Flour ☛ Vitamin K = 0 mcg; Serving size: 1 cup, 103 g

Chicken Meatless ☛ Vitamin K = 0 mcg; Serving size: 1 cup, 168 g

Chicken Meatless Breaded Fried ☛ Vitamin K = 0 mcg; Serving size: 1 cup, diced, 130 g

Chickpea Flour (Besan) ☛ Vitamin K = 8.4 mcg; Serving size: 1 cup, 92 g

ChickPeas—Mature Seeds Canned Drained Rinsed In Tap Water ☛ Vitamin K = 8.6 mcg; Serving size: 1 can drained, rinsed, 254 g

ChickPeas—Mature Seeds Canned Drained Solids ☛ Vitamin K = 8.6 mcg; Serving size: 1 can drained, 253 g

ChickPeas—Mature Seeds Raw ☛ Vitamin K = 18 mcg; Serving size: 1 cup, 200 g

ChickPeas—Mature Seeds—Cooked Boiled ((With Salt)) ☛ Vitamin K = 6.6 mcg; Serving size: 1 cup, 164 g

ChickPeas—(Garbanzo Beans) (Cooked) ☛ Vitamin K = 6.6 mcg; Serving size: 1 cup, 164 g

ChickPeas—Canned Drained—Cooked without Fat ☛ Vitamin K = 6.7 mcg; Serving size: 1 cup, 180 g

ChickPeas—Canned Drained Made With Oil ☛ Vitamin K = 21.1 mcg; Serving size: 1 cup, 180 g

ChickPeas—Dry—Cooked—Cooked without Fat ☛ Vitamin K = 7.2 mcg; Serving size: 1 cup, 180 g

ChickPeas—Dry—Cooked Made With Animal Fat Or Meat Drippings ☛ Vitamin K = 6.7 mcg; Serving size: 1 cup, 180 g

ChickPeas—Dry—Cooked Made With Margarine ☛ Vitamin K = 21.1 mcg; Serving size: 1 cup, 180 g

ChickPeas—Dry—Cooked Made With Oil ☛ Vitamin K = 22.9 mcg; Serving size: 1 cup, 180 g

Chili With Beans—Without Meat ☛ Vitamin K = 11.6 mcg; Serving size: 1 cup, 253 g

CowPeas—Common (Blackeyes Crowder Southern) Mature Seeds Raw ☞ Vitamin K = 8.4 mcg; Serving size: 1 cup, 167 g

CowPeas—Common (Blackeyes Crowder Southern) Mature Seeds—Cooked Boiled ((With Salt)) ☞ Vitamin K = 2.9 mcg; Serving size: 1 cup, 171 g

CowPeas—Dry—Cooked—Cooked with Fat ☞ Vitamin K = 18.4 mcg; Serving size: 1 cup, 180 g

CowPeas—Dry—Cooked—Cooked without Fat ☞ Vitamin K = 3.1 mcg; Serving size: 1 cup, 180 g

CowPeas—Dry—Cooked With Pork ☞ Vitamin K = 14.9 mcg; Serving size: 1 cup, 179 g

Dry-Roasted Soybeans ☞ Vitamin K = 34.4 mcg; Serving size: 1 cup, 93 g

Edamame ☞ Vitamin K = 41.4 mcg; Serving size: 1 cup, 155 g

Fava Beans—(Raw) ☞ Vitamin K = 51.5 mcg; Serving size: 1 cup, 126 g

Fava Beans—Canned Drained —Cooked with Fat ☞ Vitamin K = 19.6 mcg; Serving size: 1 cup, 180 g

Fava Beans—Dry—Cooked—Cooked with Fat ☞ Vitamin K = 20.5 mcg; Serving size: 1 cup, 180 g

Fava Beans—Dry—Cooked—Cooked without Fat ☞ Vitamin K = 5.2 mcg; Serving size: 1 cup, 180 g

Firm Tofu (With Calcium And Magnesium) ☞ Vitamin K = 3 mcg; Serving size: 1/2 cup, 126 g

Frankfurter Meatless ☞ Vitamin K = 0 mcg; Serving size: 1 cup, sliced, 140 g

Green Or Yellow Split Peas—Dry—Cooked—Cooked without Fat ☞ Vitamin K = 9 mcg; Serving size: 1 cup, 180 g

Green Or Yellow Split Peas—Dry—Cooked Made With Animal Fat Or Meat Drippings ☛ Vitamin K = 8.5 mcg; Serving size: 1 cup, 180 g

Green Or Yellow Split Peas—Dry—Cooked Made With Margarine ☛ Vitamin K = 20.7 mcg; Serving size: 1 cup, 180 g

Green Or Yellow Split Peas—Dry—Cooked Made With Oil ☛ Vitamin K = 22.1 mcg; Serving size: 1 cup, 180 g

Hummus (Commercial) ☛ Vitamin K = 3.4 mcg; Serving size: 1 tbsp, 15 g

Hummus (Homemade) ☛ Vitamin K = 0.5 mcg; Serving size: 1 tablespoon, 15 g

Kidney Beans ☛ Vitamin K = 14.9 mcg; Serving size: 1 cup, 177 g

Lentils (Cooked) ☛ Vitamin K = 3.4 mcg; Serving size: 1 cup, 198 g

Lentils Dry—Cooked—Cooked without Fat ☛ Vitamin K = 3.1 mcg; Serving size: 1 cup, 180 g

Lentils Dry—Cooked Made With Animal Fat Or Meat Drippings ☛ Vitamin K = 2.9 mcg; Serving size: 1 cup, 180 g

Lentils Dry—Cooked Made With Margarine ☛ Vitamin K = 15.1 mcg; Serving size: 1 cup, 180 g

Lentils Dry—Cooked Made With Oil ☛ Vitamin K = 16.4 mcg; Serving size: 1 cup, 180 g

Lentils Mature Seeds—Cooked Boiled ((With Salt)) ☛ Vitamin K = 3.4 mcg; Serving size: 1 cup, 198 g

Lentils Raw ☛ Vitamin K = 9.6 mcg; Serving size: 1 cup, 192 g

Lima Beans ☛ Vitamin K = 3.8 mcg; Serving size: 1 cup, 188 g

Lima Beans—Dry—Cooked—Cooked without Fat ☛ Vitamin K = 3.6 mcg; Serving size: 1 cup, 180 g

Lima Beans—Dry—Cooked Made With Animal Fat Or Meat Drippings ☞ Vitamin K = 3.4 mcg; Serving size: 1 cup, 180 g

Lima Beans—Dry—Cooked Made With Margarine ☞ Vitamin K = 16.2 mcg; Serving size: 1 cup, 180 g

Lima Beans—Dry—Cooked Made With Oil ☞ Vitamin K = 17.6 mcg; Serving size: 1 cup, 180 g

Lima Beans—Large Mature Seeds Raw ☞ Vitamin K = 10.7 mcg; Serving size: 1 cup, 178 g

Lima Beans—Large Mature Seeds—Cooked Boiled ((With Salt)) ☞ Vitamin K = 3.8 mcg; Serving size: 1 cup, 188 g

Lima Beans—Thin Seeded (Baby) Mature Seeds Raw ☞ Vitamin K = 11.9 mcg; Serving size: 1 cup, 202 g

Loaf Lentil ☞ Vitamin K = 1.6 mcg; Serving size: 1 slice (3/4" thick), 47 g

Luncheon Slices Meatless ☞ Vitamin K = 0 mcg; Serving size: 1 slice, thin, 14 g

Meat Substitute Cereal- And Vegetable Protein-Based Fried ☞ Vitamin K = 12.6 mcg; Serving size: 1 cup, cubes, 146 g

Meatballs Meatless ☞ Vitamin K = 0 mcg; Serving size: 1 cup, 144 g

Miso ☞ Vitamin K = 5 mcg; Serving size: 1 tbsp, 17 g

Mung Beans—(Cooked) ☞ Vitamin K = 5.5 mcg; Serving size: 1 cup, 202 g

Mung Beans—Dry—Cooked—Cooked with Fat ☞ Vitamin K = 17.8 mcg; Serving size: 1 cup, 180 g

Mung Beans—Dry—Cooked—Cooked without Fat ☞ Vitamin K = 4.9 mcg; Serving size: 1 cup, 180 g

Mung Beans—Mature Seeds Raw ☞ Vitamin K = 18.6 mcg; Serving size: 1 cup, 207 g

Mung Beans—Mature Seeds—Cooked Boiled ((With Salt)) ☛ Vitamin K = 5.5 mcg; Serving size: 1 cup, 202 g

Mungo Beans—(Cooked) ☛ Vitamin K = 4.9 mcg; Serving size: 1 cup, 180 g

Mungo Beans—Mature Seeds—Cooked Boiled ((With Salt)) ☛ Vitamin K = 4.9 mcg; Serving size: 1 cup, 180 g

Natto ☛ Vitamin K = 40.4 mcg; Serving size: 1 cup, 175 g

Navy Beans ☛ Vitamin K = 1.1 mcg; Serving size: 1 cup, 182 g

Noodles Chinese Cellophane Or Long Rice (Mung Beans) Dehydrated ☛ Vitamin K = 0 mcg; Serving size: 1 cup, 140 g

Peanut—All Types Dry-Roasted ((With Salt)) ☛ Vitamin K = 0 mcg; Serving size: 1 oz, 28.4 g

Peanut—All Types Oil-Roasted ((With Salt)) ☛ Vitamin K = 0 mcg; Serving size: 1 cup, chopped, 144 g

Peanut—All Types Oil-Roasted ((Without Salt)) ☛ Vitamin K = 0 mcg; Serving size: 1 cup,, 144 g

Peanut—All Types—Cooked Boiled ((With Salt)) ☛ Vitamin K = 0 mcg; Serving size: 1 cup in shell, edible yield, 63 g

Peanut—Butter (Chunk Style) ☛ Vitamin K = 0.2 mcg; Serving size: 2 tbsp, 32 g

Peanut—Butter (Smooth) ☛ Vitamin K = 0 mcg; Serving size: 2 tbsp, 32 g

Peanut—Butter Chunk Style ((With Salt)) ☛ Vitamin K = 0.2 mcg; Serving size: 2 tbsp, 32 g

Peanut—Butter Chunky Vitamin And Mineral Fortified ☛ Vitamin K = 0.2 mcg; Serving size: 2 tbsp, 32 g

Peanut—Butter Smooth Reduced Fat ☛ Vitamin K = 0.2 mcg; Serving size: 2 tbsp, 36 g

Peanut—Butter Smooth Style ((With Salt)) ☛ Vitamin K = 0.1 mcg; Serving size: 2 tbsp, 32 g

Peanut—Butter Smooth Vitamin And Mineral Fortified ☛ Vitamin K = 0.2 mcg; Serving size: 2 tbsp, 32 g

Peanut—Flour Defatted ☛ Vitamin K = 0 mcg; Serving size: 1 cup, 60 g

Peanut—Spanish Raw ☛ Vitamin K = 0 mcg; Serving size: 1 cup, 146 g

Peanut—Spread Reduced Sugar ☛ Vitamin K = 0.2 mcg; Serving size: 2 tbsp, 31 g

Peanut—Virginia Raw ☛ Vitamin K = 0 mcg; Serving size: 1 cup, 146 g

Peas—Dry—Cooked With Pork ☛ Vitamin K = 20.1 mcg; Serving size: 1 cup, 197 g

Peas—Green Split Mature Seeds Raw ☛ Vitamin K = 31.3 mcg; Serving size: 1 cup, 197 g

Peas—Split Mature Seeds—Cooked Boiled ((With Salt)) ☛ Vitamin K = 9.8 mcg; Serving size: 1 cup, 196 g

Pink Beans—Canned Drained —Cooked with Fat ☛ Vitamin K = 21.1 mcg; Serving size: 1 cup, 180 g

Pink Beans—Canned Drained —Cooked without Fat ☛ Vitamin K = 6.7 mcg; Serving size: 1 cup, 180 g

Pink Beans—Dry—Cooked—Cooked with Fat ☛ Vitamin K = 22 mcg; Serving size: 1 cup, 180 g

Pink Beans—Dry—Cooked—Cooked without Fat ☛ Vitamin K = 6.7 mcg; Serving size: 1 cup, 180 g

Pinto Beans—(Cooked) ☛ Vitamin K = 6 mcg; Serving size: 1 cup, 171 g

Pinto Calico Or Red Mexican Beans—Canned Drained —Cooked without Fat ☛ Vitamin K = 6.3 mcg; Serving size: 1 cup, 180 g

Pinto Calico Or Red Mexican Beans—Canned Drained Made With Animal Fat Or Meat Drippings ☞ Vitamin K = 5.9 mcg; Serving size: 1 cup, 180 g

Pinto Calico Or Red Mexican Beans—Canned Drained Made With Margarine ☞ Vitamin K = 19.3 mcg; Serving size: 1 cup, 180 g

Pinto Calico Or Red Mexican Beans—Canned Drained Made With Oil ☞ Vitamin K = 20.7 mcg; Serving size: 1 cup, 180 g

Pinto Calico Or Red Mexican Beans—Dry—Cooked—Cooked without Fat ☞ Vitamin K = 6.3 mcg; Serving size: 1 cup, 180 g

Pinto Calico Or Red Mexican Beans—Dry—Cooked Made With Animal Fat Or Meat Drippings ☞ Vitamin K = 5.9 mcg; Serving size: 1 cup, 180 g

Pinto Calico Or Red Mexican Beans—Dry—Cooked Made With Margarine ☞ Vitamin K = 19.8 mcg; Serving size: 1 cup, 180 g

Pinto Calico Or Red Mexican Beans—Dry—Cooked Made With Oil ☞ Vitamin K = 21.4 mcg; Serving size: 1 cup, 180 g

Raw Peanuts ☞ Vitamin K = 0 mcg; Serving size: 1 oz, 28.4 g

Red Kidney Beans—Canned Drained —Cooked without Fat ☞ Vitamin K = 12.2 mcg; Serving size: 1 cup, 180 g

Red Kidney Beans—Canned Drained Made With Oil ☞ Vitamin K = 26.3 mcg; Serving size: 1 cup, 180 g

Red Kidney Beans—Dry—Cooked—Cooked without Fat ☞ Vitamin K = 15.1 mcg; Serving size: 1 cup, 180 g

Red Kidney Beans—Dry—Cooked Made With Animal Fat Or Meat Drippings ☞ Vitamin K = 14 mcg; Serving size: 1 cup, 180 g

Red Kidney Beans—Dry—Cooked Made With Margarine ☞ Vitamin K = 27.5 mcg; Serving size: 1 cup, 180 g

Red Kidney Beans—Dry—Cooked Made With Oil ☞ Vitamin K = 29 mcg; Serving size: 1 cup, 180 g

Refried Beans—Canned Fat-Free ☞ Vitamin K = 4.6 mcg; Serving size: 1 cup, 231 g

Refried Beans—Canned Traditional Style (Includes USDA Commodity) ☞ Vitamin K = 5 mcg; Serving size: 1 cup, 238 g

Refried Beans—Made With Animal Fat Or Meat Drippings ☞ Vitamin K = 6.3 mcg; Serving size: 1 cup, 253 g

Refried Beans—Made With Margarine ☞ Vitamin K = 18 mcg; Serving size: 1 cup, 253 g

Refried Beans—Made With Oil ☞ Vitamin K = 19.2 mcg; Serving size: 1 cup, 253 g

Refried Beans—With Cheese ☞ Vitamin K = 5.3 mcg; Serving size: 1 cup, 253 g

Refried Beans—With Meat ☞ Vitamin K = 6.1 mcg; Serving size: 1 cup, 253 g

Sandwich Spread Meatless ☞ Vitamin K = 0 mcg; Serving size: 1 tbsp, 15 g

Sausage Meatless ☞ Vitamin K = 0 mcg; Serving size: 1 link, 25 g

Soft Tofu ☞ Vitamin K = 2.4 mcg; Serving size: 1 piece (2-1/2 inch x 2-3/4 inch x 1 inch), 120 g

Soy—Flour Defatted ☞ Vitamin K = 4.3 mcg; Serving size: 1 cup, 105 g

Soy—Flour Full-Fat Raw ☞ Vitamin K = 58.8 mcg; Serving size: 1 cup, stirred, 84 g

Soy—Flour Full-Fat Roasted ☞ Vitamin K = 60.4 mcg; Serving size: 1 cup, stirred, 85 g

Soy—Flour Low-Fat ☞ Vitamin K = 3.4 mcg; Serving size: 1 cup, stirred, 88 g

Soy—Milk (All Flavors) Nonfat With Added Calcium Vitamins A And D ☞ Vitamin K = 5.6 mcg; Serving size: 1 cup, 243 g

Soy—Milk Chocolate And Other Flavors Light With Added Calcium Vitamins A And D ☞ Vitamin K = 8.7 mcg; Serving size: 1 cup, 243 g

Soy—Milk Chocolate Nonfat With Added Calcium Vitamins A And D ☞ Vitamin K = 8.7 mcg; Serving size: 1 cup, 243 g

Soy—Milk Chocolate Unfortified ☞ Vitamin K = 7.3 mcg; Serving size: 1 cup, 243 g

Soy—Milk Original And Vanilla Light With Added Calcium Vitamins A And D ☞ Vitamin K = 3.9 mcg; Serving size: 1 cup, 243 g

Soy—Milk Original And Vanilla With Added Calcium Vitamins A And D ☞ Vitamin K = 7.3 mcg; Serving size: 1 cup, 243 g

Soy—Protein Concentrate Produced By Acid Wash ☞ Vitamin K = 0 mcg; Serving size: 1 oz, 28.4 g

Soy—Protein Concentrate Produced By Alcohol Extraction ☞ Vitamin K = 0 mcg; Serving size: 1 oz, 28.4 g

Soy—Protein Isolate Potassium Type ☞ Vitamin K = 0 mcg; Serving size: 1 oz, 28.4 g

Soy—Protein Powder (Isolate) ☞ Vitamin K = 0 mcg; Serving size: 1 oz, 28.4 g

Soy—Sauce ☞ Vitamin K = 0 mcg; Serving size: 1 tbsp, 16 g

Soy—Sauce Made From Hydrolyzed Vegetable Protein ☞ Vitamin K = 0 mcg; Serving size: 1 tbsp, 18 g

SoyBeans—Curd Breaded Fried ☞ Vitamin K = 1.5 mcg; Serving size: 1 slice (2-3/4" x 1" x 1/2"), 29 g

SoyBeans—Curd Cheese ☞ Vitamin K = 10.4 mcg; Serving size: 1 cup, 225 g

SoyBeans—Dry—Cooked—Cooked with Fat ☞ Vitamin K = 47.3 mcg; Serving size: 1 cup, 180 g

SoyBeans—Dry—Cooked—Cooked without Fat ☞ Vitamin K = 34.4 mcg; Serving size: 1 cup, 180 g

SoyBeans—Mature Seeds Raw ☞ Vitamin K = 87.4 mcg; Serving size: 1 cup, 186 g

SoyBeans—Mature Seeds Roasted Salted ☞ Vitamin K = 86.7 mcg; Serving size: 1 cup, 172 g

SoyBeans—Mature Seeds—Cooked Boiled ((With Salt)) ☞ Vitamin K = 33 mcg; Serving size: 1 cup, 172 g

Soyburger Meatless With Cheese On Bun ☞ Vitamin K = 9 mcg; Serving size: 1 sandwich, 140 g

Split Peas ☞ Vitamin K = 9.8 mcg; Serving size: 1 cup, 196 g

Tamari ☞ Vitamin K = 0 mcg; Serving size: 1 tbsp, 18 g

Tofu Extra Firm Prepared With Nigari ☞ Vitamin K = 2.5 mcg; Serving size: 1/5 block, 91 g

Tofu Fried ☞ Vitamin K = 2.2 mcg; Serving size: 1 oz, 28.4 g

Tofu Prepared With Calcium ☞ Vitamin K = 3 mcg; Serving size: 1/2 cup, 124 g

Tofu Yogurt ☞ Vitamin K = 9.2 mcg; Serving size: 1 cup, 262 g

Unsalted Peanut—Butter (Smooth) ☞ Vitamin K = 0.1 mcg; Serving size: 2 tbsp, 32 g

Vanilla Soy—Milk ☞ Vitamin K = 7.3 mcg; Serving size: 1 cup, 243 g

Vegetarian Chili Made With Meat Substitute ☞ Vitamin K = 13 mcg; Serving size: 1 cup, 254 g

Vegetarian Fillets ☞ Vitamin K = 0 mcg; Serving size: 1 fillet, 85 g

Vegetarian Meatloaf Or Patties ☛ Vitamin K = 0 mcg; Serving size: 1 slice, 56 g

Vegetarian Pot Pie ☛ Vitamin K = 26.1 mcg; Serving size: 1 pie, 227 g

Vegetarian Stew ☛ Vitamin K = 41.2 mcg; Serving size: 1 cup, 247 g

Vegetarian Stroganoff ☛ Vitamin K = 46.1 mcg; Serving size: 1 box (3.2 oz), dry, yields, 466 g

Veggie Burgers ☛ Vitamin K = 2.9 mcg; Serving size: 1 pattie, 70 g

Vermicelli Made From Soy ☛ Vitamin K = 5.3 mcg; Serving size: 1 cup, 140 g

VitaSoy—Usa Organic Nasoya Sprouted Tofu Plus Super Firm ☛ Vitamin K = 12.5 mcg; Serving size: 3 oz, 85 g

White Beans—Canned Drained —Cooked without Fat ☛ Vitamin K = 7.9 mcg; Serving size: 1 cup, 180 g

White Beans—Canned Drained Made With Oil ☛ Vitamin K = 22.3 mcg; Serving size: 1 cup, 180 g

White Beans—Dry—Cooked—Cooked without Fat ☛ Vitamin K = 6.3 mcg; Serving size: 1 cup, 180 g

White Beans—Dry—Cooked Made With Animal Fat Or Meat Drippings ☛ Vitamin K = 5.9 mcg; Serving size: 1 cup, 180 g

White Beans—Dry—Cooked Made With Margarine ☛ Vitamin K = 19.3 mcg; Serving size: 1 cup, 180 g

White Beans—Dry Cooked Made With Oil ☛ Vitamin K = 20.7 mcg; Serving size: 1 cup, 180 g

Yellow Canary Or Peruvian Beans—Dry—Cooked—Cooked without Fat ☛ Vitamin K = 6.3 mcg; Serving size: 1 cup, 180 g

Yellow Canary Or Peruvian Beans—Dry—Cooked Made With Animal Fat Or Meat Drippings ☛ Vitamin K = 5.9 mcg; Serving size: 1 cup, 180 g

Yellow Canary Or Peruvian Beans—Dry—Cooked Made With Margarine ☞ Vitamin K = 19.1 mcg; Serving size: 1 cup, 180 g

Yellow Canary Or Peruvian Beans—Dry—Cooked Made With Oil ☞ Vitamin K = 20.7 mcg; Serving size: 1 cup, 180 g

14

BEVERAGES

Abbott Eas Soy Protein Powder ☛ Vitamin K = 1.2 mcg; Serving size: 1 scoop, 44 g

Abbott Eas Whey Protein Powder ☛ Vitamin K = 0.2 mcg; Serving size: 2 scoop, 39 g

Abbott Ensure Nutritional Shake Ready-To-Drink ☛ Vitamin K = 21.3 mcg; Serving size: 8 fl oz, 254 g

Abbott Ensure Plus Ready-To-Drink ☛ Vitamin K = 19.9 mcg; Serving size: 1 cup, 252 g

Acai Berry Drink—Enriched ☛ Vitamin K = 44.4 mcg; Serving size: 8 fl oz, 266 g

Alcoholic Beverage—Beer Light Higher Alcohol ☛ Vitamin K = 0 mcg; Serving size: 12 fl oz, 356 g

Alcoholic Beverage—Beer Light Low Carb ☛ Vitamin K = 0 mcg; Serving size: 1 fl oz, 29.5 g

Alcoholic Beverage—Creme De Menthe 72 Proof ☛ Vitamin K = 0 mcg; Serving size: 1 fl oz, 33.6 g

Alcoholic Beverage—Daiquiri—Prepared-From-Recipe ☛ Vitamin K = 0 mcg; Serving size: 1 fl oz, 30.2 g

Alcoholic Beverage—Distilled All (Gin Rum Vodka Whiskey) 80 Proof ☛ Vitamin K = 0 mcg; Serving size: 1 fl oz, 27.8 g

Alcoholic Beverage—Malt Beer Hard Lemonade ☛ Vitamin K = 0 mcg; Serving size: fl oz, 335 g

Alcoholic Beverage—Pina Colada—Prepared-From-Recipe ☛ Vitamin K = 0 mcg; Serving size: 1 fl oz, 31.4 g

Alcoholic Beverage—Rice (Sake) ☛ Vitamin K = 0 mcg; Serving size: 1 fl oz, 29.1 g

Alcoholic Beverage—Whiskey Sour—Prepared From Item 14028 ☛ Vitamin K = 0 mcg; Serving size: 1 fl oz, 30.4 g

Alcoholic Beverage—Whiskey Sour—Prepared With Water— Whiskey And Powder Mix ☛ Vitamin K = 0 mcg; Serving size: 1 fl oz, 29.4 g

Alcoholic Beverage—Wine Cooking ☛ Vitamin K = 0 mcg; Serving size: 1 tsp, 4.9 g

Alcoholic Beverage—Wine Light ☛ Vitamin K = 0 mcg; Serving size: 1 fl oz, 29.5 g

Alcoholic Malt Beverage Higher Alcohol Sweetened ☛ Vitamin K = 0 mcg; Serving size: 1 fl oz, 30 g

Amber Hard Cider ☛ Vitamin K = 3.9 mcg; Serving size: 12 fl oz, 355 g

Black Tea—(Brewed) ☛ Vitamin K = 0 mcg; Serving size: 1 fl oz, 29.6 g

Black Tea—(Ready To Drink) ☛ Vitamin K = 0 mcg; Serving size: 16 fl oz, 473 g

Bottled Water ☛ Vitamin K = 0 mcg; Serving size: 1 fl oz, 29.6 g

Carbonated—Beverage Chocolate-Flavored Soda ☛ Vitamin K = 0 mcg; Serving size: 1 fl oz, 31 g

Chocolate Syrup ☛ Vitamin K = 0.2 mcg; Serving size: 1 serving 2 tbsp, 39 g

Chocolate-Flavor Beverage Mix—For Milk Powder With Added Nutrients ☛ Vitamin K = 0.2 mcg; Serving size: 1 serving, 22 g

Coffee ☛ Vitamin K = 0 mcg; Serving size: 1 fl oz, 29.6 g

Coffee—And Cocoa Instant Decaffeinated With Whitener And Reduced Calorie Sweetener ☛ Vitamin K = 0.1 mcg; Serving size: 1 tsp dry, 6.4 g

Coffee—Bottled/canned Light ☛ Vitamin K = 0 mcg; Serving size: 1 fl oz, 30 g

Coffee—Brewed Blend Of Regular And Decaffeinated ☛ Vitamin K = 0 mcg; Serving size: 1 fl oz, 30 g

Coffee—Cafe Mocha Decaffeinated With Non-Dairy Milk ☛ Vitamin K = 0.4 mcg; Serving size: 1 fl oz, 31 g

Coffee—Cafe Mocha With Non-Dairy Milk ☛ Vitamin K = 0.4 mcg; Serving size: 1 fl oz, 31 g

Coffee—Cappuccino Decaffeinated With Non-Dairy Milk ☛ Vitamin K = 0.2 mcg; Serving size: 1 fl oz, 30 g

Coffee—Cappuccino With Non-Dairy Milk ☛ Vitamin K = 0.2 mcg; Serving size: 1 fl oz, 30 g

Coffee—Cream Liqueur ☛ Vitamin K = 0.4 mcg; Serving size: 1 fl oz, 31.1 g

Coffee—Iced Cafe Mocha Decaffeinated With Non-Dairy Milk ☛ Vitamin K = 0.2 mcg; Serving size: 1 fl oz, 31 g

Coffee—Iced Cafe Mocha With Non-Dairy Milk ☛ Vitamin K = 0.2 mcg; Serving size: 1 fl oz, 31 g

Coffee—Iced Latte Decaffeinated With Non-Dairy Milk ☛ Vitamin K = 0.2 mcg; Serving size: 1 fl oz, 30 g

Coffee—Iced Latte Decaffeinated With Non-Dairy Milk Flavored ☞ Vitamin K = 0.2 mcg; Serving size: 1 fl oz, 31 g

Coffee—Iced Latte With Non-Dairy Milk ☞ Vitamin K = 0.2 mcg; Serving size: 1 fl oz, 30 g

Coffee—Iced Latte With Non-Dairy Milk Flavored ☞ Vitamin K = 0.2 mcg; Serving size: 1 fl oz, 31 g

Coffee—Instant Decaffeinated Powder ☞ Vitamin K = 0 mcg; Serving size: 1 tsp rounded, 1.8 g

Coffee—Instant Mocha Sweetened ☞ Vitamin K = 0.2 mcg; Serving size: 1 serving 2 tbsp, 13 g

Coffee—Instant Regular Half The Caffeine ☞ Vitamin K = 0 mcg; Serving size: 1 tsp, 1 g

Coffee—Instant Regular Powder ☞ Vitamin K = 0 mcg; Serving size: 1 tsp, 1 g

Coffee—Instant With Whitener Reduced Calorie ☞ Vitamin K = 0.1 mcg; Serving size: 1 tsp dry, 1.7 g

Coffee—Latte Decaffeinated With Non-Dairy Milk ☞ Vitamin K = 0.4 mcg; Serving size: 1 fl oz, 30 g

Coffee—Latte Decaffeinated With Non-Dairy Milk Flavored ☞ Vitamin K = 0.4 mcg; Serving size: 1 fl oz, 31 g

Coffee—Latte With Non-Dairy Milk ☞ Vitamin K = 0.4 mcg; Serving size: 1 fl oz, 30 g

Coffee—Latte With Non-Dairy Milk Flavored ☞ Vitamin K = 0.4 mcg; Serving size: 1 fl oz, 31 g

Coffee—Substitute Cereal Grain Beverage Powder ☞ Vitamin K = 0 mcg; Serving size: 1 tsp (1 serving), 3 g

Cranberry Juice Cocktail Bottled ☞ Vitamin K = 0.3 mcg; Serving size: 1 fl oz, 31.6 g

Cranberry Juice Cocktail Bottled Reduced Calorie With Calcium Saccharin And Corn Sweetener ☛ Vitamin K = 0.1 mcg; Serving size: 1 fl oz, 29.6 g

Cranberry Juice Cocktail Frozen Concentrate—Prepared With Water ☛ Vitamin K = 0 mcg; Serving size: 1 fl oz, 29.6 g

Cranberry-Apple Juice Drink—Bottled ☛ Vitamin K = 0.2 mcg; Serving size: 1 fl oz, 30.6 g

Cranberry-Apple Juice Drink—Reduced Calorie With Vitamin C Added ☛ Vitamin K = 2.6 mcg; Serving size: 1 cup (8 fl oz), 240 g

Dairy Drink—Mix Chocolate Reduced Calorie With Low-Calorie Sweeteners Powder ☛ Vitamin K = 0.2 mcg; Serving size: 1 packet (.75 oz), 21 g

Energy Drink ☛ Vitamin K = 0 mcg; Serving size: 8 fl oz, 240 g

Espresso ☛ Vitamin K = 0 mcg; Serving size: 1 fl oz, 29.6 g

Fruit And Vegetable Smoothie ☛ Vitamin K = 21 mcg; Serving size: 1 fl oz, 27 g

Fruit And Vegetable Smoothies—Added Protein ☛ Vitamin K = 19.4 mcg; Serving size: 1 fl oz, 27 g

Fruit Flavored Drink—Containing Less Than 3% Fruit Juice With High Vitamin C ☛ Vitamin K = 0 mcg; Serving size: 1 cup (8 fl oz), 238 g

Fruit Flavored Drink—Less Than 3% Juice Not Enriched With Vitamin C ☛ Vitamin K = 0 mcg; Serving size: 1 cup (8 fl oz), 238 g

Fruit Flavored Drink—Reduced Sugar Greater Than 3% Fruit Juice High Vitamin C Added Calcium ☛ Vitamin K = 0 mcg; Serving size: 8 fl oz, 240 g

Fruit Juice Drink—Greater Than 3% Fruit Juice High Vitamin C And Added Thiamin ☛ Vitamin K = 0 mcg; Serving size: 8 fl oz, 237 g

Fruit Juice Drink—Greater Than 3% Juice High Vitamin C ☛ Vitamin K = 0 mcg; Serving size: 1 cup (8 fl oz), 238 g

Fruit Juice Drink—Noncitrus Carbonated ☛ Vitamin K = 0.4 mcg; Serving size: 1 fl oz (no ice), 31 g

Fruit Smoothies—Juice Drink—No Dairy ☛ Vitamin K = 0.2 mcg; Serving size: 1 fl oz, 27 g

Fruit Smoothies—Light ☛ Vitamin K = 0.9 mcg; Serving size: 1 fl oz, 27 g

Fruit Smoothies—With Whole Fruit And Dairy ☛ Vitamin K = 0.9 mcg; Serving size: 1 fl oz, 27 g

Fruit Smoothies—With Whole Fruit And Dairy Added Protein ☛ Vitamin K = 1 mcg; Serving size: 1 fl oz, 27 g

Fruit Smoothies—With Whole Fruit No Dairy ☛ Vitamin K = 1.2 mcg; Serving size: 1 fl oz, 27 g

Fruit Smoothies—With Whole Fruit No Dairy Added Protein ☛ Vitamin K = 1.1 mcg; Serving size: 1 fl oz, 27 g

Grape Juice Drink—Canned ☛ Vitamin K = 0.1 mcg; Serving size: 1 fl oz, 31.3 g

Grape Juice Drink—Light ☛ Vitamin K = 0 mcg; Serving size: 1 fl oz (no ice), 30 g

Green Tea ☛ Vitamin K = 0 mcg; Serving size: 16 fl oz, 473 g

Irish Coffee ☛ Vitamin K = 0.1 mcg; Serving size: 1 fl oz, 30 g

Lemonade—Flavor Drink—Powder ☛ Vitamin K = 0.3 mcg; Serving size: 1 serving, 18 g

Licuado Or Batido ☛ Vitamin K = 0.1 mcg; Serving size: 1 fl oz, 27 g

Malted Drink—Mix Chocolate Powder ☛ Vitamin K = 0.5 mcg; Serving size: 1 serving (3 heaping tsp or 1 envelope), 21 g

Malted Drink—Mix Natural Powder Dairy Based. ☛ Vitamin K = 1.1 mcg; Serving size: 1 serving (3 heaping tsp or 1 envelope), 21 g

Malted Drink—Mix Natural Powder—Prepared With Whole Milk ☛ Vitamin K = 1.3 mcg; Serving size: 1 cup (8 fl oz), 265 g

Milk And Soy Chocolate Drink ☛ Vitamin K = 40.1 mcg; Serving size: 8 fl oz, 237 g

Mixed Vegetable And Fruit Juice Drink—With Added Nutrients ☛ Vitamin K = 1.2 mcg; Serving size: 8 fl oz, 247 g

Nestle Boost Plus Nutritional Drink—Ready-To-Drink ☛ Vitamin K = 29.2 mcg; Serving size: 1 bottle, 237 g

Nutritional Drink—Or Shake High Protein Ready-To-Drink—(Slim Fast) ☛ Vitamin K = 16.1 mcg; Serving size: 1 cup, 248 g

Nutritional Drink—Or Shake Ready-To-Drink—(Carnation Instant Breakfast) ☛ Vitamin K = 29.8 mcg; Serving size: 1 cup, 248 g

Nutritional Drink—Or Shake Ready-To-Drink—(Kellogg's Special K Protein) ☛ Vitamin K = 2 mcg; Serving size: 1 fl oz, 32 g

Nutritional Shake Mix High Protein Powder ☛ Vitamin K = 12.5 mcg; Serving size: 1 tbsp, 10 g

Oatmeal Beverage With Milk ☛ Vitamin K = 0.5 mcg; Serving size: 1 cup, 248 g

Oatmeal Beverage With Water ☛ Vitamin K = 0 mcg; Serving size: 1 fl oz, 31 g

Ocean Spray Cranberry-Apple Juice Drink—Bottled ☛ Vitamin K = 2.7 mcg; Serving size: 8 fl oz, 249 g

Orange And Apricot Juice Drink—Canned ☛ Vitamin K = 0 mcg; Serving size: 1 fl oz, 31.2 g

Orange Juice Drink ☛ Vitamin K = 0 mcg; Serving size: 1 cup, 249 g

Protein Powder—Soy Based ☛ Vitamin K = 0 mcg; Serving size: 1

scoop, 45 g

Protein Powder—Whey Based 🐾 Vitamin K = 0 mcg; Serving size: 1/3 cup, 32 g

Red Wine 🐾 Vitamin K = 0.1 mcg; Serving size: 1 fl oz, 29.4 g

Slimfast Meal Replacement High Protein Shake Ready-To-Drink—3-2-1 Plan 🐾 Vitamin K = 19.2 mcg; Serving size: 1 bottle, 295 g

Tap Water 🐾 Vitamin K = 0 mcg; Serving size: 1 fl oz, 29.6 g

Tea—Green Brewed Regular 🐾 Vitamin K = 0 mcg; Serving size: 1 cup, 245 g

Tea—Green Instant Decaffeinated Lemon Unsweetened Enriched With Vitamin C 🐾 Vitamin K = 0 mcg; Serving size: 2 tbsp, 4.5 g

Tea—Green Ready To Drink—Ginseng And Honey Sweetened 🐾 Vitamin K = 0 mcg; Serving size: 1 cup, 260 g

Tea—Green Ready-To-Drink—Sweetened 🐾 Vitamin K = 0 mcg; Serving size: 1 cup, 270 g

Tea—Herb Brewed Chamomile 🐾 Vitamin K = 0 mcg; Serving size: 1 fl oz, 29.6 g

Tea—Herb Other Than Chamomile Brewed 🐾 Vitamin K = 0 mcg; Serving size: 1 fl oz, 29.6 g

Tea—Hibiscus Brewed 🐾 Vitamin K = 0 mcg; Serving size: 8 fl oz, 237 g

Tea—Hot Chai With Milk 🐾 Vitamin K = 0 mcg; Serving size: 1 fl oz, 30 g

Whey Protein Powder—Isolate 🐾 Vitamin K = 40 mcg; Serving size: 3 scoop, 86 g

White Wine 🐾 Vitamin K = 0.1 mcg; Serving size: 1 fl oz, 29.4 g

Wine Non-Alcoholic 🐾 Vitamin K = 0 mcg; Serving size: 1 fl oz, 29 g

15

BREAKFAST CEREALS

Alpen ☞ Vitamin K = 1.4 mcg; Serving size: 2/3 cup, 55 g

Barbaras Puffins Original ☞ Vitamin K = 0.2 mcg; Serving size: 3/4 cup, 27 g

Cereal—(General Mills 25% Less Sugar Cocoa Puffs) ☞ Vitamin K = 0.5 mcg; Serving size: 1 cup, 32 g

Cereal—(General Mills 25% Less Sugar Trix) ☞ Vitamin K = 0.4 mcg; Serving size: 1 cup, 30 g

Cereal—(General Mills Basic 4) ☞ Vitamin K = 0.9 mcg; Serving size: 1 cup, 55 g

Cereal—(General Mills Boo Berry) ☞ Vitamin K = 0.5 mcg; Serving size: 1 cup, 33 g

Cereal—(General Mills Cheerios Apple Cinnamon) ☞ Vitamin K = 1.2 mcg; Serving size: 1 cup, 40 g

Cereal—(General Mills Cheerios Banana Nut) ☞ Vitamin K = 0.4 mcg; Serving size: 1 cup, 37 g

Cereal—(General Mills Cheerios Berry Burst) ☞ Vitamin K = 1.5 mcg;

Serving size: 1 cup, 36 g

Cereal—(General Mills Cheerios Chocolate) ☞ Vitamin K = 0.6 mcg; Serving size: 1 cup, 36 g

Cereal—(General Mills Cheerios Frosted) ☞ Vitamin K = 0.6 mcg; Serving size: 1 cup, 37 g

Cereal—(General Mills Cheerios Fruity) ☞ Vitamin K = 0.3 mcg; Serving size: 1 cup, 36 g

Cereal—(General Mills Cheerios Honey Nut) ☞ Vitamin K = 0.9 mcg; Serving size: 1 cup, 37 g

Cereal—(General Mills Cheerios Multigrain) ☞ Vitamin K = 0.5 mcg; Serving size: 1 cup, 30 g

Cereal—(General Mills Cheerios Oat Cluster Crunch) ☞ Vitamin K = 0.5 mcg; Serving size: 1 cup, 36 g

Cereal—(General Mills Cheerios Protein) ☞ Vitamin K = 0.4 mcg; Serving size: 1 cup, 28 g

Cereal—(General Mills Cheerios Yogurt Burst) ☞ Vitamin K = 0.7 mcg; Serving size: 1 cup, 40 g

Cereal—(General Mills Cheerios) ☞ Vitamin K = 0 mcg; Serving size: 10 cheerios, 1 g

Cereal—(General Mills Chex Chocolate) ☞ Vitamin K = 2.1 mcg; Serving size: 1 cup, 43 g

Cereal—(General Mills Chex Cinnamon) ☞ Vitamin K = 2.1 mcg; Serving size: 1 cup, 39 g

Cereal—(General Mills Chex Corn) ☞ Vitamin K = 0 mcg; Serving size: 1 piece, 0 g

Cereal—(General Mills Chex Honey Nut) ☞ Vitamin K = 0 mcg; Serving size: 1 piece, 0 g

Cereal—(General Mills Chex Rice) ☞ Vitamin K = 0.3 mcg; Serving size: 1 cup, 27 g

Cereal—(General Mills Cinnamon Toast Crunch) ☞ Vitamin K = 3.8 mcg; Serving size: 1 cup, 40 g

Cereal—(General Mills Cocoa Puffs) ☞ Vitamin K = 0.8 mcg; Serving size: 1 cup, 36 g

Cereal—(General Mills Cookie Crisp) ☞ Vitamin K = 0.5 mcg; Serving size: 1 cup, 35 g

Cereal—(General Mills Count Chocula) ☞ Vitamin K = 0.6 mcg; Serving size: 1 cup, 36 g

Cereal—(General Mills Frankenberry) ☞ Vitamin K = 0.4 mcg; Serving size: 1 cup, 33 g

Cereal—(General Mills Golden Grahams) ☞ Vitamin K = 0.8 mcg; Serving size: 1 cup, 40 g

Cereal—(General Mills Honey Nut Clusters) ☞ Vitamin K = 0.6 mcg; Serving size: 1 cup, 55 g

Cereal—(General Mills Kix Berry Berry) ☞ Vitamin K = 0.2 mcg; Serving size: 1 cup, 33 g

Cereal—(General Mills Lucky Charms Chocolate) ☞ Vitamin K = 0.6 mcg; Serving size: 1 cup, 37 g

Cereal—(General Mills Lucky Charms) ☞ Vitamin K = 0.5 mcg; Serving size: 1 cup, 36 g

Cereal—(General Mills Oatmeal—Crisp With Almonds) ☞ Vitamin K = 1 mcg; Serving size: 1 cup, 60 g

Cereal—(General Mills Oatmeal—Crisp With Raisins) ☞ Vitamin K = 1.2 mcg; Serving size: 1 cup, 62 g

Cereal—(General Mills Reese's Puffs) ☞ Vitamin K = 0.7 mcg; Serving size: 1 cup, 40 g

Cereal—(General Mills Trix) ☞ Vitamin K = 0.4 mcg; Serving size: 1

cup, 32 g

Cereal—(Kashi Heart To Heart Oat Flakes And Blueberry Clusters) ☛ Vitamin K = 1 mcg; Serving size: 1 cup, 55 g

Cereal—(Kellogg's Cinnabon) ☛ Vitamin K = 0.7 mcg; Serving size: 1 cup, 30 g

Cereal—(Kellogg's Cocoa Krispies) ☛ Vitamin K = 0 mcg; Serving size: 1 cup, 41 g

Cereal—(Kellogg's Corn Flakes) ☛ Vitamin K = 0 mcg; Serving size: 1 cup, 28 g

Cereal—(Kellogg's Corn Pops) ☛ Vitamin K = 0 mcg; Serving size: 1 cup, 29 g

Cereal—(Kellogg's Crispix) ☛ Vitamin K = 0 mcg; Serving size: 1 cup, 29 g

Cereal—(Kellogg's Froot Loops Marshmallow) ☛ Vitamin K = 0.2 mcg; Serving size: 1 cup, 29 g

Cereal—(Kellogg's Frosted Flakes Reduced Sugar) ☛ Vitamin K = 0 mcg; Serving size: 1 cup, 31 g

Cereal—(Kellogg's Frosted Flakes) ☛ Vitamin K = 0.1 mcg; Serving size: 1 cup, 41 g

Cereal—(Kellogg's Frosted Krispies) ☛ Vitamin K = 0 mcg; Serving size: 1 cup, 40 g

Cereal—(Kellogg's Honey Crunch Corn Flakes) ☛ Vitamin K = 0.1 mcg; Serving size: 1 cup, 40 g

Cereal—(Kellogg's Honey Smacks) ☛ Vitamin K = 1 mcg; Serving size: 1 cup, 36 g

Cereal—(Kellogg's Low Fat Granola With Raisins) ☛ Vitamin K = 1.6 mcg; Serving size: 1 cup, 90 g

Cereal—(Kellogg's Low Fat Granola) ☛ Vitamin K = 1.3 mcg; Serving size: 1 cup, 98 g

Cereal—(Kellogg's Product 19) ☛ Vitamin K = 0.1 mcg; Serving size: 1 cup, 30 g

Cereal—(Kellogg's Rice Krispies Treats Cereal) ☛ Vitamin K = 0.4 mcg; Serving size: 1 cup, 40 g

Cereal—(Kellogg's Rice Krispies) ☛ Vitamin K = 0 mcg; Serving size: 1 cup, 26 g

Cereal—(Kellogg's Smart Start Strong) ☛ Vitamin K = 0.6 mcg; Serving size: 1 cup, 50 g

Cereal—(Kellogg's Special K Blueberry) ☛ Vitamin K = 2.1 mcg; Serving size: 1 cup, 40 g

Cereal—(Kellogg's Special K Low Fat Granola) ☛ Vitamin K = 1.4 mcg; Serving size: 1 cup, 104 g

Cereal—(Kellogg's Special K) ☛ Vitamin K = 0 mcg; Serving size: 1 cup, 31 g

Cereal—(Malt-O-Meal Blueberry Muffin Tops) ☛ Vitamin K = 0.8 mcg; Serving size: 1 cup, 40 g

Cereal—(Malt-O-Meal Crispy Rice) ☛ Vitamin K = 0 mcg; Serving size: 1 cup, 28 g

Cereal—(Malt-O-Meal Golden Puffs) ☛ Vitamin K = 0.9 mcg; Serving size: 1 cup, 32 g

Cereal—(Malt-O-Meal Honey Graham Squares) ☛ Vitamin K = 0.8 mcg; Serving size: 1 cup, 40 g

Cereal—(Malt-O-Meal Honey Nut Toasty O's) ☛ Vitamin K = 0.9 mcg; Serving size: 1 cup, 38 g

Cereal—(Malt-O-Meal Toasted Oat Cereal) ☛ Vitamin K = 0.4 mcg; Serving size: 1 cup, 22 g

Cereal—(Nature Valley Granola) ☛ Vitamin K = 1.1 mcg; Serving size:

1 cup, 82 g

Cereal—(Post Alpha-Bits) ☞ Vitamin K = 0.4 mcg; Serving size: 1 cup (1 nlea serving for adults), 30 g

Cereal—(Post Bran Flakes) ☞ Vitamin K = 0.4 mcg; Serving size: 3/4 cup, 30 g

Cereal—(Post Cocoa Pebbles) ☞ Vitamin K = 0.4 mcg; Serving size: 3/4 cup, 29 g

Cereal—(Post Fruity Pebbles) ☞ Vitamin K = 0.4 mcg; Serving size: 3/4 cup, 27 g

Cereal—(Post Golden Crisp) ☞ Vitamin K = 0.2 mcg; Serving size: 3/4 cup, 27 g

Cereal—(Post Grape-Nuts Cereal) ☞ Vitamin K = 1.2 mcg; Serving size: 1/2 cup, 58 g

Cereal—(Post Grape-Nuts Flakes) ☞ Vitamin K = 0.8 mcg; Serving size: 3/4 cup, 29 g

Cereal—(Post Great Grains—Banana Nut Crunch) ☞ Vitamin K = 2.1 mcg; Serving size: 1 cup, 59 g

Cereal—(Post Great Grains—Cranberry Almond Crunch) ☞ Vitamin K = 1 mcg; Serving size: 3/4 cup, 48 g

Cereal—(Post Honey Bunches Of Oats—Honey Roasted) ☞ Vitamin K = 0.9 mcg; Serving size: 3/4 cup, 30 g

Cereal—(Post Honey Bunches Of Oats—Pecan Bunches) ☞ Vitamin K = 0.4 mcg; Serving size: 3/4 cup, 29 g

Cereal—(Post Honey Bunches Of Oats—With Almonds) ☞ Vitamin K = 1 mcg; Serving size: 3/4 cup, 32 g

Cereal—(Post Honey Nut Shredded Wheat) ☞ Vitamin K = 0.9 mcg; Serving size: 1 cup, 59 g

Cereal—(Post Honeycomb Cereal) ☞ Vitamin K = 0.2 mcg; Serving size: 1 (1/2) cup, 32 g

Cereal—(Post Raisin Bran Cereal) ☞ Vitamin K = 1.1 mcg; Serving size: 1 cup, 59 g

Cereal—(Post Selects Blueberry Morning) ☞ Vitamin K = 7 mcg; Serving size: 1 (1/4) cup, 55 g

Cereal—(Post Selects Maple Pecan Crunch) ☞ Vitamin K = 1.9 mcg; Serving size: 3/4 cup, 52 g

Cereal—(Post Shredded Wheat Lightly Frosted Spoon-Size) ☞ Vitamin K = 0.5 mcg; Serving size: 1 cup, 52 g

Cereal—(Post Shredded Wheat N Bran Spoon-Size) ☞ Vitamin K = 1.2 mcg; Serving size: 1 (1/4) cup, 59 g

Cereal—(Post Shredded Wheat Original Big Biscuit) ☞ Vitamin K = 0.7 mcg; Serving size: 2 biscuits, 47 g

Cereal—(Post Shredded Wheat Original Spoon-Size) ☞ Vitamin K = 0.7 mcg; Serving size: 1 cup, 49 g

Cereal—(Post Waffle Crisp) ☞ Vitamin K = 0.4 mcg; Serving size: 1 cup, 30 g

Cereal—(Quaker 100% Natural Granola Oats—Wheat And Honey) ☞ Vitamin K = 3.4 mcg; Serving size: 1/2 cup, 48 g

Cereal—(Quaker Instant Oatmeal—Fruit And Cream Variety Dry) ☞ Vitamin K = 0.7 mcg; Serving size: 1 packet, 35 g

Cereal—(Quaker King Vitaman) ☞ Vitamin K = 0.1 mcg; Serving size: 1 (1/2) cup, 31 g

Cereal—(Quaker Oats Capn Crunch With Crunchberries) ☞ Vitamin K = 0.2 mcg; Serving size: 3/4 cup, 26 g

Cereal—(Quaker Oats Capn Crunch) ☞ Vitamin K = 0.2 mcg; Serving size: 3/4 cup, 27 g

Cereal—(Quaker Oats Capn Crunchs Peanut Butter Crunch) ☞

Vitamin K = 0.1 mcg; Serving size: 3/4 cup, 27 g

Cereal—(Quaker Oats Christmas Crunch) ☛ Vitamin K = 0.3 mcg; Serving size: 3/4 cup, 26 g

Cereal—(Quaker Oats Corn Grits—Instant Cheddar Cheese Flavor Dry) ☛ Vitamin K = 0.1 mcg; Serving size: 1 packet, 28 g

Cereal—(Quaker Oats Corn Grits—Instant Plain Dry) ☛ Vitamin K = 0 mcg; Serving size: 1 packet, 29 g

Cereal—(Quaker Oats Corn Grits—Instant Plain—Made (Microwaved Or Boiling Water Added) Without Salt) ☛ Vitamin K = 0 mcg; Serving size: 1 cup, 219 g

Cereal—(Quaker Oats Crunchy Bran) ☛ Vitamin K = 0.1 mcg; Serving size: 3/4 cup, 27 g

Cereal—(Quaker Oats Honey Graham Oh!s) ☛ Vitamin K = 0.2 mcg; Serving size: 3/4 cup, 27 g

Cereal—(Quaker Oats Instant Oatmeal—Cinnamon-Spice Dry) ☛ Vitamin K = 0.8 mcg; Serving size: 1 packet, 43 g

Cereal—(Quaker Oats Instant Oatmeal—Raisin And Spice Dry) ☛ Vitamin K = 1 mcg; Serving size: 1 packet, 43 g

Cereal—(Quaker Oats Instant Oatmeal—Raisins Dates And Walnuts Dry) ☛ Vitamin K = 0.7 mcg; Serving size: 1 packet, 37 g

Cereal—(Quaker Oats Low Fat 100% Natural Granola With Raisins) ☛ Vitamin K = 1.7 mcg; Serving size: 2/3 cup, 55 g

Cereal—(Quaker Oats Multigrain Oatmeal—Dry) ☛ Vitamin K = 1.5 mcg; Serving size: 1/2 cup, 40 g

Cereal—(Quaker Oats Oatmeal—Squares Cinnamon) ☛ Vitamin K = 0.9 mcg; Serving size: 1 cup, 56 g

Cereal—(Quaker Oats Oatmeal—Squares) ☛ Vitamin K = 0.9 mcg; Serving size: 1 cup, 56 g

Cereal—(Quaker Oats Puffed Rice) ☛ Vitamin K = 0 mcg; Serving size: 3/4 cup, 14 g

Cereal—(Quaker Oats Puffed Wheat) ☛ Vitamin K = 0.3 mcg; Serving size: 1 cup, 15 g

Cereal—(Quaker Oats Quick Oats—Dry) ☛ Vitamin K = 0.8 mcg; Serving size: 1/2 cup, 40 g

Cereal—(Quaker Oats Sweet Crunch/quisp) ☛ Vitamin K = 0.1 mcg; Serving size: 1 cup, 27 g

Cereal—(Quaker Oats Toasted Multigrain Crisps) ☛ Vitamin K = 1.2 mcg; Serving size: 1 (1/4) cup, 57 g

Cereal—Corn Flakes ☛ Vitamin K = 0 mcg; Serving size: 1 cup, 25 g

Cereal—Crispy Brown Rice ☛ Vitamin K = 0 mcg; Serving size: 1 cup, 32 g

Cereal—Frosted Corn Flakes ☛ Vitamin K = 0.1 mcg; Serving size: 1 cup, 40 g

Cereal—Frosted Rice ☛ Vitamin K = 0 mcg; Serving size: 1 cup, 45 g

Cereal—Granola ☛ Vitamin K = 2 mcg; Serving size: 1 cup, 111 g

Cereal—Muesli ☛ Vitamin K = 1.4 mcg; Serving size: 1 cup, 85 g

Cereal—Puffed Wheat Sweetened ☛ Vitamin K = 1.1 mcg; Serving size: 1 cup, 38 g

Cereal—Rice Flakes ☛ Vitamin K = 0 mcg; Serving size: 1 cup, 27 g

Chocolate-Flavored Frosted Puffed Corn ☛ Vitamin K = 0.2 mcg; Serving size: 1 cup, 30 g

Corn Grits—White Regular And Quick Enriched Cooked With Water With Salt ☛ Vitamin K = 0 mcg; Serving size: 1 cup, 257 g

Corn Grits—White Regular And Quick Enriched Dry ☛ Vitamin K = 0 mcg; Serving size: 1 tbsp, 9.7 g

Corn Grits—Yellow Regular And Quick Unenriched Dry ☛ Vitamin K = 0 mcg; Serving size: 1 tbsp, 9.7 g

Corn Grits—Yellow Regular Quick Enriched Cooked With Water With Salt ☛ Vitamin K = 0 mcg; Serving size: 1 cup, 233 g

Cornmeal—Mush —Cooked with Fat ☛ Vitamin K = 2.2 mcg; Serving size: 1 cup, cooked, 240 g

Cornmeal—Mush—Cooked without Fat ☛ Vitamin K = 0 mcg; Serving size: 1 cup, cooked, 240 g

Cornmeal—Puerto Rican Style ☛ Vitamin K = 0.5 mcg; Serving size: 1 cup, cooked, 240 g

Cream Of Rice Cooked With Water With Salt ☛ Vitamin K = 0 mcg; Serving size: 1 cup, 244 g

Cream Of Rice Dry ☛ Vitamin K = 0 mcg; Serving size: 1/4 cup, 45 g

Cream Of Rye ☛ Vitamin K = 1.7 mcg; Serving size: 1 cup, cooked, 240 g

Cream Of Wheat—1 Minute Cook Time Cooked With Water Microwaved Without Salt ☛ Vitamin K = 0 mcg; Serving size: 1 cup, 237 g

Cream Of Wheat—1 Minute Cook Time Cooked With Water Stove-Top Without Salt ☛ Vitamin K = 0 mcg; Serving size: 1 cup, 245 g

Cream Of Wheat—1 Minute Cook Time Dry ☛ Vitamin K = 0 mcg; Serving size: 3 tablespoon (1 serving), 33 g

Cream Of Wheat—2 1/2 Minute Cook Time Cooked With Water Microwaved Without Salt ☛ Vitamin K = 0 mcg; Serving size: 1 cup, 231 g

Cream Of Wheat—2 1/2 Minute Cook Time Cooked With Water Stove-Top Without Salt ☛ Vitamin K = 0 mcg; Serving size: 1 cup, 244 g

Cream Of Wheat—2 1/2 Minute Cook Time Dry ☛ Vitamin K = 0 mcg; Serving size: 3 tablespoon, 33 g

Cream Of Wheat—Instant Dry ☛ Vitamin K = 0.1 mcg; Serving size: 1 tbsp, 11.5 g

Cream Of Wheat—Instant—Made With Water Without Salt ☛ Vitamin K = 0.2 mcg; Serving size: 1 cup, 241 g

Cream Of Wheat—Instant—Prepared With Milk —Cooked with Fat ☛ Vitamin K = 3.1 mcg; Serving size: 1 cup, cooked, 240 g

Cream Of Wheat—Instant—Prepared With Milk—Cooked without Fat ☛ Vitamin K = 0.5 mcg; Serving size: 1 cup, cooked, 240 g

Cream Of Wheat—Instant—Prepared With Non-Dairy Milk — Cooked with Fat ☛ Vitamin K = 4.6 mcg; Serving size: 1 cup, cooked, 240 g

Cream Of Wheat—Instant—Prepared With Non-Dairy Milk— Cooked without Fat ☛ Vitamin K = 1.9 mcg; Serving size: 1 cup, cooked, 240 g

Cream Of Wheat—Instant—Prepared With Water —Cooked with Fat ☛ Vitamin K = 2.9 mcg; Serving size: 1 cup, cooked, 240 g

Cream Of Wheat—Instant—Prepared With Water—Cooked without Fat ☛ Vitamin K = 0.2 mcg; Serving size: 1 cup, cooked, 240 g

Cream Of Wheat—Regular (10 Minute) Cooked With Water With Salt ☛ Vitamin K = 0.3 mcg; Serving size: 1 cup (1 serving), 251 g

Cream Of Wheat—Regular (10 Minute) Cooked With Water Without Salt ☛ Vitamin K = 0.3 mcg; Serving size: 1 cup (1 serving), 251 g

Cream Of Wheat—Regular 10 Minute Cooking Dry ☛ Vitamin K = 0.1 mcg; Serving size: 1 tbsp, 10.6 g

Cream Of Wheat—Regular Or Quick—Prepared With Milk — Cooked with Fat ☛ Vitamin K = 2.9 mcg; Serving size: 1 cup, cooked, 240 g

Cream Of Wheat—Regular Or Quick—Prepared With Milk—Cooked without Fat ☛ Vitamin K = 0.7 mcg; Serving size: 1 cup, cooked, 240 g

Cream Of Wheat—Regular Or Quick—Prepared With Non-Dairy Milk —Cooked with Fat ☛ Vitamin K = 4.6 mcg; Serving size: 1 cup, cooked, 240 g

Cream Of Wheat—Regular Or Quick—Prepared With Non-Dairy Milk—Cooked without Fat ☛ Vitamin K = 2.4 mcg; Serving size: 1 cup, cooked, 240 g

Cream Of Wheat—Regular Or Quick—Prepared With Water —Cooked with Fat ☛ Vitamin K = 2.4 mcg; Serving size: 1 cup, cooked, 240 g

Cream Of Wheat—Regular Or Quick—Prepared With Water—Cooked without Fat ☛ Vitamin K = 0.2 mcg; Serving size: 1 cup, cooked, 240 g

Familia ☛ Vitamin K = 4.6 mcg; Serving size: 1 cup, 122 g

Farina Enriched Assorted Brands Including Cream Of Wheat—Quick (1-3 Minutes) Cooked With Wat ☛ Vitamin K = 0 mcg; Serving size: 1 cup, 240 g

Farina Enriched Assorted Brands Including Cream Of Wheat—Quick (1-3 Minutes) Dry ☛ Vitamin K = 0 mcg; Serving size: 1 tbsp, 11 g

Farina Enriched Cooked With Water With Salt ☛ Vitamin K = 0 mcg; Serving size: 1 cup, 233 g

Frosted Oat Cereal—With Marshmallows ☛ Vitamin K = 0.4 mcg; Serving size: 3/4 cup, 30 g

General Mills Cheerios ☛ Vitamin K = 0.6 mcg; Serving size: 1 cup, 28 g

Granola Homemade ☛ Vitamin K = 6.5 mcg; Serving size: 1 cup, 122 g

Grits—Instant—Prepared With Milk —Cooked with Fat ☞ Vitamin K = 3.8 mcg; Serving size: 1 cup, cooked, 240 g

Grits—Instant—Prepared With Milk—Cooked without Fat ☞ Vitamin K = 0.5 mcg; Serving size: 1 cup, cooked, 240 g

Grits—Instant—Prepared With Non-Dairy Milk —Cooked with Fat ☞ Vitamin K = 5.3 mcg; Serving size: 1 cup, cooked, 240 g

Grits—Instant—Prepared With Water —Cooked with Fat ☞ Vitamin K = 3.6 mcg; Serving size: 1 cup, cooked, 240 g

Grits—Instant—Prepared With Water—Cooked without Fat ☞ Vitamin K = 0 mcg; Serving size: 1 cup, cooked, 240 g

Grits—Regular Or Quick—Prepared With Milk —Cooked with Fat ☞ Vitamin K = 2.6 mcg; Serving size: 1 cup, cooked, 240 g

Grits—Regular Or Quick—Prepared With Milk—Cooked without Fat ☞ Vitamin K = 0.5 mcg; Serving size: 1 cup, cooked, 240 g

Grits—Regular Or Quick—Prepared With Non-Dairy Milk — Cooked with Fat ☞ Vitamin K = 4.3 mcg; Serving size: 1 cup, cooked, 240 g

Grits—Regular Or Quick—Prepared With Non-Dairy Milk— Cooked without Fat ☞ Vitamin K = 2.2 mcg; Serving size: 1 cup, cooked, 240 g

Grits—Regular Or Quick—Prepared With Water —Cooked with Fat ☞ Vitamin K = 2.2 mcg; Serving size: 1 cup, cooked, 240 g

Grits—Regular Or Quick—Prepared With Water—Cooked without Fat ☞ Vitamin K = 0 mcg; Serving size: 1 cup, cooked, 240 g

Grits—With Cheese —Cooked with Fat ☞ Vitamin K = 2.6 mcg; Serving size: 1 cup, cooked, 240 g

Grits—With Cheese—Cooked without Fat ☞ Vitamin K = 0.7 mcg; Serving size: 1 cup, cooked, 240 g

Health Valley Fiber 7 Flakes ☛ Vitamin K = 0.7 mcg; Serving size: 3/4 cup, 31 g

Hominy Cooked —Cooked with Fat ☛ Vitamin K = 2.4 mcg; Serving size: 1 cup, 170 g

Hominy Cooked—Cooked without Fat ☛ Vitamin K = 0.3 mcg; Serving size: 1 cup, 165 g

Instant Grits—(Made with Vegetable Fat) ☛ Vitamin K = 1.7 mcg; Serving size: 1 cup, cooked, 240 g

Malt-O-Meal Apple Zings ☛ Vitamin K = 0 mcg; Serving size: 1 cup, 33 g

Malt-O-Meal Berry Colossal Crunch ☛ Vitamin K = 0 mcg; Serving size: 3/4 cup, 30 g

Malt-O-Meal Blueberry Mini Spooners ☛ Vitamin K = 0 mcg; Serving size: 1 cup, 55 g

Malt-O-Meal Blueberry Muffin Tops Cereal ☛ Vitamin K = 0.5 mcg; Serving size: 3/4 cup, 30 g

Malt-O-Meal Chocolate Dry ☛ Vitamin K = 0 mcg; Serving size: 3 tbsp, 35 g

Malt-O-Meal Chocolate Marshmallow Mateys ☛ Vitamin K = 0 mcg; Serving size: 3/4 cup, 30 g

Malt-O-Meal Chocolate—Made With Water Without Salt ☛ Vitamin K = 0 mcg; Serving size: 1 serving (3 dry cereal plus 1 cup water), 268 g

Malt-O-Meal Cinnamon Toasters ☛ Vitamin K = 0.5 mcg; Serving size: 3/4 cup, 30 g

Malt-O-Meal Coco-Roos ☛ Vitamin K = 0 mcg; Serving size: 3/4 cup, 30 g

Malt-O-Meal Cocoa Dyno-Bites ☛ Vitamin K = 0 mcg; Serving size: 3/4 cup, 29 g

Malt-O-Meal Colossal Crunch ☞ Vitamin K = 0 mcg; Serving size: 3/4 cup, 30 g

Malt-O-Meal Corn Bursts ☞ Vitamin K = 0 mcg; Serving size: 1 cup, 31 g

Malt-O-Meal Crispy Rice ☞ Vitamin K = 0 mcg; Serving size: 1 (1/4) cup, 33 g

Malt-O-Meal Farina Hot Wheat Cereal—Dry ☞ Vitamin K = 0 mcg; Serving size: 3 tbsp, 35 g

Malt-O-Meal Frosted Flakes ☞ Vitamin K = 0.1 mcg; Serving size: 3/4 cup, 31 g

Malt-O-Meal Frosted Mini Spooners ☞ Vitamin K = 0.9 mcg; Serving size: 1 cup, 55 g

Malt-O-Meal Fruity Dyno-Bites ☞ Vitamin K = 0.1 mcg; Serving size: 3/4 cup, 27 g

Malt-O-Meal Golden Puffs ☞ Vitamin K = 0.3 mcg; Serving size: 3/4 cup, 27 g

Malt-O-Meal Honey Graham Squares ☞ Vitamin K = 0.4 mcg; Serving size: 3/4 cup, 30 g

Malt-O-Meal Honey Nut Scooters ☞ Vitamin K = 0 mcg; Serving size: 1 cup, 30 g

Malt-O-Meal Maple & Brown Sugar Hot Wheat Cereal—Dry ☞ Vitamin K = 0 mcg; Serving size: 1/4 cup, 45 g

Malt-O-Meal Marshmallow Mateys ☞ Vitamin K = 0.3 mcg; Serving size: 1 cup, 30 g

Malt-O-Meal Oat Blenders With Honey ☞ Vitamin K = 0.1 mcg; Serving size: 3/4 cup, 30 g

Malt-O-Meal Oat Blenders With Honey & Almonds ☞ Vitamin K = 0 mcg; Serving size: 3/4 cup, 30 g

Malt-O-Meal Original Plain Dry ☞ Vitamin K = 0 mcg; Serving size: 3 tbsp, 35 g

Malt-O-Meal Original Plain—Made With Water Without Salt ☞ Vitamin K = 0 mcg; Serving size: 1 serving (3 t dry cereal plus 1 cup water), 268 g

Malt-O-Meal Raisin Bran Cereal ☞ Vitamin K = 0.2 mcg; Serving size: 1 cup, 59 g

Malt-O-Meal Tootie Fruities ☞ Vitamin K = 0 mcg; Serving size: 1 cup, 32 g

Masa Harina Cooked ☞ Vitamin K = 0 mcg; Serving size: 1 cup, cooked, 240 g

Millet Puffed ☞ Vitamin K = 0.3 mcg; Serving size: 1 cup, 21 g

Moms Best Honey Nut Toasty Os ☞ Vitamin K = 0 mcg; Serving size: 1 cup, 30 g

Moms Best Sweetened Wheat-Fuls ☞ Vitamin K = 0.8 mcg; Serving size: 1 cup, 55 g

Natures Path Organic Flax Plus Flakes ☞ Vitamin K = 0.1 mcg; Serving size: 3/4 cup, 30 g

Natures Path Organic Flax Plus Pumpkin Granola ☞ Vitamin K = 14.4 mcg; Serving size: 3/4 cup, 55 g

Oat Bran Flakes Health Valley ☞ Vitamin K = 0.9 mcg; Serving size: 1 cup, 50 g

Oatmeal— Instant Plain—Prepared With Milk —Cooked with Fat ☞ Vitamin K = 4.8 mcg; Serving size: 1 cup, cooked, 240 g

Oatmeal—From Fast Food Fruit Flavored ☞ Vitamin K = 2.2 mcg; Serving size: 1 cup, cooked, 240 g

Oatmeal—From Fast Food Maple Flavored ☞ Vitamin K = 1.2 mcg; Serving size: 1 cup, cooked, 240 g

Oatmeal—From Fast Food Other Flavors ☞ Vitamin K = 1.2 mcg; Serving size: 1 cup, cooked, 240 g

Oatmeal—From Fast Food Plain ☞ Vitamin K = 1.2 mcg; Serving size: 1 cup, cooked, 240 g

Oatmeal—Instant Fruit Flavored —Cooked with Fat ☞ Vitamin K = 4.1 mcg; Serving size: 1 cup, cooked, 240 g

Oatmeal—Instant Fruit Flavored—Cooked without Fat ☞ Vitamin K = 1 mcg; Serving size: 1 cup, cooked, 240 g

Oatmeal—Instant Maple Flavored —Cooked with Fat ☞ Vitamin K = 4.1 mcg; Serving size: 1 cup, cooked, 240 g

Oatmeal—Instant Maple Flavored—Cooked without Fat ☞ Vitamin K = 1 mcg; Serving size: 1 cup, cooked, 240 g

Oatmeal—Instant Other Flavors —Cooked with Fat ☞ Vitamin K = 4.1 mcg; Serving size: 1 cup, cooked, 240 g

Oatmeal—Instant Other Flavors—Cooked without Fat ☞ Vitamin K = 1 mcg; Serving size: 1 cup, cooked, 240 g

Oatmeal—Instant Plain—Prepared With Milk—Cooked without Fat ☞ Vitamin K = 1.2 mcg; Serving size: 1 cup, cooked, 240 g

Oatmeal—Instant Plain—Prepared With Non-Dairy Milk —Cooked with Fat ☞ Vitamin K = 6 mcg; Serving size: 1 cup, cooked, 240 g

Oatmeal—Instant Plain—Prepared With Non-Dairy Milk—Cooked without Fat ☞ Vitamin K = 2.6 mcg; Serving size: 1 cup, cooked, 240 g

Oatmeal—Instant Plain—Prepared With Water —Cooked with Fat ☞ Vitamin K = 4.3 mcg; Serving size: 1 cup, cooked, 240 g

Oatmeal—Instant Plain—Prepared With Water—Cooked without Fat ☞ Vitamin K = 1 mcg; Serving size: 1 cup, cooked, 240 g

Oatmeal—Made With Milk And Sugar Puerto Rican Style ☞ Vitamin K = 1 mcg; Serving size: 1 cup, cooked, 240 g

Oatmeal—Multigrain —Cooked with Fat ☛ Vitamin K = 3.6 mcg; Serving size: 1 cup, cooked, 240 g

Oatmeal—Multigrain—Cooked without Fat ☛ Vitamin K = 1.4 mcg; Serving size: 1 cup, cooked, 240 g

Oatmeal—Reduced Sugar Flavored —Cooked with Fat ☛ Vitamin K = 4.3 mcg; Serving size: 1 cup, cooked, 240 g

Oatmeal—Reduced Sugar Flavored—Cooked without Fat ☛ Vitamin K = 1 mcg; Serving size: 1 cup, cooked, 240 g

Oatmeal—Reduced Sugar Plain —Cooked with Fat ☛ Vitamin K = 4.3 mcg; Serving size: 1 cup, cooked, 240 g

Oatmeal—Reduced Sugar Plain—Cooked without Fat ☛ Vitamin K = 1 mcg; Serving size: 1 cup, cooked, 240 g

Oatmeal—Regular Or Quick—Prepared With Milk —Cooked with Fat ☛ Vitamin K = 3.4 mcg; Serving size: 1 cup, cooked, 240 g

Oatmeal—Regular Or Quick—Prepared With Milk—Cooked without Fat ☛ Vitamin K = 1.2 mcg; Serving size: 1 cup, cooked, 240 g

Oatmeal—Regular Or Quick—Prepared With Non-Dairy Milk — Cooked with Fat ☛ Vitamin K = 5 mcg; Serving size: 1 cup, cooked, 240 g

Oatmeal—Regular Or Quick—Prepared With Non-Dairy Milk— Cooked without Fat ☛ Vitamin K = 2.9 mcg; Serving size: 1 cup, cooked, 240 g

Oatmeal—Regular Or Quick—Prepared With Water —Cooked with Fat ☛ Vitamin K = 3.1 mcg; Serving size: 1 cup, cooked, 240 g

Oatmeal—Regular Or Quick—Prepared With Water—Cooked without Fat ☛ Vitamin K = 0.7 mcg; Serving size: 1 cup, cooked, 240 g

Oats—Instant Fortified Maple And Brown Sugar Dry ☛ Vitamin K = 0.6 mcg; Serving size: 1 packet, 43 g

Oats—Instant Fortified Plain Dry ☛ Vitamin K = 0.5 mcg; Serving size: 1 packet, 28 g

Oats—Instant Fortified Plain—Made With Water ☛ Vitamin K = 0.9 mcg; Serving size: 1 cup, cooked, 234 g

Oats—Instant Fortified With Cinnamon And Spice Dry ☛ Vitamin K = 0.9 mcg; Serving size: 1 packet, 45 g

Oats—Instant Fortified With Cinnamon And Spice—Made With Water ☛ Vitamin K = 1.2 mcg; Serving size: 1 cup, 240 g

Oats—Instant Fortified With Raisins And Spice—Made With Water ☛ Vitamin K = 1.2 mcg; Serving size: 1 cup, 240 g

Oats—Regular And Quick Not Fortified Dry ☛ Vitamin K = 1.6 mcg; Serving size: 1 cup, 81 g

Ralston Corn Biscuits ☛ Vitamin K = 0 mcg; Serving size: 1 cup (nlea serving), 30 g

Ralston Corn Flakes ☛ Vitamin K = 0 mcg; Serving size: 1 cup, 28 g

Ralston Crisp Rice ☛ Vitamin K = 0 mcg; Serving size: 1 (1/4) cup, 33 g

Ralston Crispy Hexagons ☛ Vitamin K = 0 mcg; Serving size: 1 cup, 29 g

Ralston Enriched Bran Flakes ☛ Vitamin K = 0.8 mcg; Serving size: 1 serving (nlea serving size = 0.75 cup), 29 g

Ralston Tasteeos ☛ Vitamin K = 0.4 mcg; Serving size: 1 cup, 28 g

Rice Cream Of— Cooked —Cooked with Fat ☛ Vitamin K = 2.2 mcg; Serving size: 1 cup, cooked, 240 g

Rice Cream Of—Cooked—Cooked without Fat ☛ Vitamin K = 0 mcg; Serving size: 1 cup, cooked, 240 g

Rice Cream Of—Cooked—Prepared With Milk ☛ Vitamin K = 2.6 mcg; Serving size: 1 cup, cooked, 240 g

Sun Country Kretschmer Honey Crunch Wheat Germ ☛ Vitamin K = 0.5 mcg; Serving size: 2 tbsp, 14 g

Toasted Wheat Germ ☛ Vitamin K = 1.1 mcg; Serving size: 1 oz, 28.4 g

Uncle Sam Cereal ☛ Vitamin K = 1 mcg; Serving size: 3/4 cup, 55 g

Upma Indian Breakfast Dish ☛ Vitamin K = 9.2 mcg; Serving size: 1 cup, cooked, 170 g

Weetabix Whole Grain Cereal ☛ Vitamin K = 0.6 mcg; Serving size: 2 biscuits, 35 g

Wheat Cereal—Chocolate Flavored Cooked ☛ Vitamin K = 1 mcg; Serving size: 1 cup, cooked, 240 g

Wheat Cream Of Cooked—Prepared With Milk And Sugar Puerto Rican Style ☛ Vitamin K = 0.5 mcg; Serving size: 1 cup, cooked, 245 g

Wheatena Cooked With Water With Salt ☛ Vitamin K = 1 mcg; Serving size: 1 cup, 243 g

Wheatena Dry ☛ Vitamin K = 0.9 mcg; Serving size: 1/3 cup, 40 g

White Cornmeal—(Grits) ☛ Vitamin K = 0 mcg; Serving size: 1 cup, 257 g

Whole Wheat Cereal—Cooked —Cooked with Fat ☛ Vitamin K = 3.1 mcg; Serving size: 1 cup, cooked, 240 g

Whole Wheat Cereal—Cooked—Cooked without Fat ☛ Vitamin K = 0.7 mcg; Serving size: 1 cup, cooked, 240 g

Whole Wheat Hot Natural Cereal—Cooked With Water With Salt ☛ Vitamin K = 1 mcg; Serving size: 1 cup, 242 g

Whole Wheat Hot Natural Cereal—Cooked With Water Without Salt ☛ Vitamin K = 1 mcg; Serving size: 1 cup, 242 g

Whole Wheat Hot Natural Cereal—Dry ☛ Vitamin K = 2.3 mcg; Serving size: 1 cup, 94 g

16

DAIRY AND EGG PRODUCTS

Almond Milk—Unsweetened ☞ Vitamin K = 0 mcg; Serving size: 1 cup, 244 g

Beverage Instant Breakfast Powder—Chocolate Not Reconstituted ☞ Vitamin K = 6.7 mcg; Serving size: 1 tbsp, 7.4 g

Beverage Instant Breakfast Powder—Chocolate Sugar-Free Not Reconstituted ☞ Vitamin K = 6.7 mcg; Serving size: 1 tbsp, 5.6 g

Buttermilk ☞ Vitamin K = 0.7 mcg; Serving size: 1 cup, 245 g

ButterMilk—Fat-free (Skim) ☞ Vitamin K = 0.2 mcg; Serving size: 1 cup, 244 g

ButterMilk—Reduced Fat—(1%) ☞ Vitamin K = 0.2 mcg; Serving size: 1 cup, 244 g

Camembert ☞ Vitamin K = 0.6 mcg; Serving size: 1 oz, 28.4 g

Cheddar Cheese—(Non-Fat Or Fat-free) ☞ Vitamin K = 0.2 mcg; Serving size: 1 serving, 28 g

Cheese—American ☞ Vitamin K = 3.8 mcg; Serving size: 1 cup, 113 g

Cheese—American Cheddar Imitation ☛ Vitamin K = 0.6 mcg; Serving size: 1 slice, 21 g

Cheese—American Cheese—Spread ☛ Vitamin K = 2.5 mcg; Serving size: 1 cup, diced, 140 g

Cheese—Blue ☛ Vitamin K = 0.7 mcg; Serving size: 1 oz, 28.4 g

Cheese—Brick Cheese ☛ Vitamin K = 3.3 mcg; Serving size: 1 cup, diced, 132 g

Cheese—Brie ☛ Vitamin K = 0.7 mcg; Serving size: 1 oz, 28.4 g

Cheese—Cheddar ☛ Vitamin K = 3.2 mcg; Serving size: 1 cup, diced, 132 g

Cheese—Cheddar ☛ Vitamin K = 0.2 mcg; Serving size: 1 cracker-size slice, 9 g

Cheese—Cheddar Reduced Fat— ☛ Vitamin K = 0.3 mcg; Serving size: 1 slice, 21 g

Cheese—Colby ☛ Vitamin K = 3.6 mcg; Serving size: 1 cup, diced, 132 g

Cheese—Colby Jack ☛ Vitamin K = 0.2 mcg; Serving size: 1 cracker-size slice, 9 g

Cheese—Cottage Cheese—(Blended With Fruit) ☛ Vitamin K = 0.5 mcg; Serving size: 4 oz, 113 g

Cheese—Cottage Cheese—(Blended) ☛ Vitamin K = 0 mcg; Serving size: 4 oz, 113 g

Cheese—Cottage Cheese—With Gelatin Dessert ☛ Vitamin K = 0 mcg; Serving size: 1 cup, 240 g

Cheese—Cottage Cheese—With Gelatin Dessert And Fruit ☛ Vitamin K = 2.2 mcg; Serving size: 1 cup, 240 g

Cheese—Cottage Cheese—With Gelatin Dessert And Vegetables ☛ Vitamin K = 6.2 mcg; Serving size: 1 cup, 240 g

Cheese—Cottage Reduced Fat—1% Milkfat Lactose Reduced ☛ Vitamin K = 0.1 mcg; Serving size: 4 oz, 113 g

Cheese—Cottage Reduced Fat—1% Milkfat No Sodium Added ☛ Vitamin K = 0.1 mcg; Serving size: 4 oz, 113 g

Cheese—Cottage Reduced Fat—1% Milkfat With Vegetables ☛ Vitamin K = 2.9 mcg; Serving size: 4 oz, 113 g

Cheese—Cottage Reduced Fat—With Fruit ☛ Vitamin K = 1.4 mcg; Serving size: 1 cup, 226 g

Cheese—Cottage With Vegetables ☛ Vitamin K = 12.4 mcg; Serving size: 4 oz, 113 g

Cheese—Cream Cheese ☛ Vitamin K = 0.3 mcg; Serving size: 1 tbsp, 14.5 g

Cheese—Cream Reduced Fat— ☛ Vitamin K = 0.2 mcg; Serving size: 1 tbsp, 15 g

Cheese—Dry White Queso Seco ☛ Vitamin K = 1.5 mcg; Serving size: 1 cup grated, 97 g

Cheese—Edam ☛ Vitamin K = 0.7 mcg; Serving size: 1 oz, 28.4 g

Cheese—Fat-free Cream ☛ Vitamin K = 0 mcg; Serving size: 1 tbsp, 18 g

Cheese—Fatfree Swiss Cheese ☛ Vitamin K = 0.1 mcg; Serving size: 1 serving, 28 g

Cheese—Feta ☛ Vitamin K = 2.7 mcg; Serving size: 1 cup, crumbled, 150 g

Cheese—Fontina ☛ Vitamin K = 3.4 mcg; Serving size: 1 cup, diced, 132 g

Cheese—Food Pasteurized Process American Without Added Vitamin D ☛ Vitamin K = 2.9 mcg; Serving size: 1 cup, 113 g

Cheese—Goat ☞ Vitamin K = 3.4 mcg; Serving size: 1 cup, crumbled, 140 g

Cheese—Goat Semisoft Type ☞ Vitamin K = 0.7 mcg; Serving size: 1 oz, 28.4 g

Cheese—Gouda ☞ Vitamin K = 0.7 mcg; Serving size: 1 oz, 28.4 g

Cheese—Gouda Or Edam ☞ Vitamin K = 0.2 mcg; Serving size: 1 cracker-size slice, 9 g

Cheese—Grated Parmesan (Hard) ☞ Vitamin K = 0.5 mcg; Serving size: 1 oz, 28.4 g

Cheese—Grated Parmesan—(Low-Sodium) ☞ Vitamin K = 2 mcg; Serving size: 1 cup, grated, 100 g

Cheese—Gruyere ☞ Vitamin K = 0.8 mcg; Serving size: 1 oz, 28.4 g

Cheese—Hard Goat ☞ Vitamin K = 0.9 mcg; Serving size: 1 oz, 28.4 g

Cheese—Limburger ☞ Vitamin K = 3.1 mcg; Serving size: 1 cup, 134 g

Cheese—Low-Sodium Cheddar ☞ Vitamin K = 3.6 mcg; Serving size: 1 cup, diced, 132 g

Cheese—Mexican Blend Cheese ☞ Vitamin K = 0.7 mcg; Serving size: 1/4 cup shredded, 28 g

Cheese—Mexican Blend Reduced Fat— ☞ Vitamin K = 0.5 mcg; Serving size: 1 oz, 28.4 g

Cheese—Mexican Queso Anejo ☞ Vitamin K = 3.3 mcg; Serving size: 1 cup, crumbled, 132 g

Cheese—Mexican Queso Asadero ☞ Vitamin K = 3.2 mcg; Serving size: 1 cup, diced, 132 g

Cheese—Monterey ☞ Vitamin K = 3.3 mcg; Serving size: 1 cup, diced, 132 g

Cheese—Monterey Reduced Fat— ☞ Vitamin K = 2.4 mcg; Serving size: 1 cup, diced, 132 g

Cheese—Mozzarella ☞ Vitamin K = 2.6 mcg; Serving size: 1 cup, shredded, 112 g

Cheese—Mozzarella (Hard) ☞ Vitamin K = 0.7 mcg; Serving size: 1 oz, 28.4 g

Cheese—Mozzarella (Lowfat) ☞ Vitamin K = 0.5 mcg; Serving size: 1 oz, 28.4 g

Cheese—Mozzarella Reduced Moisture Part-Skim Shredded ☞ Vitamin K = 1.1 mcg; Serving size: 1 cup, 86 g

Cheese—Mozzarella Reduced Sodium ☞ Vitamin K = 2.4 mcg; Serving size: 1 cup, diced, 132 g

Cheese—Mozzarella—(Non-Fat Or Fat-free) ☞ Vitamin K = 1.8 mcg; Serving size: 1 cup, shredded, 113 g

Cheese—Muenster ☞ Vitamin K = 3.3 mcg; Serving size: 1 cup, diced, 132 g

Cheese—Muenster Reduced Fat— ☞ Vitamin K = 1.7 mcg; Serving size: 1 cup, shredded, 113 g

Cheese—Neufchatel ☞ Vitamin K = 0.5 mcg; Serving size: 1 oz, 28.4 g

Cheese—Nonfat American Cheese ☞ Vitamin K = 0 mcg; Serving size: 1 serving, 19 g

Cheese—Nonfat Cottage ☞ Vitamin K = 0 mcg; Serving size: 1 cup (not packed), 145 g

Cheese—Parmesan Dry Grated Reduced Fat— ☞ Vitamin K = 1.7 mcg; Serving size: 1 cup, 100 g

Cheese—Parmesan—Topping Fat-free ☞ Vitamin K = 0 mcg; Serving size: 1 tablespoon, 5 g

Cheese—Pasteurized Process American Reduced Fat— ☛ Vitamin K = 3.8 mcg; Serving size: 1 cup, diced, 140 g

Cheese—Pasteurized Process American Without Added Vitamin D ☛ Vitamin K = 0.7 mcg; Serving size: 1 oz, 28.4 g

Cheese—Pasteurized Process Cheddar Or American Reduced Sodium ☛ Vitamin K = 3.6 mcg; Serving size: 1 cup, diced, 140 g

Cheese—Port De Salut ☛ Vitamin K = 3.2 mcg; Serving size: 1 cup, diced, 132 g

Cheese—Processed American Cheese ☛ Vitamin K = 1.1 mcg; Serving size: 1 oz, 28.4 g

Cheese—Processed Pimento Cheese ☛ Vitamin K = 4.1 mcg; Serving size: 1 cup, diced, 140 g

Cheese—Processed Swiss Cheese ☛ Vitamin K = 3.1 mcg; Serving size: 1 cup, diced, 140 g

Cheese—Product Pasteurized Process American Reduced Fat— Fortified With Vitamin D ☛ Vitamin K = 0.5 mcg; Serving size: 1 slice 3/4 oz, 21 g

Cheese—Product Pasteurized Process American Vitamin D Fortified ☛ Vitamin K = 0.6 mcg; Serving size: 1 slice (2/3 oz), 19 g

Cheese—Provolone ☛ Vitamin K = 2.9 mcg; Serving size: 1 cup, diced, 132 g

Cheese—Puerto Rican White Cheese ☛ Vitamin K = 1.4 mcg; Serving size: 1 cup, 128 g

Cheese—Reduced Fat— Cheddar ☛ Vitamin K = 0.8 mcg; Serving size: 1 cup, diced, 132 g

Cheese—Reduced Fat—Cottage (1%) ☛ Vitamin K = 0.1 mcg; Serving size: 4 oz, 113 g

Cheese—Reduced Fat—Cottage (2%) ☞ Vitamin K = 0 mcg; Serving size: 4 oz, 113 g

Cheese—Ricotta ☞ Vitamin K = 1.4 mcg; Serving size: 1/2 cup, 124 g

Cheese—Ricotta ☞ Vitamin K = 2.2 mcg; Serving size: 1 cup, 246 g

Cheese—Romano ☞ Vitamin K = 0.6 mcg; Serving size: 1 oz, 28.4 g

Cheese—Sauce Prepared From Recipe ☞ Vitamin K = 0.3 mcg; Serving size: 2 tbsp, 30 g

Cheese—Sharp Cheddar Cheese ☞ Vitamin K = 0.5 mcg; Serving size: 1 slice (2/3 oz), 19 g

Cheese—Soft Goat Cheese ☞ Vitamin K = 0.5 mcg; Serving size: 1 oz, 28.4 g

Cheese—Souffle ☞ Vitamin K = 1 mcg; Serving size: 1 cup, 95 g

Cheese—Spread American Or Cheddar Cheese—Base Reduced Fat — ☞ Vitamin K = 0 mcg; Serving size: 1 piece, 21 g

Cheese—Spread Cream Cheese—Base ☞ Vitamin K = 0.7 mcg; Serving size: 1 oz, 28.4 g

Cheese—Substitute Mozzarella ☞ Vitamin K = 1.1 mcg; Serving size: 1 cup, shredded, 113 g

Cheese—Swiss ☞ Vitamin K = 1.8 mcg; Serving size: 1 cup, diced, 132 g

Cheese—Swiss Reduced Fat— ☞ Vitamin K = 0.1 mcg; Serving size: 1 slice (1 oz), 28 g

Cheese—Swiss Reduced Sodium ☞ Vitamin K = 0.7 mcg; Serving size: 1 slice, 28 g

Cheese—With Nuts ☞ Vitamin K = 0.3 mcg; Serving size: 1 tablespoon, 15 g

Chicken Or Turkey Souffle ☞ Vitamin K = 1.1 mcg; Serving size: 1 cup, 159 g

Chocolate Milk—Made From Dry Mix With Fat-free Milk ☞ Vitamin K = 0.2 mcg; Serving size: 1 cup, 248 g

Chocolate Milk—Made From Dry Mix With Fat-free Milk— (Nesquik) ☞ Vitamin K = 0.2 mcg; Serving size: 1 cup, 248 g

Chocolate Milk—Made From Dry Mix With Non-Dairy Milk ☞ Vitamin K = 3.7 mcg; Serving size: 1 cup, 248 g

Chocolate Milk—Made From Dry Mix With Non-Dairy Milk— (Nesquik) ☞ Vitamin K = 3.7 mcg; Serving size: 1 cup, 248 g

Chocolate Milk—Made From Dry Mix With Reduced Fat—Milk ☞ Vitamin K = 0.5 mcg; Serving size: 1 cup, 248 g

Chocolate Milk—Made From Dry Mix With Reduced Fat—Milk ☞ Vitamin K = 0.2 mcg; Serving size: 1 cup, 248 g

Chocolate Milk—Made From Dry Mix With Reduced Fat—Milk— (Nesquik) ☞ Vitamin K = 0.5 mcg; Serving size: 1 cup, 248 g

Chocolate Milk—Made From Dry Mix With Reduced Fat—Milk— (Nesquik) ☞ Vitamin K = 0.2 mcg; Serving size: 1 cup, 248 g

Chocolate Milk—Made From Dry Mix With Whole Milk ☞ Vitamin K = 0.7 mcg; Serving size: 1 cup, 248 g

Chocolate Milk—Made From Dry Mix With Whole Milk—(Nesquik) ☞ Vitamin K = 0.7 mcg; Serving size: 1 cup, 248 g

Chocolate Milk—Made From Light Syrup With Fat-free Milk ☞ Vitamin K = 0 mcg; Serving size: 1 cup, 248 g

Chocolate Milk—Made From Light Syrup With Non-Dairy Milk ☞ Vitamin K = 3.2 mcg; Serving size: 1 cup, 248 g

Chocolate Milk—Made From Light Syrup With Reduced Fat—Milk ☞ Vitamin K = 0.5 mcg; Serving size: 1 cup, 248 g

Chocolate Milk—Made From Light Syrup With Reduced Fat—Milk
☛ Vitamin K = 0.2 mcg; Serving size: 1 cup, 248 g

Chocolate Milk—Made From Light Syrup With Whole Milk ☛
Vitamin K = 0.7 mcg; Serving size: 1 cup, 248 g

Chocolate Milk—Made From No Sugar Added Dry Mix With Fat-free
Milk— (Nesquik) ☛ Vitamin K = 0 mcg; Serving size: 1 cup, 248 g

Chocolate Milk—Made From No Sugar Added Dry Mix With Non-
Dairy Milk—(Nesquik) ☛ Vitamin K = 3.5 mcg; Serving size: 1 cup,
248 g

Chocolate Milk—Made From No Sugar Added Dry Mix With
Reduced Fat—Milk—(Nesquik) ☛ Vitamin K = 0.5 mcg; Serving size:
1 cup, 248 g

Chocolate Milk—Made From No Sugar Added Dry Mix With
Reduced Fat—Milk—(Nesquik) ☛ Vitamin K = 0.2 mcg; Serving size:
1 cup, 248 g

Chocolate Milk—Made From No Sugar Added Dry Mix With Whole
Milk—(Nesquik) ☛ Vitamin K = 0.7 mcg; Serving size: 1 cup, 248 g

Chocolate Milk—Made From Reduced Sugar Mix With Fat-free Milk
☛ Vitamin K = 0 mcg; Serving size: 1 cup, 248 g

Chocolate Milk—Made From Reduced Sugar Mix With Non-Dairy
Milk ☛ Vitamin K = 3.5 mcg; Serving size: 1 cup, 248 g

Chocolate Milk—Made From Reduced Sugar Mix With Reduced Fat
—Milk ☛ Vitamin K = 0.5 mcg; Serving size: 1 cup, 248 g

Chocolate Milk—Made From Reduced Sugar Mix With Reduced Fat
—Milk ☛ Vitamin K = 0.2 mcg; Serving size: 1 cup, 248 g

Chocolate Milk—Made From Reduced Sugar Mix With Whole Milk
☛ Vitamin K = 0.7 mcg; Serving size: 1 cup, 248 g

Chocolate Milk—Made From Sugar Free Syrup With Fat-free Milk ☛
Vitamin K = 0 mcg; Serving size: 1 cup, 248 g

Chocolate Milk—Made From Sugar Free Syrup With Non-Dairy Milk ☞ Vitamin K = 3.5 mcg; Serving size: 1 cup, 248 g

Chocolate Milk—Made From Sugar Free Syrup With Reduced Fat—Milk ☞ Vitamin K = 0.5 mcg; Serving size: 1 cup, 248 g

Chocolate Milk—Made From Sugar Free Syrup With Reduced Fat—Milk ☞ Vitamin K = 0.2 mcg; Serving size: 1 cup, 248 g

Chocolate Milk—Made From Sugar Free Syrup With Whole Milk ☞ Vitamin K = 0.7 mcg; Serving size: 1 cup, 248 g

Chocolate Milk—Made From Syrup With Fat-free Milk ☞ Vitamin K = 0 mcg; Serving size: 1 cup, 248 g

Chocolate Milk—Made From Syrup With Non-Dairy Milk ☞ Vitamin K = 3.2 mcg; Serving size: 1 cup, 248 g

Chocolate Milk—Made From Syrup With Reduced Fat—Milk ☞ Vitamin K = 0.5 mcg; Serving size: 1 cup, 248 g

Chocolate Milk—Made From Syrup With Reduced Fat—Milk ☞ Vitamin K = 0.2 mcg; Serving size: 1 cup, 248 g

Chocolate Milk—Made From Syrup With Whole Milk ☞ Vitamin K = 0.7 mcg; Serving size: 1 cup, 248 g

Chocolate Milk—Ready To Drink Reduced Fat— ☞ Vitamin K = 0 mcg; Serving size: 1 fl oz, 31 g

Chocolate Milk—Ready To Drink Reduced Fat—(Nesquik) ☞ Vitamin K = 0.2 mcg; Serving size: 1 cup, 248 g

Chocolate Milk—Ready To Drink Reduced Fat—No Sugar Added (Nesquik) ☞ Vitamin K = 0.2 mcg; Serving size: 1 cup, 248 g

Cottage Cheese—Farmer's ☞ Vitamin K = 1.1 mcg; Serving size: 1 cup, 210 g

Cream Substitute—Liquid Light ☞ Vitamin K = 0.3 mcg; Serving size: 1 fl oz, 30 g

Cream Substitute—Powdered Light ☛ Vitamin K = 3.7 mcg; Serving size: 1 cup, 94 g

Cream—Cream Substitute—Flavored Liquid ☛ Vitamin K = 0.5 mcg; Serving size: 1 tbsp, 15 g

Cream—Cream Substitute—Flavored Powdered ☛ Vitamin K = 1.1 mcg; Serving size: 4 tsp, 12 g

Cream—Cream Substitute—Powdered ☛ Vitamin K = 1.6 mcg; Serving size: 1 cup, 94 g

Cream—Cultured Sour Cream ☛ Vitamin K = 0.2 mcg; Serving size: 1 tbsp, 12 g

Cream—Fat-free Sour Cream ☛ Vitamin K = 0 mcg; Serving size: 1 tablespoon, 12 g

Cream—Half And Half Cream ☛ Vitamin K = 0.4 mcg; Serving size: 1 fl oz, 30.2 g

Cream—Half And Half Fat-free ☛ Vitamin K = 0.1 mcg; Serving size: 2 tbsp, 29 g

Cream—Heavy Whipping Cream ☛ Vitamin K = 3.8 mcg; Serving size: 1 cup, whipped, 120 g

Cream—Imitation Sour Cream ☛ Vitamin K = 1.4 mcg; Serving size: 1 oz, 28.4 g

Cream—Light Cream (Coffe Cream) ☛ Vitamin K = 0.5 mcg; Serving size: 1 fl oz, 30 g

Cream—Light Whipping Cream ☛ Vitamin K = 3.2 mcg; Serving size: 1 cup, whipped, 120 g

Cream—Reduced Fat— Sour Cream ☛ Vitamin K = 0.1 mcg; Serving size: 1 tablespoon, 12 g

Cream—Reduced Fat—Sour Cream ☛ Vitamin K = 0.1 mcg; Serving size: 1 tbsp, 15 g

Cream—Sour Cream Light ☛ Vitamin K = 0.1 mcg; Serving size: 1 tablespoon, 12 g

Cream—Whipped Cream ☛ Vitamin K = 1.1 mcg; Serving size: 1 cup, 60 g

Cream—Whipped Cream Substitute—Dietetic Made From Powdered Mix ☛ Vitamin K = 0 mcg; Serving size: 1 cup, 80 g

Dehydrated Milk ☛ Vitamin K = 0.7 mcg; Serving size: 1/4 cup, 32 g

Dessert Topping—Powdered ☛ Vitamin K = 4.3 mcg; Serving size: 1 (1/2) oz, 43 g

Dessert Topping—Powdered 1.5 Ounce Prepared With 1/2 Cup Milk ☛ Vitamin K = 2.2 mcg; Serving size: 1 cup, 80 g

Dessert Topping—Pressurized ☛ Vitamin K = 3.9 mcg; Serving size: 1 cup, 70 g

Dessert Topping—Semi Solid Frozen ☛ Vitamin K = 4.7 mcg; Serving size: 1 cup, 75 g

Dried Eggs ☛ Vitamin K = 1 mcg; Serving size: 1 cup, sifted, 85 g

Dried Sweet Whey Powder ☛ Vitamin K = 0.1 mcg; Serving size: 1 cup, 145 g

Dried Whey Powder (Acid) ☛ Vitamin K = 0 mcg; Serving size: 1 cup, 57 g

Duck Egg Cooked ☛ Vitamin K = 0.4 mcg; Serving size: 1 egg, 70 g

Dulce De Leche ☛ Vitamin K = 0.2 mcg; Serving size: 1 tbsp, 19 g

Egg Benedict ☛ Vitamin K = 5.2 mcg; Serving size: 1 medium egg, 149 g

Egg Casserole With Bread Cheese—Milk—And Meat ☛ Vitamin K = 0.7 mcg; Serving size: 1 cup, 164 g

Egg Creamed ☛ Vitamin K = 0.8 mcg; Serving size: 1 medium egg, 139 g

Egg Deviled ☛ Vitamin K = 3.3 mcg; Serving size: 1/2 small egg, 24 g

Egg Duck Whole Fresh Raw ☛ Vitamin K = 0.3 mcg; Serving size: 1 egg, 70 g

Egg Goose Whole Fresh Raw ☛ Vitamin K = 0.6 mcg; Serving size: 1 egg, 144 g

Egg Omelet ☛ Vitamin K = 0.7 mcg; Serving size: 1 tbsp, 15 g

Egg White Cooked Cooked with Fat ☛ Vitamin K = 1.4 mcg; Serving size: 1 small egg white, 24 g

Egg White Cooked Cooked without Fat ☛ Vitamin K = 0 mcg; Serving size: 1 small egg white, 24 g

Egg White Dried ☛ Vitamin K = 0 mcg; Serving size: 1 oz, 28 g

Egg White Omelet Scrambled Or Fried With Cheese—And Meat Cooked without Fat ☛ Vitamin K = 0.1 mcg; Serving size: 1 small egg, 41 g

Egg White Omelet Scrambled Or Fried With Cheese—And Vegetables Cooked with Fat ☛ Vitamin K = 3.9 mcg; Serving size: 1 small egg, 42 g

Egg White Omelet Scrambled Or Fried With Cheese—And Vegetables Cooked without Fat ☛ Vitamin K = 0.5 mcg; Serving size: 1 small egg, 39 g

Egg White Omelet Scrambled Or Fried With Cheese—Cooked with Fat ☛ Vitamin K = 2.2 mcg; Serving size: 1 small egg, 28 g

Egg White Omelet Scrambled Or Fried With Cheese—Cooked without Fat ☛ Vitamin K = 0.1 mcg; Serving size: 1 small egg, 26 g

Egg White Omelet Scrambled Or Fried With Cheese—Meat And

Vegetables Cooked with Fat ➨ Vitamin K = 3.7 mcg; Serving size: 1 small egg, 43 g

Egg White Omelet Scrambled Or Fried With Cheese—Meat And Vegetables Cooked without Fat ➨ Vitamin K = 0.3 mcg; Serving size: 1 small egg, 41 g

Egg White Omelet Scrambled Or Fried With Meat And Vegetables Cooked with Fat ➨ Vitamin K = 3.5 mcg; Serving size: 1 small egg, 39 g

Egg Whole Baked Cooked with Fat ➨ Vitamin K = 2.6 mcg; Serving size: 1 small, 47 g

Egg Whole Baked Cooked without Fat ➨ Vitamin K = 0.1 mcg; Serving size: 1 small, 33 g

Egg Whole Boiled Or Poached ➨ Vitamin K = 0.1 mcg; Serving size: 1 small, 37 g

Egg Whole Fried With Animal Fat Or Meat Drippings ➨ Vitamin K = 0.1 mcg; Serving size: 1 small, 35 g

Egg Whole Fried With Butter ➨ Vitamin K = 0.3 mcg; Serving size: 1 small, 35 g

Egg Whole Fried With Margarine ➨ Vitamin K = 2.6 mcg; Serving size: 1 small, 35 g

Egg Whole Fried With Oil ➨ Vitamin K = 3.1 mcg; Serving size: 1 small, 35 g

Egg Yolk Dried ➨ Vitamin K = 1 mcg; Serving size: 1 cup, sifted, 67 g

Egg Yolk Only Cooked Cooked with Fat ➨ Vitamin K = 1.2 mcg; Serving size: 1 small egg yolk, 13 g

Egg Yolk Only Cooked Cooked without Fat ➨ Vitamin K = 0.1 mcg; Serving size: 1 small egg yolk, 13 g

Egg Yolks (Raw) ➨ Vitamin K = 0.1 mcg; Serving size: 1 large, 17 g

Eggnog ➨ Vitamin K = 0.8 mcg; Serving size: 1 cup, 254 g

Eggnog Reduced Fat—/ Light ☛ Vitamin K = 0.5 mcg; Serving size: 1 cup, 256 g

Eggs (Raw) ☛ Vitamin K = 0.2 mcg; Serving size: 1 large, 50 g

Eggs A La Malaguena Puerto Rican Style ☛ Vitamin K = 11.7 mcg; Serving size: 1 medium egg, 117 g

Eggs Scrambled Frozen Mixture ☛ Vitamin K = 0.5 mcg; Serving size: 1 oz, 28.4 g

Evaporated Milk ☛ Vitamin K = 0 mcg; Serving size: 1 fl oz, 31.9 g

Fat-free Ice Cream—No Sugar Added Flavors Other Than Chocolate ☛ Vitamin K = 0 mcg; Serving size: 1/2 cup, 68 g

Fried Eggs ☛ Vitamin K = 2.6 mcg; Serving size: 1 large, 46 g

Ghee (Clarified Butter) ☛ Vitamin K = 1.1 mcg; Serving size: 1 tbsp, 12.8 g

Goat Milk ☛ Vitamin K = 0.1 mcg; Serving size: 1 fl oz, 30.5 g

Goose Egg Cooked ☛ Vitamin K = 0.7 mcg; Serving size: 1 egg, 144 g

Grated Parmesan ☛ Vitamin K = 1.7 mcg; Serving size: 1 cup, 100 g

Hard Boiled Eggs ☛ Vitamin K = 0.4 mcg; Serving size: 1 cup, chopped, 136 g

Hot Chocolate / Cocoa Prepared With Dry Mix And Non-Dairy Milk ☛ Vitamin K = 3.5 mcg; Serving size: 1 cup, 248 g

Hot Chocolate / Cocoa Prepared With Dry Mix And Reduced Fat—Milk ☛ Vitamin K = 0.7 mcg; Serving size: 1 cup, 248 g

Hot Chocolate / Cocoa Prepared With Dry Mix And Reduced Fat—Milk ☛ Vitamin K = 0.5 mcg; Serving size: 1 cup, 248 g

Hot Cocoa ☛ Vitamin K = 0.5 mcg; Serving size: 1 cup, 250 g

Huevos Rancheros ☛ Vitamin K = 5.7 mcg; Serving size: 1 egg, ns as to size, 118 g

Ice Cream—Bar Cake Covered ☛ Vitamin K = 4.2 mcg; Serving size: 1 bar, 59 g

Ice Cream—Bar Or Stick Chocolate Covered ☛ Vitamin K = 0.7 mcg; Serving size: 1 bar, 50 g

Ice Cream—Bar Or Stick Chocolate Ice Cream—Chocolate Covered ☛ Vitamin K = 0.7 mcg; Serving size: 1 bar, 49 g

Ice Cream—Bar Or Stick Rich Chocolate Ice Cream—Thick Chocolate Covering ☛ Vitamin K = 2.7 mcg; Serving size: 1 bar, 81 g

Ice Cream—Bar Or Stick Rich Ice Cream—Thick Chocolate Covering ☛ Vitamin K = 2.1 mcg; Serving size: 1 bar, 81 g

Ice Cream—Bar Or Stick With Fruit ☛ Vitamin K = 1.2 mcg; Serving size: 1 bar, 41 g

Ice Cream—Bar Stick Or Nugget With Crunch Coating ☛ Vitamin K = 21.2 mcg; Serving size: 26 pieces, 95 g

Ice Cream—Cone Chocolate Covered Or Dipped Chocolate Ice Cream ☛ Vitamin K = 1.1 mcg; Serving size: 1 cone, 78 g

Ice Cream—Cone Chocolate Covered Or Dipped Flavors Other Than Chocolate ☛ Vitamin K = 0.7 mcg; Serving size: 1 cone and single dip, 78 g

Ice Cream—Cone Chocolate Covered With Nuts Chocolate Ice Cream ☛ Vitamin K = 0.9 mcg; Serving size: 1 cone, 78 g

Ice Cream—Cone Chocolate Covered With Nuts Flavors Other Than Chocolate ☛ Vitamin K = 1.1 mcg; Serving size: 1 unit, 96 g

Ice Cream—Cone No Topping Chocolate Ice Cream ☛ Vitamin K = 0.8 mcg; Serving size: 1 cone and single dip (or 1 small cone), 78 g

Ice Cream—Cone No Topping Flavors Other Than Chocolate ☛ Vitamin K = 0.3 mcg; Serving size: 1 cone and single dip (or 1 small cone), 78 g

Ice Cream—Cone With Nuts Chocolate Ice Cream ☞ Vitamin K = 0.6 mcg; Serving size: 1 cone, 78 g

Ice Cream—Cone With Nuts Flavors Other Than Chocolate ☞ Vitamin K = 0.2 mcg; Serving size: 1 cone, 78 g

Ice Cream—Cookie Sandwich ☞ Vitamin K = 1.1 mcg; Serving size: 1 serving, 82 g

Ice Cream—Fried ☞ Vitamin K = 7.3 mcg; Serving size: 1 cup, 133 g

Ice Cream—Light Soft Serve Chocolate ☞ Vitamin K = 1.2 mcg; Serving size: 1 medium, 298 g

Ice Cream—Pie No Crust ☞ Vitamin K = 5.6 mcg; Serving size: 1 pie (8" dia), 794 g

Ice Cream—Pie With Cookie Crust Fudge Topping And Whipped Cream ☞ Vitamin K = 90 mcg; Serving size: 1 pie (8" dia), 1836 g

Ice Cream—Sandwich ☞ Vitamin K = 0.9 mcg; Serving size: 1 serving, 70 g

Ice Cream—Sandwich Prepared With Light Chocolate Ice Cream ☞ Vitamin K = 0.5 mcg; Serving size: 1 sandwich, 68 g

Ice Cream—Sandwich Vanilla Light No Sugar Added ☞ Vitamin K = 0.4 mcg; Serving size: 1 serving, 70 g

Ice Cream—Soda Chocolate ☞ Vitamin K = 0.2 mcg; Serving size: 1 soda (10 fl oz), 240 g

Ice Cream—Soda Flavors Other Than Chocolate ☞ Vitamin K = 0.2 mcg; Serving size: 1 soda (10 fl oz), 240 g

Ice Cream—Sundae Chocolate Or Fudge Topping With Whipped Cream ☞ Vitamin K = 2.3 mcg; Serving size: 1 sundae, 165 g

Ice Cream—Sundae Fruit Topping With Whipped Cream ☞ Vitamin K = 1.3 mcg; Serving size: 1 sundae, 165 g

Ice Cream—Sundae Fudge Topping With Cake With Whipped Cream ☞ Vitamin K = 3.7 mcg; Serving size: 1 sundae, 175 g

Ice Cream—Sundae Not Fruit Or Chocolate Topping With Whipped Cream ☞ Vitamin K = 1 mcg; Serving size: 1 sundae, 165 g

Ice Cream—Sundae Prepackaged Type Flavors Other Than Chocolate ☞ Vitamin K = 0.4 mcg; Serving size: 1 sundae (6 fl oz), 131 g

Imitation Cheese—American Or Cheddar Reduced Cholesterol ☞ Vitamin K = 3.1 mcg; Serving size: 1 cup, shredded, 113 g

Low-Fat Milk—1% ☞ Vitamin K = 0.2 mcg; Serving size: 1 cup, 244 g

Low-Fat Milk—2% ☞ Vitamin K = 0.5 mcg; Serving size: 1 cup, 244 g

Low-Fat Yogurt ☞ Vitamin K = 0.3 mcg; Serving size: 1 container (6 oz), 170 g

Milk—ButterMilk—Dried ☞ Vitamin K = 0.1 mcg; Serving size: 1/4 cup, 30 g

Milk—ButterMilk—Fluid Cultured Reduced Fat— ☞ Vitamin K = 0.2 mcg; Serving size: 1 cup, 245 g

Milk—Canned Evaporated With Added Vitamin D And Without Added Vitamin A ☞ Vitamin K = 0.2 mcg; Serving size: 1 fl oz, 31.5 g

Milk—Chocolate Fluid Commercial Reduced Fat— With Added Calcium ☞ Vitamin K = 0.5 mcg; Serving size: 1 cup, 250 g

Milk—Chocolate Fluid Commercial Whole With Added Vitamin A And Vitamin D ☞ Vitamin K = 0.8 mcg; Serving size: 1 cup, 250 g

Milk—Chocolate Reduced Fat—With Added Vitamin A And Vitamin D ☞ Vitamin K = 0.3 mcg; Serving size: 1 cup, 250 g

Milk—Dessert Bar Frozen Made From Reduced Fat—Milk ☞ Vitamin K = 0.4 mcg; Serving size: 1 bar, 68 g

Milk—Dessert Bar Or Stick Frozen With Coconut ☞ Vitamin K = 0.1 mcg; Serving size: 1 fruit stix bar (4 fl oz), 129 g

Milk—Dessert Sandwich Bar Frozen Made From Reduced Fat—Milk ☞ Vitamin K = 0.4 mcg; Serving size: 1 weight watchers sandwich bar (2.75 fl oz plus 2 wafers), 64 g

Milk—Dessert Sandwich Bar Frozen With Low-Calorie Sweetener Made From Reduced Fat—Milk ☞ Vitamin K = 0.9 mcg; Serving size: 1 eskimo pie sandwich (3.2 fl oz), 59 g

Milk—Dry Reconstituted Whole ☞ Vitamin K = 0.7 mcg; Serving size: 1 cup, 244 g

Milk—Dry Whole Without Added Vitamin D ☞ Vitamin K = 2.8 mcg; Serving size: 1 cup, 128 g

Milk—Evaporated 2% Fat With Added Vitamin A And Vitamin D ☞ Vitamin K = 0.5 mcg; Serving size: 1 cup, 252 g

Milk—Evaporated Reduced Fat—(2%) ☞ Vitamin K = 0.5 mcg; Serving size: 1 cup, 252 g

Milk—Filled Fluid With Lauric Acid Oil ☞ Vitamin K = 2 mcg; Serving size: 1 cup, 244 g

Milk—Fluid 1% Fat Without Added Vitamin A And Vitamin D ☞ Vitamin K = 0.2 mcg; Serving size: 1 cup, 244 g

Milk—Nonfat Fluid With Added Nonfat Milk—Solids Vitamin A And Vitamin D (Fat-free Or Skim) ☞ Vitamin K = 0 mcg; Serving size: 1 cup, 245 g

Milk—Nonfat Fluid Without Added Vitamin A And Vitamin D (Fat-free Or Skim) ☞ Vitamin K = 0 mcg; Serving size: 1 cup, 245 g

Milk—Reduced Fat—Fluid 2% Milkfat Without Added Vitamin A And Vitamin D ☞ Vitamin K = 0.5 mcg; Serving size: 1 cup, 246 g

Milk—Reduced Sodium Fluid ☞ Vitamin K = 0.7 mcg; Serving size: 1 cup, 244 g

Milk—Shake Bottled Chocolate ☞ Vitamin K = 0.1 mcg; Serving size: 1 fl oz, 31 g

Milk—Shake Home Recipe Chocolate ☞ Vitamin K = 0.1 mcg; Serving size: 1 fl oz, 28 g

Milk—Shake Home Recipe Chocolate Light ☞ Vitamin K = 0.1 mcg; Serving size: 1 fl oz, 28 g

Milk—Shake Home Recipe Flavors Other Than Chocolate ☞ Vitamin K = 0.1 mcg; Serving size: 1 fl oz, 28 g

Milk—Shake Home Recipe Flavors Other Than Chocolate Light ☞ Vitamin K = 0.1 mcg; Serving size: 1 fl oz, 28 g

Milk—Shake With Malt ☞ Vitamin K = 0.1 mcg; Serving size: 1 fl oz, 28 g

Milk—Shakes Thick Chocolate ☞ Vitamin K = 0.1 mcg; Serving size: 1 fl oz, 28.4 g

Milk—Shakes Thick Vanilla ☞ Vitamin K = 0.1 mcg; Serving size: 1 fl oz, 28.4 g

Milk—Whole 3.25% Milkfat Without Added Vitamin A And Vitamin D ☞ Vitamin K = 0.7 mcg; Serving size: 1 cup, 244 g

Mozzarella (Hard And Lowfat) ☞ Vitamin K = 1.7 mcg; Serving size: 1 cup, diced, 132 g

Protein Supplement Milk—Based Muscle Milk—Light Powder ☞ Vitamin K = 0.3 mcg; Serving size: 2 scoops, 50 g

Protein Supplement Milk—Based Muscle Milk—Powder ☞ Vitamin K = 0.1 mcg; Serving size: 1 tbsp, 11 g

Quail Egg Canned ☞ Vitamin K = 0 mcg; Serving size: 1 egg, 9 g

Reddi Wip Fat-free Whipped Topping ☞ Vitamin K = 0 mcg; Serving size: 1 tablespoon, 4 g

Rice Dessert Bar Frozen Chocolate Nondairy Chocolate Covered ☞ Vitamin K = 1.9 mcg; Serving size: 1 bar (4 oz), 113 g

Rice Dessert Bar Frozen Flavors Other Than Chocolate Nondairy Carob Covered ☛ Vitamin K = 1.1 mcg; Serving size: 1 bar (4 oz), 113 g

Rice Frozen Dessert Nondairy Flavors Other Than Chocolate ☛ Vitamin K = 4.6 mcg; Serving size: 1 cup, 172 g

Ripe Plantain Omelet Puerto Rican Style ☛ Vitamin K = 9.9 mcg; Serving size: 1 medium egg, 79 g

Salted Butter ☛ Vitamin K = 0.4 mcg; Serving size: 1 pat (1 inch sq, 1/3 inch high), 5 g

Scrambled Eggs ☛ Vitamin K = 2.4 mcg; Serving size: 1 large, 61 g

Scrambled Eggs With Jerked Beef Puerto Rican Style ☛ Vitamin K = 1.4 mcg; Serving size: 1 cup, 140 g

Seafood Souffle ☛ Vitamin K = 1.1 mcg; Serving size: 1 cup, 159 g

Shredded Parmesan ☛ Vitamin K = 0.1 mcg; Serving size: 1 tbsp, 5 g

Shrimp-Egg Patty ☛ Vitamin K = 5.5 mcg; Serving size: 1 patty (about 2" dia), 18 g

Skim Milk ☛ Vitamin K = 0 mcg; Serving size: 1 cup, 245 g

Soft Serve Chocolate Ice Cream ☛ Vitamin K = 0.8 mcg; Serving size: 1/2 cup, 86 g

Squash Summer—Souffle ☛ Vitamin K = 3.1 mcg; Serving size: 1 cup, 136 g

Squash Winter Souffle ☛ Vitamin K = 5.2 mcg; Serving size: 1 cup, 157 g

Strawberry Milk—Fat-free ☛ Vitamin K = 0 mcg; Serving size: 1 fl oz, 31 g

Strawberry Milk—Non-Dairy ☛ Vitamin K = 3.5 mcg; Serving size: 1 cup, 248 g

Strawberry Milk—Reduced Fat— ☛ Vitamin K = 0.5 mcg; Serving size: 1 cup, 248 g

Strawberry Milk—Reduced Fat— ☛ Vitamin K = 0.2 mcg; Serving size: 1 cup, 248 g

Strawberry Milk—Whole ☛ Vitamin K = 0.7 mcg; Serving size: 1 cup, 248 g

Sweet Whey Fluid ☛ Vitamin K = 0 mcg; Serving size: 1 cup, 246 g

Sweetened Condensed Milk ☛ Vitamin K = 0.2 mcg; Serving size: 1 fl oz, 38.2 g

Tofu Frozen Dessert Chocolate ☛ Vitamin K = 5.9 mcg; Serving size: 1 cup, 164 g

Tofu Frozen Dessert Flavors Other Than Chocolate ☛ Vitamin K = 5.4 mcg; Serving size: 1 cup, 164 g

Unsalted Butter ☛ Vitamin K = 0.4 mcg; Serving size: 1 pat (1 inch sq, 1/3 inch high), 5 g

Whole Milk ☛ Vitamin K = 0.7 mcg; Serving size: 1 cup, 244 g

Yogurt—Chocolate Nonfat Milk ☛ Vitamin K = 0 mcg; Serving size: 1 container (6 oz), 170 g

Yogurt—Coconut Milk ☛ Vitamin K = 0 mcg; Serving size: 1 6 oz container, 170 g

Yogurt—Frozen Chocolate Reduced Fat—Milk ☛ Vitamin K = 0.6 mcg; Serving size: 1 cup, 200 g

Yogurt—Frozen Chocolate-Coated ☛ Vitamin K = 0.1 mcg; Serving size: 1 bar, 41 g

Yogurt—Frozen Cone Chocolate ☛ Vitamin K = 0.9 mcg; Serving size: 1 small cone, 78 g

Yogurt—Fruit Reduced Fat—With Reduced Calorie Sweetener ☛ Vitamin K = 2 mcg; Serving size: 1 container (6 oz), 170 g

Yogurt—Fruit Reduced Fat—With Reduced Calorie Sweetener Fortified With Vitamin D ☛ Vitamin K = 2 mcg; Serving size: 1 container (6 oz), 170 g

Yogurt—Fruit Variety Nonfat ☛ Vitamin K = 1.9 mcg; Serving size: 1 container (6 oz), 170 g

Yogurt—Fruit Variety Nonfat Fortified With Vitamin D ☛ Vitamin K = 1.9 mcg; Serving size: 1 container (6 oz), 170 g

Yogurt—Greek Reduced Fat—Milk—Fruit ☛ Vitamin K = 0 mcg; Serving size: 1 tube, 57 g

Yogurt—Greek Whole Milk—Flavors Other Than Fruit ☛ Vitamin K = 0.6 mcg; Serving size: 1 5.3 oz container, 150 g

Yogurt—Liquid ☛ Vitamin K = 0.1 mcg; Serving size: 1 bottle, 93 g

Yogurt—Nonfat Milk—Flavors Other Than Fruit ☛ Vitamin K = 0.2 mcg; Serving size: 1 4 oz container, 113 g

Yogurt—Nonfat Milk—Fruit ☛ Vitamin K = 0.2 mcg; Serving size: 1 4 oz container, 113 g

Yogurt—Reduced Fat—Milk—Flavors Other Than Fruit ☛ Vitamin K = 0.1 mcg; Serving size: 1 tube, 64 g

Yogurt—Reduced Fat—Milk—Fruit ☛ Vitamin K = 0.1 mcg; Serving size: 1 tube, 64 g

Yogurt—Vanilla Flavor Reduced Fat—Milk—Sweetened With Reduced Calorie Sweetener ☛ Vitamin K = 0.2 mcg; Serving size: 1 container, 170 g

Yogurt—Whole Milk—Flavors Other Than Fruit ☛ Vitamin K = 0.2 mcg; Serving size: 1 4 oz container, 113 g

Yogurt—Whole Milk—Fruit ☛ Vitamin K = 0.2 mcg; Serving size: 1 4 oz container, 113 g

17

FAST-FOOD ITEMS

Bacon And Cheese Sandwich—With Spread ☞ Vitamin K = 9.1 mcg; Serving size: 1 sandwich, 121 g

Bacon And Egg Sandwich ☞ Vitamin K = 3.4 mcg; Serving size: 1 sandwich, 177 g

Bacon Breaded Fried Chicken Fillet And Tomato Club With Lettuce And Spread ☞ Vitamin K = 33.1 mcg; Serving size: 1 sandwich, 227 g

Bacon Cheeseburger—1 Large Patty With Condiments On Bun From Fast Food / Restaurant ☞ Vitamin K = 33.2 mcg; Serving size: 1 (1/3 lb) cheeseburger, 335 g

Bacon Cheeseburger—1 Medium Patty Plain On Bun From Fast Food / Restaurant ☞ Vitamin K = 7.1 mcg; Serving size: 1 (1/4 lb) bacon cheeseburger, 170 g

Bacon Cheeseburger—1 Medium Patty Plain On White Bun ☞ Vitamin K = 4.9 mcg; Serving size: 1 (1/4 lb) bacon cheeseburger, 180 g

Bacon Cheeseburger—1 Medium Patty With Condiments On Bun From Fast Food / Restaurant ☞ Vitamin K = 9.8 mcg; Serving size: 1 (1/4 lb) bacon cheeseburger, 240 g

Bacon Cheeseburger—1 Medium Patty With Condiments On Wheat Bun ☞ Vitamin K = 19.2 mcg; Serving size: 1 (1/4 lb) bacon cheeseburger, 240 g

Bacon Cheeseburger—1 Medium Patty With Condiments On White Bun ☞ Vitamin K = 18.7 mcg; Serving size: 1 (1/4 lb) bacon cheeseburger, 240 g

Bacon Cheeseburger—1 Medium Patty With Condiments On Whole Wheat Bun ☞ Vitamin K = 19.2 mcg; Serving size: 1 (1/4 lb) bacon cheeseburger, 240 g

Bacon Cheeseburger—1 Small Patty With Condiments On Bun From Fast Food / Restaurant ☞ Vitamin K = 8 mcg; Serving size: 1 bacon cheeseburger, 160 g

Bacon Cheeseburger—1 Small Patty With Condiments On Bun From Fast Food / Restaurant (Wendy's Jr. Bacon Cheeseburger) ☞ Vitamin K = 5.7 mcg; Serving size: 1 wendy's jr. bacon cheeseburger, 150 g

Bacon Chicken And Tomato Club Sandwich—On Multigrain Roll With Lettuce And Spread ☞ Vitamin K = 9.5 mcg; Serving size: 1 sandwich, 194 g

Bacon Lettuce And Tomato Sandwich—With Spread ☞ Vitamin K = 26.2 mcg; Serving size: 1 sandwich, 164 g

Bacon Lettuce Tomato And Cheese Submarine Sandwich—With Spread ☞ Vitamin K = 28.9 mcg; Serving size: 1 submarine, 260 g

Bacon On Biscuit ☞ Vitamin K = 3.3 mcg; Serving size: 1 sandwich, 93 g

Bacon Sandwich—With Spread ☞ Vitamin K = 7.5 mcg; Serving size: 1 sandwich, 91 g

Bagel— With Breakfast Steak Egg Cheese And Condiments ☞ Vitamin K = 8.6 mcg; Serving size: 1 item, 254 g

Bagel— With Egg Sausage Patty Cheese And Condiments ☞ Vitamin K = 6.1 mcg; Serving size: 1 item, 219 g

Beef Barbecue Sandwich—Or Sloppy Joe On Bun ☞ Vitamin K = 5.2 mcg; Serving size: 1 barbecue sandwich, 186 g

Beef Barbecue Submarine Sandwich—On Bun ☞ Vitamin K = 5.2 mcg; Serving size: 1 sandwich, 192 g

Biscuit With Crispy Chicken Fillet ☞ Vitamin K = 8.7 mcg; Serving size: 1 item, 132 g

Biscuit With Egg And Bacon ☞ Vitamin K = 6.5 mcg; Serving size: 1 biscuit, 150 g

Biscuit With Egg And Ham ☞ Vitamin K = 6.6 mcg; Serving size: 1 biscuit, 182 g

Biscuit With Egg Cheese And Bacon ☞ Vitamin K = 6.1 mcg; Serving size: 1 item, 145 g

Biscuit With Gravy ☞ Vitamin K = 13.3 mcg; Serving size: 1 biscuit with gravy, 221 g

Biscuit With Ham ☞ Vitamin K = 9.2 mcg; Serving size: 1 biscuit, 162 g

Biscuit With Sausage ☞ Vitamin K = 6.1 mcg; Serving size: 1 item, 111 g

Blended Soft Serve Ice Cream With Cookies ☞ Vitamin K = 11.1 mcg; Serving size: 12 fl oz cup, 337 g

Blintz Cheese-Filled ☞ Vitamin K = 3 mcg; Serving size: 1 blintz, 70 g

Blintz Fruit-Filled ☞ Vitamin K = 3.2 mcg; Serving size: 1 blintz, 70 g

Bologna And Cheese Sandwich—With Spread ☞ Vitamin K = 8.1 mcg; Serving size: 1 sandwich, 111 g

Bologna Sandwich—With Spread ☞ Vitamin K = 7.1 mcg; Serving size: 1 sandwich, 83 g

Breadstick—Soft Prepared With Garlic And Parmesan Cheese ☞ Vitamin K = 9.1 mcg; Serving size: 1 breadstick, 43 g

Breakfast Burrito—With Egg Cheese And Sausage ☞ Vitamin K = 4.8 mcg; Serving size: 1 burrito, 109 g

Bruschetta ☞ Vitamin K = 5 mcg; Serving size: 1 slice, 43 g

Buffalo Chicken Submarine Sandwich ☞ Vitamin K = 35.5 mcg; Serving size: 1 submarine, 240 g

Buffalo Chicken Submarine Sandwich—With Cheese ☞ Vitamin K = 34.8 mcg; Serving size: 1 submarine, 260 g

Burger King—Cheeseburger ☞ Vitamin K = 7.6 mcg; Serving size: 1 item, 133 g

Burger King—Chicken Strips ☞ Vitamin K = 2.3 mcg; Serving size: 1 strip, 36 g

Burger King—Croissanwich With Egg And Cheese ☞ Vitamin K = 10.5 mcg; Serving size: 1 item, 110 g

Burger King—Croissanwich With Sausage And Cheese ☞ Vitamin K = 8.5 mcg; Serving size: 1 item, 131 g

Burger King—Croissanwich With Sausage Egg And Cheese ☞ Vitamin K = 16.2 mcg; Serving size: 1 sandwich, 171 g

Burger King—Double Whopper No Cheese ☞ Vitamin K = 52.7 mcg; Serving size: 1 item, 374 g

Burger King—Double Whopper With Cheese ☞ Vitamin K = 45.9 mcg; Serving size: 1 item, 399 g

Burger King—French Fries ☞ Vitamin K = 8.2 mcg; Serving size: 1 small serving, 74 g

Burger King—French Toast—Sticks ☞ Vitamin K = 3 mcg; Serving size: 1 stick, 21 g

Burger King—Hamburger ☞ Vitamin K = 5.4 mcg; Serving size: 1

sandwich, 99 g

Burger King—Original Chicken Sandwich ☛ Vitamin K = 47.2 mcg; Serving size: 1 sandwich, 199 g

Burger King—Premium Fish Sandwich ☛ Vitamin K = 49.5 mcg; Serving size: 1 sandwich, 220 g

Burger King—Whopper No Cheese ☛ Vitamin K = 56.7 mcg; Serving size: 1 item, 291 g

Burger King—Whopper With Cheese ☛ Vitamin K = 60.4 mcg; Serving size: 1 item, 316 g

Burrito—Taco Or Quesadilla—With Egg ☛ Vitamin K = 7.2 mcg; Serving size: 1 small, 110 g

Burrito—Taco Or Quesadilla—With Egg And Breakfast Meat ☛ Vitamin K = 6.9 mcg; Serving size: 1 small, 123 g

Burrito—Taco Or Quesadilla—With Egg And Potato ☛ Vitamin K = 8.9 mcg; Serving size: 1 small, 127 g

Burrito—Taco Or Quesadilla—With Egg Beans And Breakfast Meat ☛ Vitamin K = 9 mcg; Serving size: 1 small, 150 g

Burrito—Taco Or Quesadilla—With Egg Potato—And Breakfast Meat ☛ Vitamin K = 8.9 mcg; Serving size: 1 small, 144 g

Burrito—Taco Or Quesadilla—With Egg Potato—And Breakfast Meat From Fast Food ☛ Vitamin K = 7.6 mcg; Serving size: 1 small, 144 g

Burrito—With Beans And Beef ☛ Vitamin K = 5.8 mcg; Serving size: 1 item, 241 g

Burrito—With Beans And Cheese ☛ Vitamin K = 5.9 mcg; Serving size: 1 each burrito, 185 g

Burrito—With Beans Cheese And Beef ☛ Vitamin K = 14.7 mcg; Serving size: 1 burrito, 241 g

Cheese Pizza ☛ Vitamin K = 7.2 mcg; Serving size: 1 slice, 107 g

Cheeseburger—1 Large Patty Plain On Bun From Fast Food / Restaurant ☛ Vitamin K = 6.2 mcg; Serving size: 1 (1/3 lb) cheeseburger, 200 g

Cheeseburger—1 Large Patty With Condiments On Bun From Fast Food / Restaurant ☛ Vitamin K = 33.7 mcg; Serving size: 1 (1/3 lb) cheeseburger, 315 g

Cheeseburger—1 Medium Patty Plain On Wheat Bun ☛ Vitamin K = 5.4 mcg; Serving size: 1 (1/4 lb) cheeseburger, 165 g

Cheeseburger—1 Medium Patty Plain On White Bun ☛ Vitamin K = 5 mcg; Serving size: 1 (1/4 lb) cheeseburger, 165 g

Cheeseburger—1 Medium Patty Plain On Whole Wheat Bun ☛ Vitamin K = 5.4 mcg; Serving size: 1 cheeseburger, 165 g

Cheeseburger—1 Medium Patty With Condiments On Wheat Bun ☛ Vitamin K = 19.4 mcg; Serving size: 1 (1/4 lb) cheeseburger, 225 g

Cheeseburger—1 Medium Patty With Condiments On White Bun ☛ Vitamin K = 18.9 mcg; Serving size: 1 (1/4 lb) cheeseburger, 225 g

Cheeseburger—1 Medium Patty With Condiments On Whole Wheat Bun ☛ Vitamin K = 19.4 mcg; Serving size: 1 (1/4 lb) cheeseburger, 225 g

Cheeseburger—1 Miniature Patty On Miniature Bun From School ☛ Vitamin K = 2.6 mcg; Serving size: 1 miniature, 60 g

Cheeseburger—1 Miniature Patty Plain On Miniature Bun From Fast Food / Restaurant ☛ Vitamin K = 2.1 mcg; Serving size: 1 miniature, 60 g

Cheeseburger—1 Miniature Patty With Condiments On Miniature Bun From Fast Food / Restaurant ☛ Vitamin K = 7.6 mcg; Serving size: 1 miniature, 75 g

Cheeseburger—1 Small Patty Plain On Wheat Bun ☞ Vitamin K = 4.6 mcg; Serving size: 1 cheeseburger, 140 g

Cheeseburger—1 Small Patty Plain On White Bun ☞ Vitamin K = 4.3 mcg; Serving size: 1 cheeseburger, 140 g

Cheeseburger—1 Small Patty With Condiments On Bun From Fast Food / Restaurant (Burger King—Whopper Jr. With Cheese) ☞ Vitamin K = 17.5 mcg; Serving size: 1 burger king whopper jr, 170 g

Cheeseburger—1 Small Patty With Condiments On Bun From Fast Food / Restaurant (Wendy's Jr. Cheeseburger—Deluxe) ☞ Vitamin K = 16.5 mcg; Serving size: 1 wendy's jr. cheeseburger deluxe, 160 g

Cheeseburger—1 Small Patty With Condiments On Wheat Bun ☞ Vitamin K = 18.3 mcg; Serving size: 1 cheeseburger, 195 g

Cheeseburger—1 Small Patty With Condiments On White Bun ☞ Vitamin K = 17.9 mcg; Serving size: 1 cheeseburger, 195 g

Cheeseburger—1 Small Patty With Condiments On Whole Wheat Bun ☞ Vitamin K = 18.3 mcg; Serving size: 1 cheeseburger, 195 g

Cheeseburger—Double Regular Patty And Bun With Condiments ☞ Vitamin K = 7.3 mcg; Serving size: 1 sandwich, 155 g

Cheeseburger—Double Regular Patty; With Condiments ☞ Vitamin K = 7.3 mcg; Serving size: 1 sandwich, 155 g

Cheeseburger—Nfs ☞ Vitamin K = 18.9 mcg; Serving size: 1 cheese-burger, 225 g

Cheeseburger—On Bun From School ☞ Vitamin K = 5.3 mcg; Serving size: 1 cheeseburger, 115 g

Cheeseburger—Single Large Patty; Plain ☞ Vitamin K = 8.4 mcg; Serving size: 1 sandwich, 182 g

Cheeseburger—Single Large Patty; With Condiments ☞ Vitamin K = 8.8 mcg; Serving size: 1 item, 199 g

Cheeseburger—Single Large Patty; With Condiments Vegetables And Mayonnaise ☞ Vitamin K = 30.5 mcg; Serving size: 1 sandwich, 215 g

Cheeseburger—Single Regular Patty With Condiments ☞ Vitamin K = 7 mcg; Serving size: 1 item, 127 g

Cheeseburger—Single Regular Patty With Condiments And Vegetables ☞ Vitamin K = 4.8 mcg; Serving size: 1 sandwich, 115 g

Cheeseburger—Single Regular Patty; Plain ☞ Vitamin K = 3.8 mcg; Serving size: 1 sandwich, 91 g

Chicken Barbecue Sandwich ☞ Vitamin K = 3.3 mcg; Serving size: 1 sandwich, 239 g

Chicken Breaded And Fried Boneless Pieces Plain ☞ Vitamin K = 6.7 mcg; Serving size: 6 pieces, 96 g

Chicken Fillet Breaded Fried Sandwich—With Cheese Lettuce Tomato And Spread ☞ Vitamin K = 10.6 mcg; Serving size: 1 sandwich, 241 g

Chicken Fillet Broiled Sandwich—On Oat Bran Bun With Lettuce Tomato Spread ☞ Vitamin K = 18 mcg; Serving size: 1 burger king sandwich, 155 g

Chicken Fillet Sandwich—Plain With Pickles ☞ Vitamin K = 15.9 mcg; Serving size: 1 sandwich, 187 g

Chicken Patty Sandwich—Miniature With Spread ☞ Vitamin K = 5.4 mcg; Serving size: 1 miniature sandwich, 31 g

Chicken Patty Sandwich—Or Biscuit ☞ Vitamin K = 10 mcg; Serving size: 1 sandwich, 173 g

Chicken Salad Or Chicken Spread Sandwich ☞ Vitamin K = 28.8 mcg; Serving size: 1 sandwich, 141 g

Chicken Sandwich—With Cheese And Spread ☞ Vitamin K = 8 mcg; Serving size: 1 sandwich, 136 g

Chicken Sandwich—With Spread ☛ Vitamin K = 7.3 mcg; Serving size: 1 sandwich, 112 g

Chicken Tenders ☛ Vitamin K = 2.4 mcg; Serving size: 1 strip, 30 g

Chinese Pancake ☛ Vitamin K = 0 mcg; Serving size: 1 pancake, 28 g

Coleslaw (Fast Food) ☛ Vitamin K = 135.4 mcg; Serving size: 1 cup, 191 g

Corned Beef Sandwich ☛ Vitamin K = 13.8 mcg; Serving size: 1 sandwich, 130 g

Crab Cake Sandwich—On Bun ☛ Vitamin K = 22.8 mcg; Serving size: 1 sandwich, 140 g

Crepe—Chocolate Filled ☛ Vitamin K = 1.8 mcg; Serving size: 1 crepe with filling, any size, 80 g

Crepe—Fruit Filled ☛ Vitamin K = 10.2 mcg; Serving size: 1 crepe with filling, any size, 80 g

Crepe—Plain ☛ Vitamin K = 2.3 mcg; Serving size: 1 crepe, any size, 65 g

Crispy Chicken Bacon And Tomato Club Sandwich—With Cheese Lettuce And Mayonnaise ☛ Vitamin K = 22.8 mcg; Serving size: 1 sandwich, 271 g

Croissant Sandwich—Filled With Broccoli And Cheese ☛ Vitamin K = 16.4 mcg; Serving size: 1 croissant, 113 g

Croissant Sandwich—Filled With Chicken Broccoli And Cheese Sauce ☛ Vitamin K = 9 mcg; Serving size: 1 croissant, 128 g

Croissant Sandwich—Filled With Ham And Cheese ☛ Vitamin K = 1.6 mcg; Serving size: 1 croissant, 113 g

Croissant Sandwich—With Bacon And Egg ☛ Vitamin K = 5.3 mcg; Serving size: 1 croissant, 113 g

Croissant Sandwich—With Bacon Egg And Cheese ☞ Vitamin K = 3.7 mcg; Serving size: 1 croissant, 131 g

Croissant Sandwich—With Sausage And Egg ☞ Vitamin K = 5.3 mcg; Serving size: 1 croissant, 142 g

Croissant With Egg Cheese And Bacon ☞ Vitamin K = 3.6 mcg; Serving size: 1 item, 128 g

Croissant With Egg Cheese And Ham ☞ Vitamin K = 3.3 mcg; Serving size: 1 item, 155 g

Croissant With Egg Cheese And Sausage ☞ Vitamin K = 3.1 mcg; Serving size: 1 sandwich, 171 g

Cuban Sandwich—With Spread ☞ Vitamin K = 19.1 mcg; Serving size: 1 sandwich (6" long), 255 g

Digiorno—Pizza Cheese Topping Cheese Stuffed Crust Frozen Baked ☞ Vitamin K = 13.8 mcg; Serving size: 1 slice 1/4 of pie, 164 g

Digiorno—Pizza Cheese Topping Rising Crust Frozen Baked ☞ Vitamin K = 12.6 mcg; Serving size: 1 slice 1/4 of pie, 183 g

Digiorno—Pizza Cheese Topping Thin Crispy Crust Frozen Baked ☞ Vitamin K = 6.8 mcg; Serving size: 1 slice 1/4 of pie, 161 g

Digiorno—Pizza Pepperoni Topping Cheese Stuffed Crust Frozen Baked ☞ Vitamin K = 14 mcg; Serving size: 1 slice 1/4 of pie, 179 g

Digiorno—Pizza Pepperoni Topping Rising Crust Frozen Baked ☞ Vitamin K = 15.7 mcg; Serving size: 1 slice 1/4 of pie, 207 g

Digiorno—Pizza Pepperoni Topping Thin Crispy Crust Frozen Baked ☞ Vitamin K = 7.3 mcg; Serving size: 1 slice 1/4 of pie, 145 g

Digiorno—Pizza Supreme Topping Rising Crust Frozen Baked ☞ Vitamin K = 17.3 mcg; Serving size: 1 slice 1/4 of pie, 227 g

Digiorno—Pizza Supreme Topping Thin Crispy Crust Frozen Baked ☞ Vitamin K = 8.8 mcg; Serving size: 1 slice 1/4 of pie, 155 g

Domino's—14 Inch Cheese Pizza Classic Hand-Tossed Crust ☛ Vitamin K = 5.8 mcg; Serving size: 1 slice, 108 g

Domino's—14 Inch Cheese Pizza Crunchy Thin Crust ☛ Vitamin K = 11.1 mcg; Serving size: 1 slice, 70 g

Domino's—14 Inch Cheese Pizza Ultimate Deep Dish Crust ☛ Vitamin K = 7.2 mcg; Serving size: 1 slice, 118 g

Domino's—14 Inch Extravaganzza Feast Pizza Classic Hand-Tossed Crust ☛ Vitamin K = 7.9 mcg; Serving size: 1 slice, 151 g

Domino's—14 Inch Pepperoni Pizza Classic Hand-Tossed Crust ☛ Vitamin K = 5.9 mcg; Serving size: 1 slice, 113 g

Domino's—14 Inch Pepperoni Pizza Ultimate Deep Dish Crust ☛ Vitamin K = 7.3 mcg; Serving size: 1 slice, 123 g

Dosa (Indian) Plain ☛ Vitamin K = 1.7 mcg; Serving size: 1 small, 35 g

Double Bacon Cheeseburger—2 Large Patties With Condiments On Bun From Fast Food / Restaurant ☛ Vitamin K = 17.6 mcg; Serving size: 1 sandwich, 400 g

Double Bacon Cheeseburger—2 Medium Patties Plain On Bun From Fast Food / Restaurant ☛ Vitamin K = 7.4 mcg; Serving size: 1 double bacon cheeseburger, 275 g

Double Bacon Cheeseburger—2 Medium Patties With Condiments On Bun From Fast Food / Restaurant ☛ Vitamin K = 21.1 mcg; Serving size: 1 double bacon cheeseburger, 335 g

Double Bacon Cheeseburger—2 Medium Patties With Condiments On Bun From Fast Food / Restaurant (Wendy's Baconator) ☛ Vitamin K = 21.1 mcg; Serving size: 1 wendy's baconator, 335 g

Double Bacon Cheeseburger—2 Small Patties With Condiments On Bun From Fast Food / Restaurant (Burger King—Bacon Double Cheeseburger) ☛ Vitamin K = 16.4 mcg; Serving size: 1 burger king double bacon cheeseburger, 200 g

Double Cheeseburger—2 Medium Patties Plain On Bun From Fast Food / Restaurant ☛ Vitamin K = 8.9 mcg; Serving size: 1 double cheeseburger, 235 g

Double Cheeseburger—2 Small Patties Plain On Bun From Fast Food / Restaurant ☛ Vitamin K = 5.7 mcg; Serving size: 1 double cheeseburger, 155 g

Double Hamburger 2 Medium Patties Plain On Bun From Fast Food / Restaurant ☛ Vitamin K = 6.6 mcg; Serving size: 1 double hamburger, 220 g

Double Hamburger 2 Small Patties Plain On Bun From Fast Food / Restaurant ☛ Vitamin K = 4.5 mcg; Serving size: 1 double hamburger, 135 g

Double Hamburger 2 Small Patties With Condiments On Bun From Fast Food / Restaurant ☛ Vitamin K = 18.1 mcg; Serving size: 1 double hamburger, 190 g

Egg And Cheese On Biscuit ☛ Vitamin K = 11.8 mcg; Serving size: 1 sandwich, 140 g

Egg And Steak On Biscuit ☛ Vitamin K = 12.7 mcg; Serving size: 1 sandwich, 179 g

Egg Cheese And Bacon On Bagel ☛ Vitamin K = 5.2 mcg; Serving size: 1 sandwich, 246 g

Egg Cheese And Beef On English Muffin ☛ Vitamin K = 10.3 mcg; Serving size: 1 great starts sandwich (5.2 oz), 147 g

Egg Cheese And Ham On Bagel ☛ Vitamin K = 33.8 mcg; Serving size: 1 mcdonald's sandwich, 218 g

Egg Cheese And Ham On Biscuit ☛ Vitamin K = 6.1 mcg; Serving size: 1 sandwich, 174 g

Egg Cheese And Sausage On Bun ☛ Vitamin K = 7.3 mcg; Serving size: 1 sandwich, 148 g

Egg Cheese Ham And Bacon On Bun ☛ Vitamin K = 7.9 mcg; Serving size: 1 jack-in-the-box sandwich, 226 g

Egg Extra Cheese And Extra Sausage On Bun ☛ Vitamin K = 5.1 mcg; Serving size: 1 jack-in-the-box sandwich, 213 g

Egg Salad Sandwich ☛ Vitamin K = 51.4 mcg; Serving size: 1 sandwich, 159 g

Egg Scrambled ☛ Vitamin K = 8.6 mcg; Serving size: 2 eggs, 96 g

English Muffin With Cheese And Sausage ☛ Vitamin K = 2.4 mcg; Serving size: 1 item, 108 g

English Muffin—With Egg Cheese And Canadian Bacon ☛ Vitamin K = 1 mcg; Serving size: 1 sandwich, 126 g

English Muffin—With Egg Cheese And Sausage ☛ Vitamin K = 2.5 mcg; Serving size: 1 item, 165 g

Fajita-Style Beef Sandwich—With Cheese On Pita Bread With Lettuce And Tomato ☛ Vitamin K = 10.7 mcg; Serving size: 1 pita sandwich, 175 g

Fajita-Style Chicken Sandwich—With Cheese On Pita Bread With Lettuce And Tomato ☛ Vitamin K = 7.2 mcg; Serving size: 1 pita sandwich, 207 g

Fast Food Biscuit ☛ Vitamin K = 2.5 mcg; Serving size: 1 biscuit, 55 g

Fast Food—Pizza Chain 14 Inch Pizza Cheese Topping Stuffed Crust ☛ Vitamin K = 9.7 mcg; Serving size: 1 slice 1/8 pizza, 117 g

Fast Food—Pizza Chain 14 Inch Pizza Cheese Topping Thick Crust ☛ Vitamin K = 11.5 mcg; Serving size: 1 slice, 115 g

Fast Food—Pizza Chain 14 Inch Pizza Cheese Topping Thin Crust ☛ Vitamin K = 7.4 mcg; Serving size: 1 slice, 76 g

Fast Food—Pizza Chain 14 Inch Pizza Meat And Vegetable Topping Regular Crust ☛ Vitamin K = 8.4 mcg; Serving size: 1 slice, 136 g

Fast Food—Pizza Chain 14 Inch Pizza Pepperoni Topping Thick Crust ☞ Vitamin K = 13.6 mcg; Serving size: 1 slice, 118 g

Fast Food—Pizza Chain 14 Inch Pizza Pepperoni Topping Thin Crust ☞ Vitamin K = 7.5 mcg; Serving size: 1 slice, 79 g

Fast Food—Pizza Chain 14 Inch Pizza Sausage Topping Thick Crust ☞ Vitamin K = 15 mcg; Serving size: 1 slice, 127 g

Fast Food—Pizza Chain 14 Inch Pizza Sausage Topping Thin Crust ☞ Vitamin K = 8.4 mcg; Serving size: 1 slice, 88 g

Fast Foods—Biscuit With Egg And Sausage ☞ Vitamin K = 7.1 mcg; Serving size: 1 item, 162 g

Fast Foods—Cheeseburger—Double Large Patty; With Condiments Vegetables And Mayonnaise ☞ Vitamin K = 32.7 mcg; Serving size: 1 item, 355 g

Fast Foods—Crispy Chicken Filet Sandwich—With Lettuce And Mayonnaise ☞ Vitamin K = 7 mcg; Serving size: 1 sandwich, 152 g

Fast Foods—Fried Chicken Breast Meat And Skin And Breading ☞ Vitamin K = 0 mcg; Serving size: 1 breast, with skin, 203 g

Fast Foods—Fried Chicken Breast Meat Only Skin And Breading Removed ☞ Vitamin K = 0 mcg; Serving size: 1 breast without skin, 142 g

Fast Foods—Fried Chicken Drumstick Meat And Skin With Breading ☞ Vitamin K = 0 mcg; Serving size: 1 drumstick, with skin, 75 g

Fast Foods—Fried Chicken Thigh Meat And Skin And Breading ☞ Vitamin K = 0 mcg; Serving size: 1 thigh with skin, 136 g

Fast Foods—Fried Chicken Thigh Meat Only Skin And Breading Removed ☞ Vitamin K = 0 mcg; Serving size: 1 thigh without skin, 84 g

Fast Foods—Fried Chicken Wing Meat And Skin And Breading ☞ Vitamin K = 0 mcg; Serving size: 1 wing, with skin, 58 g

Fast Foods—Fried Chicken Wing Meat Only Skin And Breading Removed ☞ Vitamin K = 0 mcg; Serving size: 1 wing without skin, 37 g

Fast Foods—Grilled Chicken Filet Sandwich—With Lettuce Tomato And Spread ☞ Vitamin K = 15.4 mcg; Serving size: 1 sandwich, 230 g

Fish Sandwich—With Tartar Sauce ☞ Vitamin K = 29.9 mcg; Serving size: 1 sandwich, 220 g

Fish Sandwich—With Tartar Sauce And Cheese ☞ Vitamin K = 10.6 mcg; Serving size: 1 sandwich, 134 g

Frankfurter Or Hot Dog Sandwich—Beef And Pork Plain On Multi-grain Bread ☞ Vitamin K = 0.6 mcg; Serving size: 1 frankfurter on bread, 93 g

Frankfurter Or Hot Dog Sandwich—Beef And Pork Plain On Multi-grain Bun ☞ Vitamin K = 1.5 mcg; Serving size: 1 frankfurter on bun, 102 g

Frankfurter Or Hot Dog Sandwich—Beef And Pork Plain On Wheat Bread ☞ Vitamin K = 1.5 mcg; Serving size: 1 frankfurter on bread, 85 g

Frankfurter Or Hot Dog Sandwich—Beef And Pork Plain On Wheat Bun ☞ Vitamin K = 3.3 mcg; Serving size: 1 frankfurter on bun, 102 g

Frankfurter Or Hot Dog Sandwich—Beef And Pork Plain On White Bread ☞ Vitamin K = 0.1 mcg; Serving size: 1 frankfurter on bread, 85 g

Frankfurter Or Hot Dog Sandwich—Beef And Pork Plain On White Bun ☞ Vitamin K = 2.3 mcg; Serving size: 1 frankfurter on bun, 102 g

Frankfurter Or Hot Dog Sandwich—Beef And Pork Plain On Whole Grain White Bread ☞ Vitamin K = 3 mcg; Serving size: 1 frankfurter on bread, 93 g

Frankfurter Or Hot Dog Sandwich—Beef And Pork Plain On Whole

Grain White Bun ☞ Vitamin K = 2.4 mcg; Serving size: 1 frankfurter on bun, 102 g

Frankfurter Or Hot Dog Sandwich—Beef And Pork Plain On Whole Wheat Bread ☞ Vitamin K = 3 mcg; Serving size: 1 frankfurter on bread, 93 g

Frankfurter Or Hot Dog Sandwich—Beef And Pork Plain On Whole Wheat Bun ☞ Vitamin K = 2.1 mcg; Serving size: 1 frankfurter on bun, 102 g

Frankfurter Or Hot Dog Sandwich—Beef Plain On Multigrain Bread ☞ Vitamin K = 1.6 mcg; Serving size: 1 frankfurter on bread, 93 g

Frankfurter Or Hot Dog Sandwich—Beef Plain On Multigrain Bun ☞ Vitamin K = 2.4 mcg; Serving size: 1 frankfurter on bun, 102 g

Frankfurter Or Hot Dog Sandwich—Beef Plain On Wheat Bread ☞ Vitamin K = 2.5 mcg; Serving size: 1 frankfurter on bread, 85 g

Frankfurter Or Hot Dog Sandwich—Beef Plain On Wheat Bun ☞ Vitamin K = 4.2 mcg; Serving size: 1 frankfurter on bun, 102 g

Frankfurter Or Hot Dog Sandwich—Beef Plain On White Bread ☞ Vitamin K = 1.1 mcg; Serving size: 1 frankfurter on bread, 85 g

Frankfurter Or Hot Dog Sandwich—Beef Plain On White Bun ☞ Vitamin K = 3.3 mcg; Serving size: 1 frankfurter on bun, 102 g

Frankfurter Or Hot Dog Sandwich—Beef Plain On Whole Grain White Bread ☞ Vitamin K = 3.8 mcg; Serving size: 1 frankfurter on bread, 93 g

Frankfurter Or Hot Dog Sandwich—Beef Plain On Whole Grain White Bun ☞ Vitamin K = 3.4 mcg; Serving size: 1 frankfurter on bun, 102 g

Frankfurter Or Hot Dog Sandwich—Beef Plain On Whole Wheat Bread ☞ Vitamin K = 3.9 mcg; Serving size: 1 frankfurter on bread, 93 g

Frankfurter Or Hot Dog Sandwich—Beef Plain On Whole Wheat Bun ☞ Vitamin K = 3.1 mcg; Serving size: 1 frankfurter on bun, 102 g

Frankfurter Or Hot Dog Sandwich—Chicken And/or Turkey Plain On Multigrain Bread ☞ Vitamin K = 0.5 mcg; Serving size: 1 frankfurter on bread, 93 g

Frankfurter Or Hot Dog Sandwich—Chicken And/or Turkey Plain On Multigrain Bun ☞ Vitamin K = 1.4 mcg; Serving size: 1 frankfurter on bun, 102 g

Frankfurter Or Hot Dog Sandwich—Chicken And/or Turkey Plain On Wheat Bread ☞ Vitamin K = 1.4 mcg; Serving size: 1 frankfurter on bread, 85 g

Frankfurter Or Hot Dog Sandwich—Chicken And/or Turkey Plain On Wheat Bun ☞ Vitamin K = 3.1 mcg; Serving size: 1 frankfurter on bun, 102 g

Frankfurter Or Hot Dog Sandwich—Chicken And/or Turkey Plain On White Bread ☞ Vitamin K = 0.1 mcg; Serving size: 1 frankfurter on bread, 85 g

Frankfurter Or Hot Dog Sandwich—Chicken And/or Turkey Plain On White Bun ☞ Vitamin K = 2.1 mcg; Serving size: 1 frankfurter on bun, 102 g

Frankfurter Or Hot Dog Sandwich—Chicken And/or Turkey Plain On Whole Grain White Bread ☞ Vitamin K = 2.8 mcg; Serving size: 1 frankfurter on bread, 93 g

Frankfurter Or Hot Dog Sandwich—Chicken And/or Turkey Plain On Whole Grain White Bun ☞ Vitamin K = 2.2 mcg; Serving size: 1 frankfurter on bun, 102 g

Frankfurter Or Hot Dog Sandwich—Chicken And/or Turkey Plain On Whole Wheat Bread ☞ Vitamin K = 2.8 mcg; Serving size: 1 frankfurter on bread, 93 g

Frankfurter Or Hot Dog Sandwich—Chicken And/or Turkey Plain

On Whole Wheat Bun 🖙 Vitamin K = 2 mcg; Serving size: 1 frankfurter on bun, 102 g

Frankfurter Or Hot Dog Sandwich—Fat-free Plain On Multigrain Bread 🖙 Vitamin K = 1.6 mcg; Serving size: 1 frankfurter on bread, 93 g

Frankfurter Or Hot Dog Sandwich—Fat-free Plain On Multigrain Bun 🖙 Vitamin K = 2.4 mcg; Serving size: 1 frankfurter on bun, 102 g

Frankfurter Or Hot Dog Sandwich—Fat-free Plain On Wheat Bread 🖙 Vitamin K = 2.5 mcg; Serving size: 1 frankfurter on bread, 85 g

Frankfurter Or Hot Dog Sandwich—Fat-free Plain On Wheat Bun 🖙 Vitamin K = 4.2 mcg; Serving size: 1 frankfurter on bun, 102 g

Frankfurter Or Hot Dog Sandwich—Fat-free Plain On White Bread 🖙 Vitamin K = 1.1 mcg; Serving size: 1 frankfurter on bread, 85 g

Frankfurter Or Hot Dog Sandwich—Fat-free Plain On White Bun 🖙 Vitamin K = 3.3 mcg; Serving size: 1 frankfurter on bun, 102 g

Frankfurter Or Hot Dog Sandwich—Fat-free Plain On Whole Grain White Bread 🖙 Vitamin K = 3.8 mcg; Serving size: 1 frankfurter on bread, 93 g

Frankfurter Or Hot Dog Sandwich—Fat-free Plain On Whole Grain White Bun 🖙 Vitamin K = 3.4 mcg; Serving size: 1 frankfurter on bun, 102 g

Frankfurter Or Hot Dog Sandwich—Fat-free Plain On Whole Wheat Bread 🖙 Vitamin K = 3.9 mcg; Serving size: 1 frankfurter on bread, 93 g

Frankfurter Or Hot Dog Sandwich—Fat-free Plain On Whole Wheat Bun 🖙 Vitamin K = 3.1 mcg; Serving size: 1 frankfurter on bun, 102 g

Frankfurter Or Hot Dog Sandwich—Meat And Poultry Plain On Multigrain Bread 🖙 Vitamin K = 0.6 mcg; Serving size: 1 frankfurter on bread, 93 g

Frankfurter Or Hot Dog Sandwich—Meat And Poultry Plain On Multigrain Bun ☞ Vitamin K = 1.4 mcg; Serving size: 1 frankfurter on bun, 102 g

Frankfurter Or Hot Dog Sandwich—Meat And Poultry Plain On Wheat Bread ☞ Vitamin K = 1.4 mcg; Serving size: 1 frankfurter on bread, 85 g

Frankfurter Or Hot Dog Sandwich—Meat And Poultry Plain On Wheat Bun ☞ Vitamin K = 3.2 mcg; Serving size: 1 frankfurter on bun, 102 g

Frankfurter Or Hot Dog Sandwich—Meat And Poultry Plain On White Bread ☞ Vitamin K = 0.1 mcg; Serving size: 1 frankfurter on bread, 85 g

Frankfurter Or Hot Dog Sandwich—Meat And Poultry Plain On White Bun ☞ Vitamin K = 2.2 mcg; Serving size: 1 frankfurter on bun, 102 g

Frankfurter Or Hot Dog Sandwich—Meat And Poultry Plain On Whole Grain White Bread ☞ Vitamin K = 2.8 mcg; Serving size: 1 frankfurter on bread, 93 g

Frankfurter Or Hot Dog Sandwich—Meat And Poultry Plain On Whole Grain White Bun ☞ Vitamin K = 2.3 mcg; Serving size: 1 frankfurter on bun, 102 g

Frankfurter Or Hot Dog Sandwich—Meat And Poultry Plain On Whole Wheat Bread ☞ Vitamin K = 2.9 mcg; Serving size: 1 frankfurter on bread, 93 g

Frankfurter Or Hot Dog Sandwich—Meat And Poultry Plain On Whole Wheat Bun ☞ Vitamin K = 2 mcg; Serving size: 1 frankfurter on bun, 102 g

Frankfurter Or Hot Dog Sandwich—Meatless On Bread With Meatless Chili ☞ Vitamin K = 1.3 mcg; Serving size: 1 frankfurter on bread, 162 g

Frankfurter Or Hot Dog Sandwich—Meatless On Bun With Meatless Chili ☞ Vitamin K = 3.4 mcg; Serving size: 1 frankfurter on bun, 179 g

Frankfurter Or Hot Dog Sandwich—Meatless Plain On Bread ☞ Vitamin K = 0.1 mcg; Serving size: 1 frankfurter on bread, 98 g

Frankfurter Or Hot Dog Sandwich—Meatless Plain On Bun ☞ Vitamin K = 2.2 mcg; Serving size: 1 frankfurter on bun, 115 g

Frankfurter Or Hot Dog Sandwich—NFS Plain On Multigrain Bun ☞ Vitamin K = 2.4 mcg; Serving size: 1 frankfurter on bun, 102 g

Frankfurter Or Hot Dog Sandwich—NFS Plain On Wheat Bread ☞ Vitamin K = 2.5 mcg; Serving size: 1 frankfurter on bread, 85 g

Frankfurter Or Hot Dog Sandwich—NFS Plain On Wheat Bun ☞ Vitamin K = 4.2 mcg; Serving size: 1 frankfurter on bun, 102 g

Frankfurter Or Hot Dog Sandwich—NFS Plain On White Bread ☞ Vitamin K = 1.1 mcg; Serving size: 1 frankfurter on bread, 85 g

Frankfurter Or Hot Dog Sandwich—NFS Plain On White Bun ☞ Vitamin K = 3.3 mcg; Serving size: 1 frankfurter on bun, 102 g

Frankfurter Or Hot Dog Sandwich—NFS Plain On Whole Grain White Bread ☞ Vitamin K = 3.8 mcg; Serving size: 1 frankfurter on bread, 93 g

Frankfurter Or Hot Dog Sandwich—NFS Plain On Whole Grain White Bun ☞ Vitamin K = 3.4 mcg; Serving size: 1 frankfurter on bun, 102 g

Frankfurter Or Hot Dog Sandwich—NFS Plain On Whole Wheat Bread ☞ Vitamin K = 3.9 mcg; Serving size: 1 frankfurter on bread, 93 g

Frankfurter Or Hot Dog Sandwich—NFS Plain On Whole Wheat Bun ☞ Vitamin K = 3.1 mcg; Serving size: 1 frankfurter on bun, 102 g

Frankfurter Or Hot Dog Sandwich—Reduced-Fat Or Light Plain On

Multigrain Bread ☛ Vitamin K = 0.7 mcg; Serving size: 1 frankfurter on bread, 93 g

Frankfurter Or Hot Dog Sandwich—Reduced-Fat Or Light Plain On Multigrain Bun ☛ Vitamin K = 1.5 mcg; Serving size: 1 frankfurter on bun, 102 g

Frankfurter Or Hot Dog Sandwich—Reduced-Fat Or Light Plain On Wheat Bread ☛ Vitamin K = 1.5 mcg; Serving size: 1 frankfurter on bread, 85 g

Frankfurter Or Hot Dog Sandwich—Reduced-Fat Or Light Plain On Wheat Bun ☛ Vitamin K = 3.3 mcg; Serving size: 1 frankfurter on bun, 102 g

Frankfurter Or Hot Dog Sandwich—Reduced-Fat Or Light Plain On White Bread ☛ Vitamin K = 0.3 mcg; Serving size: 1 frankfurter on bread, 85 g

Frankfurter Or Hot Dog Sandwich—Reduced-Fat Or Light Plain On White Bun ☛ Vitamin K = 2.3 mcg; Serving size: 1 frankfurter on bun, 102 g

Frankfurter Or Hot Dog Sandwich—Reduced-Fat Or Light Plain On Whole Grain White Bread ☛ Vitamin K = 3 mcg; Serving size: 1 frankfurter on bread, 93 g

Frankfurter Or Hot Dog Sandwich—Reduced-Fat Or Light Plain On Whole Grain White Bun ☛ Vitamin K = 2.4 mcg; Serving size: 1 frankfurter on bun, 102 g

Frankfurter Or Hot Dog Sandwich—Reduced-Fat Or Light Plain On Whole Wheat Bread ☛ Vitamin K = 3 mcg; Serving size: 1 frankfurter on bread, 93 g

Frankfurter Or Hot Dog Sandwich—Reduced-Fat Or Light Plain On Whole Wheat Bun ☛ Vitamin K = 2.2 mcg; Serving size: 1 frankfurter on bun, 102 g

Frankfurter Or Hot Dog Sandwich—With Chili On Multigrain Bread ☞ Vitamin K = 4.6 mcg; Serving size: 1 frankfurter on bread, 157 g

Frankfurter Or Hot Dog Sandwich—With Chili On Multigrain Bun ☞ Vitamin K = 5.5 mcg; Serving size: 1 frankfurter on bun, 166 g

Frankfurter Or Hot Dog Sandwich—With Chili On Wheat Bread ☞ Vitamin K = 5.4 mcg; Serving size: 1 frankfurter on bread, 149 g

Frankfurter Or Hot Dog Sandwich—With Chili On Wheat Bun ☞ Vitamin K = 7.1 mcg; Serving size: 1 frankfurter on bun, 166 g

Frankfurter Or Hot Dog Sandwich—With Chili On White Bread ☞ Vitamin K = 4 mcg; Serving size: 1 frankfurter on bread, 149 g

Frankfurter Or Hot Dog Sandwich—With Chili On White Bun ☞ Vitamin K = 6.1 mcg; Serving size: 1 frankfurter on bun, 166 g

Frankfurter Or Hot Dog Sandwich—With Chili On Whole Grain White Bread ☞ Vitamin K = 6.8 mcg; Serving size: 1 frankfurter on bread, 157 g

Frankfurter Or Hot Dog Sandwich—With Chili On Whole Grain White Bun ☞ Vitamin K = 6.3 mcg; Serving size: 1 frankfurter on bun, 166 g

Frankfurter Or Hot Dog Sandwich—With Chili On Whole Wheat Bread ☞ Vitamin K = 6.9 mcg; Serving size: 1 frankfurter on bread, 157 g

Frankfurter Or Hot Dog Sandwich—With Chili On Whole Wheat Bun ☞ Vitamin K = 7.1 mcg; Serving size: 1 frankfurter on bun, 166 g

Frankfurter Or Hot Dog Sandwich—With Meatless Chili On Multigrain Bread ☞ Vitamin K = 2.8 mcg; Serving size: 1 frankfurter on bread, 157 g

Frankfurter Or Hot Dog Sandwich—With Meatless Chili On Multigrain Bun ☞ Vitamin K = 3.7 mcg; Serving size: 1 frankfurter on bun, 166 g

Frankfurter Or Hot Dog Sandwich—With Meatless Chili On Wheat Bread ☛ Vitamin K = 3.7 mcg; Serving size: 1 frankfurter on bread, 149 g

Frankfurter Or Hot Dog Sandwich—With Meatless Chili On Wheat Bun ☛ Vitamin K = 5.3 mcg; Serving size: 1 frankfurter on bun, 166 g

Frankfurter Or Hot Dog Sandwich—With Meatless Chili On White Bread ☛ Vitamin K = 2.4 mcg; Serving size: 1 frankfurter on bread, 149 g

Frankfurter Or Hot Dog Sandwich—With Meatless Chili On White Bun ☛ Vitamin K = 4.5 mcg; Serving size: 1 frankfurter on bun, 166 g

Frankfurter Or Hot Dog Sandwich—With Meatless Chili On Whole Grain White Bread ☛ Vitamin K = 5 mcg; Serving size: 1 frankfurter on bread, 157 g

Frankfurter Or Hot Dog Sandwich—With Meatless Chili On Whole Grain White Bun ☛ Vitamin K = 4.5 mcg; Serving size: 1 frankfurter on bun, 166 g

Frankfurter Or Hot Dog Sandwich—With Meatless Chili On Whole Wheat Bread ☛ Vitamin K = 6.9 mcg; Serving size: 1 frankfurter on bread, 157 g

Frankfurter Or Hot Dog Sandwich—With Meatless Chili On Whole Wheat Bun ☛ Vitamin K = 4.3 mcg; Serving size: 1 frankfurter on bun, 166 g

French Toast—From School Nfs ☛ Vitamin K = 0.4 mcg; Serving size: 1 bite size, 10 g

French Toast—Gluten-Free ☛ Vitamin K = 3.3 mcg; Serving size: 1 slice, any size, 65 g

French Toast—Gluten-Free From Frozen ☛ Vitamin K = 0 mcg; Serving size: 1 bite size, 10 g

French Toast—Nfs ☛ Vitamin K = 3.3 mcg; Serving size: 1 slice, any size, 65 g

French Toast—Plain ☛ Vitamin K = 3.3 mcg; Serving size: 1 slice, any size, 65 g

French Toast—Plain From Fast Food / Restaurant ☛ Vitamin K = 5.8 mcg; Serving size: 1 slice, any size, 85 g

French Toast—Plain From Frozen ☛ Vitamin K = 0 mcg; Serving size: 1 bite size, 10 g

French Toast—Plain Reduced-Fat ☛ Vitamin K = 0.2 mcg; Serving size: 1 slice, any size, 65 g

French Toast—Sticks ☛ Vitamin K = 9.4 mcg; Serving size: 3 pieces, 65 g

French Toast—Sticks From School Nfs ☛ Vitamin K = 1 mcg; Serving size: 1 stick, 25 g

French Toast—Sticks Nfs ☛ Vitamin K = 2.1 mcg; Serving size: 1 stick, 25 g

French Toast—Sticks Plain From Fast Food / Restaurant ☛ Vitamin K = 4.3 mcg; Serving size: 1 stick, 25 g

French Toast—Sticks Plain From Frozen ☛ Vitamin K = 3.8 mcg; Serving size: 1 stick, 45 g

French Toast—Sticks Whole Grain ☛ Vitamin K = 3.5 mcg; Serving size: 1 stick, 45 g

French Toast—Whole Grain ☛ Vitamin K = 5 mcg; Serving size: 1 slice, any size, 65 g

French Toast—Whole Grain From Fast Food / Restaurant ☛ Vitamin K = 8.3 mcg; Serving size: 1 slice, any size, 85 g

French Toast—Whole Grain From Frozen ☛ Vitamin K = 0.3 mcg; Serving size: 1 bite size, 10 g

French Toast—Whole Grain Reduced-Fat ☞ Vitamin K = 2 mcg; Serving size: 1 slice, any size, 65 g

Fried Bread Puerto Rican Style ☞ Vitamin K = 7.8 mcg; Serving size: 2 fritters with syrup (4" x 2-1/2" x 3-1/4"), 110 g

Fried Egg Sandwich ☞ Vitamin K = 2.5 mcg; Serving size: 1 sandwich, 96 g

Griddle Cake Sandwich—Egg Cheese And Bacon ☞ Vitamin K = 3.5 mcg; Serving size: 1 item 6.1 oz, 174 g

Griddle Cake Sandwich—Egg Cheese And Sausage ☞ Vitamin K = 3.6 mcg; Serving size: 1 item, 199 g

Griddle Cake Sandwich—Sausage ☞ Vitamin K = 1.4 mcg; Serving size: 1 item, 135 g

Grilled Chicken Bacon And Tomato Club Sandwich—With Cheese Lettuce And Mayonnaise ☞ Vitamin K = 23.3 mcg; Serving size: 1 sandwich, 268 g

Gyro Sandwich—(Pita Bread Beef Lamb Onion Condiments) With Tomato And Spread ☞ Vitamin K = 14.8 mcg; Serving size: 1 gyro, 390 g

Ham And Cheese On English Muffin ☞ Vitamin K = 0.7 mcg; Serving size: 1 jimmy dean sandwich, 57 g

Ham And Cheese Sandwich—On Bun With Lettuce And Spread ☞ Vitamin K = 16 mcg; Serving size: 1 sandwich, 154 g

Ham And Cheese Sandwich—With Lettuce And Spread ☞ Vitamin K = 10.9 mcg; Serving size: 1 sandwich, 155 g

Ham And Cheese Sandwich—With Spread Grilled ☞ Vitamin K = 10.2 mcg; Serving size: 1 sandwich, 141 g

Ham And Egg Sandwich ☞ Vitamin K = 2.6 mcg; Serving size: 1 sandwich, 124 g

Ham And Tomato Club Sandwich—With Lettuce And Spread ☛ Vitamin K = 44.2 mcg; Serving size: 1 sandwich, 254 g

Ham Salad Sandwich ☛ Vitamin K = 28.5 mcg; Serving size: 1 sandwich, 141 g

Ham Sandwich—With Lettuce And Spread ☛ Vitamin K = 9.9 mcg; Serving size: 1 sandwich, 127 g

Ham Sandwich—With Spread ☛ Vitamin K = 10.6 mcg; Serving size: 1 sandwich, 112 g

Hamburger 1 Medium Patty Plain On Wheat Bun ☛ Vitamin K = 4.9 mcg; Serving size: 1 hamburger, 145 g

Hamburger 1 Medium Patty Plain On White Bun ☛ Vitamin K = 4.5 mcg; Serving size: 1 hamburger, 145 g

Hamburger 1 Medium Patty Plain On Whole Wheat Bun ☛ Vitamin K = 4.9 mcg; Serving size: 1 hamburger, 145 g

Hamburger 1 Medium Patty With Condiments On Wheat Bun ☛ Vitamin K = 18.4 mcg; Serving size: 1 hamburger, 200 g

Hamburger 1 Medium Patty With Condiments On White Bun ☛ Vitamin K = 18 mcg; Serving size: 1 hamburger, 200 g

Hamburger 1 Medium Patty With Condiments On Whole Wheat Bun ☛ Vitamin K = 18.4 mcg; Serving size: 1 hamburger, 200 g

Hamburger 1 Miniature Patty On Miniature Bun From School ☛ Vitamin K = 2.5 mcg; Serving size: 1 miniature hamburger, 50 g

Hamburger 1 Miniature Patty Plain On Miniature Bun From Fast Food / Restaurant ☛ Vitamin K = 1.9 mcg; Serving size: 1 miniature hamburger, 50 g

Hamburger 1 Miniature Patty With Condiments On Miniature Bun From Fast Food / Restaurant ☛ Vitamin K = 7.3 mcg; Serving size: 1 miniature hamburger, 65 g

Hamburger 1 Small Patty Plain On Wheat Bun ☞ Vitamin K = 4 mcg; Serving size: 1 hamburger, 115 g

Hamburger 1 Small Patty Plain On White Bun ☞ Vitamin K = 3.7 mcg; Serving size: 1 hamburger, 115 g

Hamburger 1 Small Patty Plain On Whole Wheat Bun ☞ Vitamin K = 4 mcg; Serving size: 1 hamburger, 115 g

Hamburger 1 Small Patty With Condiments On Bun From Fast Food / Restaurant (Burger King—Whopper Jr.) ☞ Vitamin K = 17.1 mcg; Serving size: 1 burger king whopper jr, 150 g

Hamburger 1 Small Patty With Condiments On White Bun ☞ Vitamin K = 17.5 mcg; Serving size: 1 hamburger, 175 g

Hamburger 1 Small Patty With Condiments On Whole Wheat Bun ☞ Vitamin K = 17.9 mcg; Serving size: 1 hamburger, 175 g

Hamburger Large Single Patty With Condiments ☞ Vitamin K = 8.6 mcg; Serving size: 1 item, 171 g

Hamburger Nfs ☞ Vitamin K = 18 mcg; Serving size: 1 hamburger, 200 g

Hamburger On Bun From School ☞ Vitamin K = 4.7 mcg; Serving size: 1 hamburger, 95 g

Hamburger—Double Large Patty; With Condiments Vegetables And Mayonnaise ☞ Vitamin K = 52.7 mcg; Serving size: 1 item, 374 g

Hamburger—Single Large Patty; With Condiments Vegetables And Mayonnaise ☞ Vitamin K = 35.3 mcg; Serving size: 1 item, 247 g

Hamburger—Single Regular Patty; Plain ☞ Vitamin K = 3.8 mcg; Serving size: 1 sandwich, 78 g

Hamburger—Single Regular Patty; With Condiments ☞ Vitamin K = 4.8 mcg; Serving size: 1 sandwich, 97 g

Hors D'oeuvres With Spread ☞ Vitamin K = 0.9 mcg; Serving size: 1 hors d'oeuvre, 23 g

Hot Ham And Cheese Sandwich—On Bun ☞ Vitamin K = 23.3 mcg; Serving size: 1 sandwich, 162 g

Hush Puppies ☞ Vitamin K = 0.7 mcg; Serving size: 1 piece, 22 g

KFC—Coleslaw ☞ Vitamin K = 79.4 mcg; Serving size: 1 package, 112 g

KFC—Crispy Chicken Strips ☞ Vitamin K = 4.4 mcg; Serving size: 1 strip, 47 g

KFC—Popcorn Chicken ☞ Vitamin K = 1.1 mcg; Serving size: 1 piece, 6.4 g

Little Caesar's—14 Inch Cheese Pizza Large Deep Dish Crust ☞ Vitamin K = 6.9 mcg; Serving size: 1 slice, 102 g

Little Caesar's—14 Inch Cheese Pizza Thin Crust ☞ Vitamin K = 4.6 mcg; Serving size: 1 slice, 48 g

Little Caesar's—14 Inch Original Round Cheese Pizza Regular Crust ☞ Vitamin K = 5.3 mcg; Serving size: 1 slice, 89 g

Little Caesar's—14 Inch Original Round Meat And Vegetable Pizza Regular Crust ☞ Vitamin K = 6.6 mcg; Serving size: 1 slice, 115 g

Little Caesar's—14 Inch Original Round Pepperoni Pizza Regular Crust ☞ Vitamin K = 5.3 mcg; Serving size: 1 slice, 90 g

Little Caesar's—14 Inch Pepperoni Pizza Large Deep Dish Crust ☞ Vitamin K = 7.4 mcg; Serving size: 1 slice, 104 g

McDonald's—Filet-O-Fish ☞ Vitamin K = 6.6 mcg; Serving size: 1 sandwich, 134 g

McDonald's—French Fries ☞ Vitamin K = 11.4 mcg; Serving size: 1 small serving, 71 g

McDonald's—Southern Style Chicken Biscuit ☞ Vitamin K = 8.7 mcg; Serving size: 1 biscuit regular size biscuit, 132 g

Meat Sandwich—Nfs ☛ Vitamin K = 7.1 mcg; Serving size: 1 sandwich, 83 g

Meat Spread Or Potted Meat Sandwich ☛ Vitamin K = 1 mcg; Serving size: 1 sandwich, 107 g

Midnight Sandwich—With Spread ☛ Vitamin K = 17.1 mcg; Serving size: 1 sandwich, 201 g

Miniature Cinnamon Rolls ☛ Vitamin K = 3.5 mcg; Serving size: 1 each, 25 g

Nachos—With Cheese ☛ Vitamin K = 15.4 mcg; Serving size: 1 serving, 80 g

Nachos—With Cheese Beans Ground Beef And Tomatoes ☛ Vitamin K = 12 mcg; Serving size: 1 serving, 222 g

Onion Rings Breaded And Fried ☛ Vitamin K = 65.3 mcg; Serving size: 1 package (18 onion rings), 117 g

Pancakes—Buckwheat ☛ Vitamin K = 1.1 mcg; Serving size: 1 miniature/bite size pancake, 10 g

Pancakes—Cornmeal ☛ Vitamin K = 0.5 mcg; Serving size: 1 miniature/bite size pancake, 10 g

Pancakes—From School Nfs ☛ Vitamin K = 0.6 mcg; Serving size: 1 miniature/bite size pancake, 10 g

Pancakes—Nfs ☛ Vitamin K = 1 mcg; Serving size: 1 miniature/bite size pancake, 10 g

Pancakes—Plain ☛ Vitamin K = 1 mcg; Serving size: 1 miniature/bite size pancake, 10 g

Pancakes—Plain From Fast Food / Restaurant ☛ Vitamin K = 1.4 mcg; Serving size: 1 miniature/bite size pancake, 10 g

Pancakes—Plain Reduced-Fat From Fozen ☛ Vitamin K = 0.7 mcg; Serving size: 1 miniature/bite size pancake, 10 g

Pancakes—Pumpkin ☛ Vitamin K = 1.1 mcg; Serving size: 1 miniature/bite size pancake, 10 g

Pancakes—Whole Grain ☛ Vitamin K = 1 mcg; Serving size: 1 miniature/bite size pancake, 10 g

Pancakes—Whole Grain And Nuts From Fast Food / Restaurant ☛ Vitamin K = 1.3 mcg; Serving size: 1 miniature/bite size pancake, 10 g

Pancakes—Whole Grain From Fast Food / Restaurant ☛ Vitamin K = 1.4 mcg; Serving size: 1 miniature/bite size pancake, 10 g

Pancakes—Whole Grain From Frozen ☛ Vitamin K = 0.6 mcg; Serving size: 1 miniature/bite size pancake, 10 g

Pancakes—Whole Grain Reduced-Fat ☛ Vitamin K = 0.7 mcg; Serving size: 1 miniature/bite size pancake, 10 g

Pancakes—Whole Grain Reduced-Fat From Frozen ☛ Vitamin K = 0.6 mcg; Serving size: 1 miniature/bite size pancake, 10 g

Pancakes—With Chocolate ☛ Vitamin K = 0.9 mcg; Serving size: 1 miniature/bite size pancake, 10 g

Pancakes—With Chocolate From Fast Food / Restaurant ☛ Vitamin K = 1.3 mcg; Serving size: 1 miniature/bite size pancake, 10 g

Pancakes—With Chocolate From Frozen ☛ Vitamin K = 0.7 mcg; Serving size: 1 miniature/bite size pancake, 10 g

Pancakes—With Fruit ☛ Vitamin K = 1.2 mcg; Serving size: 1 miniature/bite size pancake, 10 g

Pancakes—With Fruit From Fast Food / Restaurant ☛ Vitamin K = 1.5 mcg; Serving size: 1 miniature/bite size pancake, 10 g

Pancakes—With Fruit From Frozen ☛ Vitamin K = 0.7 mcg; Serving size: 1 miniature/bite size pancake, 10 g

Papa John's—14 Inch Cheese Pizza Original Crust ☛ Vitamin K = 8.8 mcg; Serving size: 1 slice, 117 g

Papa John's—14 Inch Cheese Pizza Thin Crust ☛ Vitamin K = 4.9 mcg; Serving size: 1 slice, 87 g

Papa John's—14 Inch Pepperoni Pizza Original Crust ☛ Vitamin K = 7.5 mcg; Serving size: 1 slice, 123 g

Papa John's—14 Inch The Works Pizza Original Crust ☛ Vitamin K = 8.6 mcg; Serving size: 1 slice, 153 g

Pastrami Sandwich ☛ Vitamin K = 13.7 mcg; Serving size: 1 sandwich, 134 g

Pepperoni And Salami Submarine Sandwich—With Lettuce Tomato And Spread ☛ Vitamin K = 44.2 mcg; Serving size: 1 submarine, 240 g

Pepperoni Pizza ☛ Vitamin K = 7.1 mcg; Serving size: 1 slice, 111 g

Pig In A Blanket Frankfurter Or Hot Dog Wrapped In Dough ☛ Vitamin K = 4.1 mcg; Serving size: 1 pig in blanket, 85 g

Pizza Cheese Topping Regular Crust Frozen Cooked ☛ Vitamin K = 5.3 mcg; Serving size: 1 serving= 9 serving per 24 oz package, 81 g

Pizza Cheese Topping Rising Crust Frozen Cooked ☛ Vitamin K = 10.4 mcg; Serving size: 1 serving= 6 serving per 29.25 oz package, 139 g

Pizza Cheese Topping Thin Crust Frozen Cooked ☛ Vitamin K = 2.9 mcg; Serving size: 1 slice, 69 g

Pizza Hut—12 Inch Cheese Pizza Hand-Tossed Crust ☛ Vitamin K = 9.7 mcg; Serving size: 1 slice, 96 g

Pizza Hut—12 Inch Cheese Pizza Pan Crust ☛ Vitamin K = 15.5 mcg; Serving size: 1 slice, 100 g

Pizza Hut—12 Inch Cheese Pizza Thin N Crispy Crust ☛ Vitamin K = 5.7 mcg; Serving size: 1 slice, 69 g

Pizza Hut—12 Inch Pepperoni Pizza Hand-Tossed Crust ☛ Vitamin K = 8.2 mcg; Serving size: 1 slice, 96 g

Pizza Hut—12 Inch Pepperoni Pizza Pan Crust ☛ Vitamin K = 18.5

mcg; Serving size: 1 slice, 96 g

Pizza Hut—12 Inch Super Supreme Pizza Hand-Tossed Crust ☞ Vitamin K = 9.3 mcg; Serving size: 1 slice, 127 g

Pizza Hut—14 Inch Cheese Pizza Hand-Tossed Crust ☞ Vitamin K = 8.1 mcg; Serving size: 1 slice, 105 g

Pizza Hut—14 Inch Cheese Pizza Pan Crust ☞ Vitamin K = 19 mcg; Serving size: 1 slice, 112 g

Pizza Hut—14 Inch Cheese Pizza Thin N Crispy Crust ☞ Vitamin K = 6.1 mcg; Serving size: 1 slice, 79 g

Pizza Hut—14 Inch Pepperoni Pizza Hand-Tossed Crust ☞ Vitamin K = 9.4 mcg; Serving size: 1 slice, 110 g

Pizza Hut—14 Inch Pepperoni Pizza Pan Crust ☞ Vitamin K = 24.3 mcg; Serving size: 1 slice, 113 g

Pizza Hut—14 Inch Super Supreme Pizza Hand-Tossed Crust ☞ Vitamin K = 10 mcg; Serving size: 1 slice, 123 g

Pizza Hut—Breadstick—Parmesan Garlic ☞ Vitamin K = 9.1 mcg; Serving size: 1 breadstick, 43 g

Pizza Meat And Vegetable Topping Regular Crust Frozen Cooked ☞ Vitamin K = 11.7 mcg; Serving size: 1 serving 5 servings per 24.2 oz package, 143 g

Pizza Meat And Vegetable Topping Rising Crust Frozen Cooked ☞ Vitamin K = 11.4 mcg; Serving size: 1 serving 6 servings per 34.98 oz package, 170 g

Pizza Meat Topping Thick Crust Frozen Cooked ☞ Vitamin K = 7.8 mcg; Serving size: 1 slice 1/8 of 12 inch pizza, 103 g

Pizza Pepperoni Topping Regular Crust Frozen Cooked ☞ Vitamin K = 9 mcg; Serving size: 1/4 pizza 12 inch diameter, 127 g

Pork Barbecue Sandwich—Or Sloppy Joe On Bun ☞ Vitamin K = 3.7

mcg; Serving size: 1 barbecue sandwich, 186 g

Pork Sandwich ☛ Vitamin K = 0.1 mcg; Serving size: 1 sandwich, 136 g

Pork Sandwich—On White Roll With Onions Dill Pickles And Barbecue Sauce ☛ Vitamin K = 7.4 mcg; Serving size: 1 sandwich, 189 g

Pork Sandwich—With Gravy ☛ Vitamin K = 0.2 mcg; Serving size: 1 sandwich, 218 g

Potato—French Fried In Vegetable Oil ☛ Vitamin K = 8 mcg; Serving size: 1 serving small, 71 g

Potato—French Fries From Fresh Baked ☛ Vitamin K = 0.2 mcg; Serving size: 1 shoestring, 2 g

Potato—French Fries From Fresh Fried ☛ Vitamin K = 0.3 mcg; Serving size: 1 shoestring, 2 g

Potato—French Fries From Frozen Fried ☛ Vitamin K = 0.3 mcg; Serving size: 1 shoestring, 2 g

Potato—French Fries Nfs ☛ Vitamin K = 0.3 mcg; Serving size: 1 shoestring, 2 g

Potato—French Fries School ☛ Vitamin K = 0.2 mcg; Serving size: 1 shoestring, 2 g

Potato—French Fries With Cheese ☛ Vitamin K = 0.9 mcg; Serving size: 1 fry, any cut, 8 g

Potato—French Fries With Cheese Fast Food / Restaurant ☛ Vitamin K = 12.4 mcg; Serving size: 1 kids meal order, 107 g

Potato—French Fries With Cheese School ☛ Vitamin K = 1.2 mcg; Serving size: 1 fry, any cut, 11 g

Potato—French Fries With Chili ☛ Vitamin K = 0.7 mcg; Serving size: 1 fry, any cut, 8 g

Potato—French Fries With Chili And Cheese ☛ Vitamin K = 1 mcg;

Serving size: 1 fry, any cut, 10 g

Potato—French Fries With Chili And Cheese Fast Food / Restaurant ☞ Vitamin K = 1 mcg; Serving size: 1 fry, any cut, 10 g

Potato—French Fries With Chili Fast Food / Restaurant ☞ Vitamin K = 0.7 mcg; Serving size: 1 fry, any cut, 8 g

Potato—Hash Brown From Dry Mix ☞ Vitamin K = 28.6 mcg; Serving size: 1 cup, 160 g

Potato—Hash Brown From Fast Food With Cheese ☞ Vitamin K = 4.7 mcg; Serving size: 1 patty, 55 g

Potato—Hash Brown From Fresh ☞ Vitamin K = 24.6 mcg; Serving size: 1 cup, 160 g

Potato—Hash Brown From Fresh With Cheese ☞ Vitamin K = 21.4 mcg; Serving size: 1 cup, 160 g

Potato—Hash Brown From Restaurant With Cheese ☞ Vitamin K = 4.7 mcg; Serving size: 1 patty, 55 g

Potato—Hash Brown From School Lunch ☞ Vitamin K = 9.9 mcg; Serving size: 1 patty, 55 g

Potato—Hash Brown Nfs ☞ Vitamin K = 9.8 mcg; Serving size: 1 patty, 55 g

Potato—Hash Brown Ready-To-Heat ☞ Vitamin K = 9.8 mcg; Serving size: 1 patty, 55 g

Potato—Hash Brown Ready-To-Heat With Cheese ☞ Vitamin K – 8.5 mcg; Serving size: 1 patty, 55 g

Potato—Home Fries From Fresh ☞ Vitamin K = 29 mcg; Serving size: 1 cup, 200 g

Potato—Home Fries From Restaurant / Fast Food ☞ Vitamin K = 49 mcg; Serving size: 1 cup, 200 g

Potato—Home Fries Nfs ☞ Vitamin K = 32.4 mcg; Serving size: 1 cup,

200 g

Potato—Home Fries Ready-To-Heat ☛ Vitamin K = 32.4 mcg; Serving size: 1 cup, 200 g

Potato—Home Fries With Vegetables ☛ Vitamin K = 31.8 mcg; Serving size: 1 cup, 200 g

Potato—Mashed ☛ Vitamin K = 14.3 mcg; Serving size: 1 cup, 242 g

Potato—Patty ☛ Vitamin K = 5 mcg; Serving size: 1 patty, 55 g

Potato—Skins Nfs ☛ Vitamin K = 2.1 mcg; Serving size: skin from 1 small, 25 g

Potato—Skins With Cheese ☛ Vitamin K = 3 mcg; Serving size: skin from 1 small, 35 g

Potato—Skins With Cheese And Bacon ☛ Vitamin K = 2.8 mcg; Serving size: skin from 1 small, 35 g

Potato—Skins Without Topping ☛ Vitamin K = 2.5 mcg; Serving size: skin from 1 small, 25 g

Potato—Tots Fast Food / Restaurant ☛ Vitamin K = 17 mcg; Serving size: 1 cup, 130 g

Potato—Tots From Fresh Fried Or Baked ☛ Vitamin K = 13.8 mcg; Serving size: 1 cup, 130 g

Potato—Tots Frozen Baked ☛ Vitamin K = 3.4 mcg; Serving size: 1 cup, 130 g

Potato—Tots Frozen Fried ☛ Vitamin K = 13.8 mcg; Serving size: 1 cup, 130 g

Potato—Tots Nfs ☛ Vitamin K = 13.8 mcg; Serving size: 1 cup, 130 g

Potato—Tots School ☛ Vitamin K = 15.2 mcg; Serving size: 1 cup, 130 g

Potatoes Hash Browns Round Pieces Or Patty ☛ Vitamin K = 0.5 mcg; Serving size: 1 round piece, 5.5 g

Puerto Rican Sandwich ☛ Vitamin K = 21.4 mcg; Serving size: 1 sandwich, 160 g

Quesadilla With Chicken ☛ Vitamin K = 4.3 mcg; Serving size: 1 each quesadilla, 180 g

Reuben Sandwich—Corned Beef Sandwich—With Sauerkraut And Cheese With Spread ☛ Vitamin K = 23.7 mcg; Serving size: 1 sandwich, 181 g

Roast Beef Sandwich—Plain ☛ Vitamin K = 4.2 mcg; Serving size: 1 sandwich, 149 g

Roast Beef Sandwich—With Bacon And Cheese Sauce ☛ Vitamin K = 6.3 mcg; Serving size: 1 sandwich, 218 g

Roast Beef Sandwich—With Cheese ☛ Vitamin K = 2.7 mcg; Serving size: 1 sandwich, 190 g

Roast Beef Sandwich—With Gravy ☛ Vitamin K = 1.8 mcg; Serving size: 1 sandwich, 222 g

Roast Beef Submarine Sandwich—On Roll Au Jus ☛ Vitamin K = 4.6 mcg; Serving size: 1 sandwich, 193 g

Roast Beef Submarine Sandwich—With Cheese Lettuce Tomato And Spread ☛ Vitamin K = 30.2 mcg; Serving size: 1 submarine, 260 g

Roast Beef Submarine Sandwich—With Lettuce Tomato And Spread ☛ Vitamin K = 28.8 mcg; Serving size: 1 submarine, 240 g

Salami Sandwich—With Spread ☛ Vitamin K = 7.9 mcg; Serving size: 1 sandwich, 82 g

Sandwich—Nfs ☛ Vitamin K = 7.1 mcg; Serving size: 1 sandwich, 83 g

Sardine Sandwich—With Lettuce And Spread ☛ Vitamin K = 44.1 mcg; Serving size: 1 sandwich, 214 g

Sausage And Spaghetti Sauce Sandwich ☛ Vitamin K = 11.9 mcg; Serving size: 1 sandwich, 189 g

Sausage Pizza ☞ Vitamin K = 7.8 mcg; Serving size: 1 slice, 116 g

Sausage Sandwich ☞ Vitamin K = 0.1 mcg; Serving size: 1 sandwich, 107 g

School Lunch—Chicken Nuggets Whole Grain Breaded ☞ Vitamin K = 9.2 mcg; Serving size: 5 pieces, 88 g

School Lunch—Chicken Patty Whole Grain Breaded ☞ Vitamin K = 4.2 mcg; Serving size: 1 patty, 86 g

School Lunch—Pizza Cheese Topping Thick Crust Whole Grain Frozen Cooked ☞ Vitamin K = 7.2 mcg; Serving size: 1 slice per 1/10 pizza, 124 g

School Lunch—Pizza Cheese Topping Thin Crust Whole Grain Frozen Cooked ☞ Vitamin K = 5.5 mcg; Serving size: 1 piece 4 inchx6 inch, 130 g

School Lunch—Pizza Pepperoni Topping Thick Crust Whole Grain Frozen Cooked ☞ Vitamin K = 13.4 mcg; Serving size: 1 slice per 1/10 pizza, 124 g

School Lunch—Pizza Pepperoni Topping Thin Crust Whole Grain Frozen Cooked ☞ Vitamin K = 6.6 mcg; Serving size: 1 piece 4 inchx6 inch, 127 g

School Lunch—Pizza Sausage Topping Thick Crust Whole Grain Frozen Cooked ☞ Vitamin K = 4.3 mcg; Serving size: 1 slice per 1/10 pizza, 129 g

School Lunch—Pizza Sausage Topping Thin Crust Whole Grain Frozen Cooked ☞ Vitamin K = 7 mcg; Serving size: 1 piece 4 inch x 6 inch, 133 g

Scrambled Egg Sandwich ☞ Vitamin K = 2.5 mcg; Serving size: 1 sandwich, 112 g

Shrimp Breaded And Fried ☞ Vitamin K = 1.8 mcg; Serving size: 3 pieces shrimp, 39 g

Soft Serve Blended With Chocolate Candy ☛ Vitamin K = 2.4 mcg; Serving size: 12 fl oz cup, 348 g

Steak And Cheese Sandwich—Plain On Roll ☛ Vitamin K = 4.8 mcg; Serving size: 1 sandwich, 170 g

Steak And Cheese Submarine Sandwich—Plain On Roll ☛ Vitamin K = 5.9 mcg; Serving size: 1 submarine, 197 g

Steak And Cheese Submarine Sandwich—With Fried Peppers And Onions On Roll ☛ Vitamin K = 11.2 mcg; Serving size: 1 submarine, 260 g

Steak Sandwich—Plain On Biscuit ☛ Vitamin K = 4.5 mcg; Serving size: 1 sandwich, 142 g

Steak Sandwich—Plain On Roll ☛ Vitamin K = 3.6 mcg; Serving size: 1 sandwich, 142 g

Steak Submarine Sandwich—With Lettuce And Tomato ☛ Vitamin K = 9.5 mcg; Serving size: 1 sandwich, 186 g

Submarine Sandwich—Bacon Lettuce And Tomato On White Bread ☛ Vitamin K = 9.5 mcg; Serving size: 6 inch sub, 148 g

Submarine Sandwich—Ham On White Bread With Lettuce And Tomato ☛ Vitamin K = 8.6 mcg; Serving size: 6 inch sub, 184 g

Submarine Sandwich—Meatball Marinara On White Bread ☛ Vitamin K = 13.8 mcg; Serving size: 6 inch sub, 209 g

Submarine Sandwich—Tuna On White Bread With Lettuce And Tomato ☛ Vitamin K = 53.1 mcg; Serving size: 6 inch sub, 237 g

Taco Bell—Bean Burrito ☛ Vitamin K = 7.8 mcg; Serving size: 1 each burrito, 185 g

Taco Bell—Burrito—Supreme With Beef ☛ Vitamin K = 13 mcg; Serving size: 1 burrito, 241 g

Taco Bell—Burrito—Supreme With Chicken ☛ Vitamin K = 13.1 mcg;

Serving size: 1 item, 248 g

Taco Bell—Burrito—Supreme With Steak ☛ Vitamin K = 14.9 mcg; Serving size: 1 item, 248 g

Taco Bell—Nachos ☛ Vitamin K = 6 mcg; Serving size: 1 serving, 80 g

Taco Bell—Nachos—Supreme ☛ Vitamin K = 14.2 mcg; Serving size: 1 serving, 222 g

Taco Bell—Original Taco With Beef Cheese And Lettuce ☛ Vitamin K = 10.6 mcg; Serving size: 1 each taco, 69 g

Taco Bell—Soft Taco With Beef Cheese And Lettuce ☛ Vitamin K = 11.4 mcg; Serving size: 1 each taco, 102 g

Taco Bell—Soft Taco With Chicken Cheese And Lettuce ☛ Vitamin K = 8.5 mcg; Serving size: 1 each taco, 98 g

Taco Bell—Soft Taco With Steak ☛ Vitamin K = 26.4 mcg; Serving size: 1 item, 127 g

Taco Bell—Taco Salad ☛ Vitamin K = 57 mcg; Serving size: 1 item, 533 g

Taco With Beef Cheese And Lettuce Hard Shell ☛ Vitamin K = 10.6 mcg; Serving size: 1 each taco, 69 g

Taco With Beef Cheese And Lettuce Soft ☛ Vitamin K = 7.5 mcg; Serving size: 1 each taco, 102 g

Taco With Chicken Lettuce And Cheese Soft ☛ Vitamin K = 7.7 mcg; Serving size: 1 each taco, 98 g

Taquito Or Flauta With Egg ☛ Vitamin K = 2 mcg; Serving size: 1 small taquito, 36 g

Taquito Or Flauta With Egg And Breakfast Meat ☛ Vitamin K = 1.9 mcg; Serving size: 1 small taquito, 36 g

Tomato Sandwich ☛ Vitamin K = 21.8 mcg; Serving size: 1 sandwich, 134 g

Triple Cheeseburger—3 Medium Patties With Condiments On Bun
From Fast Food / Restaurant ☛ Vitamin K = 17.6 mcg; Serving size: 1
triple cheeseburger, 420 g

Tuna Melt Sandwich ☛ Vitamin K = 43.8 mcg; Serving size: 1 sandwich, 150 g

Tuna Salad Sandwich ☛ Vitamin K = 20.9 mcg; Serving size: 1 sandwich, 157 g

Tuna Salad Sandwich—With Lettuce ☛ Vitamin K = 23.4 mcg;
Serving size: 1 sandwich, 167 g

Turkey And Bacon Submarine Sandwich—With Cheese Lettuce
Tomato And Spread ☛ Vitamin K = 34.3 mcg; Serving size: 1 submarine, 260 g

Turkey And Bacon Submarine Sandwich—With Lettuce Tomato
And Spread ☛ Vitamin K = 35.3 mcg; Serving size: 1 submarine, 240 g

Turkey Ham And Roast Beef Club Sandwich—With Lettuce Tomato
And Spread ☛ Vitamin K = 32.9 mcg; Serving size: 1 sandwich, 240 g

Turkey Or Chicken Burger Plain On Bun From Fast Food / Restaurant
☛ Vitamin K = 2.9 mcg; Serving size: 1 sandwich, 145 g

Turkey Or Chicken Burger Plain On Wheat Bun ☛ Vitamin K = 3.3
mcg; Serving size: 1 sandwich, 145 g

Turkey Or Chicken Burger Plain On White Bun ☛ Vitamin K = 2.9
mcg; Serving size: 1 sandwich, 145 g

Turkey Or Chicken Burger With Condiments On Bun From Fast
Food / Restaurant ☛ Vitamin K = 16.4 mcg; Serving size: 1 sandwich,
200 g

Turkey Or Chicken Burger With Condiments On Wheat Bun ☛
Vitamin K = 16.8 mcg; Serving size: 1 sandwich, 200 g

Turkey Or Chicken Burger With Condiments On White Bun ☛
Vitamin K = 16.4 mcg; Serving size: 1 sandwich, 200 g

Turkey Or Chicken Burger With Condiments On Whole Wheat Bun ☛ Vitamin K = 16.8 mcg; Serving size: 1 sandwich, 200 g

Turkey Salad Or Turkey Spread Sandwich ☛ Vitamin K = 28.3 mcg; Serving size: 1 sandwich, 141 g

Turkey Sandwich—With Gravy ☛ Vitamin K = 0 mcg; Serving size: 1 sandwich, 284 g

Turkey Sandwich—With Spread ☛ Vitamin K = 10.9 mcg; Serving size: 1 sandwich, 143 g

Vanilla Light Soft-Serve Ice Cream With Cone ☛ Vitamin K = 0.6 mcg; Serving size: 1 item, 120 g

Vegetable Submarine Sandwich—With Fat-free Spread ☛ Vitamin K = 19.4 mcg; Serving size: 1 submarine, 240 g

Vegetable Submarine Sandwich—With Spread ☛ Vitamin K = 45.3 mcg; Serving size: 1 submarine, 167 g

Waffle—Chocolate ☛ Vitamin K = 1.5 mcg; Serving size: 1 miniature/bite size waffle, 10 g

Waffle—Chocolate From Fast Food / Restaurant ☛ Vitamin K = 2.3 mcg; Serving size: 1 miniature/bite size waffle, 10 g

Waffle—Chocolate From Frozen ☛ Vitamin K = 1.2 mcg; Serving size: 1 miniature/bite size waffle, 10 g

Waffle—Cinnamon ☛ Vitamin K = 1.7 mcg; Serving size: 1 miniature/bite size waffle, 10 g

Waffle—Cornmeal ☛ Vitamin K = 0 mcg; Serving size: 1 miniature/bite size waffle, 10 g

Waffle—Fruit ☛ Vitamin K = 1.8 mcg; Serving size: 1 miniature/bite size waffle, 10 g

Waffle—Fruit From Fast Food / Restaurant ☛ Vitamin K = 2.6 mcg; Serving size: 1 miniature/bite size waffle, 10 g

Waffle—Fruit From Frozen ☞ Vitamin K = 1.3 mcg; Serving size: 1 miniature/bite size waffle, 10 g

Waffle—Plain ☞ Vitamin K = 1.7 mcg; Serving size: 1 miniature/bite size waffle, 10 g

Waffle—Plain From Fast Food / Restaurant ☞ Vitamin K = 2.6 mcg; Serving size: 1 miniature/bite size waffle, 10 g

Waffle—Plain Reduced-Fat ☞ Vitamin K = 1.2 mcg; Serving size: 1 miniature/bite size waffle, 10 g

Waffle—Plain Reduced-Fat From Frozen ☞ Vitamin K = 0.5 mcg; Serving size: 1 miniature/bite size waffle, 10 g

Waffle—Whole Grain ☞ Vitamin K = 1.8 mcg; Serving size: 1 miniature/bite size waffle, 10 g

Waffle—Whole Grain From Fast Food / Restaurant ☞ Vitamin K = 2.7 mcg; Serving size: 1 miniature/bite size waffle, 10 g

Waffle—Whole Grain From Frozen ☞ Vitamin K = 0.9 mcg; Serving size: 1 miniature/bite size waffle, 10 g

Waffle—Whole Grain Fruit From Frozen ☞ Vitamin K = 0.9 mcg; Serving size: 1 miniature/bite size waffle, 10 g

Waffle—Whole Grain Reduced-Fat ☞ Vitamin K = 1.2 mcg; Serving size: 1 miniature/bite size waffle, 10 g

Wendys—Chicken Nuggets ☞ Vitamin K = 5.4 mcg; Serving size: 5 pieces, 68 g

Wendys—Classic Double With Cheese ☞ Vitamin K = 21.4 mcg; Serving size: 1 item, 310 g

Wendys—Classic Single Hamburger No Cheese ☞ Vitamin K = 19.6 mcg; Serving size: 1 item, 218 g

Wendys—Classic Single Hamburger With Cheese ☞ Vitamin K = 21.9 mcg; Serving size: 1 item, 236 g

Wendys—French Fries ☞ Vitamin K = 4.5 mcg; Serving size: 1 kid's meal serving, 71 g

Wendys—Frosty Dairy Dessert ☞ Vitamin K = 0.5 mcg; Serving size: 1 junior 6 oz. cup, 113 g

Wendys—Homestyle Chicken Fillet Sandwich ☞ Vitamin K = 24.6 mcg; Serving size: 1 item, 230 g

Wendys—Jr. Hamburger With Cheese ☞ Vitamin K = 5.4 mcg; Serving size: 1 item, 129 g

Wendys—Jr. Hamburger Without Cheese ☞ Vitamin K = 5.3 mcg; Serving size: 1 item, 117 g

Wendys—Ultimate Chicken Grill Sandwich ☞ Vitamin K = 20 mcg; Serving size: 1 item, 225 g

Wrap Sandwich—Filled With Beef Patty Cheese And Spread And/or Sauce ☞ Vitamin K = 12.7 mcg; Serving size: 1 snack wrap sandwich, 126 g

Wrap Sandwich—Filled With Meat Poultry Or Fish And Vegetables ☞ Vitamin K = 17.5 mcg; Serving size: 1 sandwich, 240 g

Wrap Sandwich—Filled With Meat Poultry Or Fish Vegetables And Cheese ☞ Vitamin K = 18.8 mcg; Serving size: 1 sandwich, 280 g

Wrap Sandwich—Filled With Meat Poultry Or Fish Vegetables And Rice ☞ Vitamin K = 74.5 mcg; Serving size: 1 sandwich, 433 g

Wrap Sandwich—Filled With Meat Poultry Or Fish Vegetables Rice And Cheese ☞ Vitamin K = 82.7 mcg; Serving size: 1 sandwich, 467 g

Wrap Sandwich—Filled With Vegetables ☞ Vitamin K = 26.8 mcg; Serving size: 1 sandwich, 273 g

Wrap Sandwich—Filled With Vegetables And Rice ☞ Vitamin K = 28.3 mcg; Serving size: 1 sandwich, 404 g

18

FATS AND OILS

Animal Fat Or Drippings ☛ Vitamin K = 1.2 mcg; Serving size: 1 cup, 205 g

Bacon Grease ☛ Vitamin K = 0 mcg; Serving size: 1 tsp, 4.3 g

Beef Tallow ☛ Vitamin K = 0 mcg; Serving size: 1 tbsp, 12.8 g

Butter Light Stick With Salt ☛ Vitamin K = 0.7 mcg; Serving size: 1 tablespoon, 14 g

Butter Light Stick Without Salt ☛ Vitamin K = 0.7 mcg; Serving size: 1 tablespoon, 14 g

Butter Replacement Without Fat Powder ☛ Vitamin K = 0 mcg; Serving size: 1 cup, 80 g

Butter Whipped Tub Salted ☛ Vitamin K = 6.9 mcg; Serving size: 1 cup, 151 g

Butter-Margarine—Blend Stick Salted ☛ Vitamin K = 113.5 mcg; Serving size: 1 cup, 227 g

Cheese Cream—Light Or Lite ☛ Vitamin K = 2.6 mcg; Serving size: 1 cup, 240 g

Cheese Spread Cream—Cheese Light Or Lite ☞ Vitamin K = 2.6 mcg; Serving size: 1 cup, 240 g

Cocoa Butter ☞ Vitamin K = 3.4 mcg; Serving size: 1 tablespoon, 13.6 g

Coffee Creamer Liquid Fat-free Flavored ☞ Vitamin K = 1.7 mcg; Serving size: 1 cup, 240 g

Cream—Half And Half ☞ Vitamin K = 3.1 mcg; Serving size: 1 cup, 240 g

Cream—Half And Half Flavored ☞ Vitamin K = 3.1 mcg; Serving size: 1 cup, 240 g

Cream—Heavy ☞ Vitamin K = 7.7 mcg; Serving size: 1 cup, 240 g

Cream—Light ☞ Vitamin K = 4.1 mcg; Serving size: 1 cup, 240 g

Cream—Whipped ☞ Vitamin K = 3.6 mcg; Serving size: 1 cup, 120 g

Creamy Dressing—Prepared With Sour Cream—And/or Buttermilk And Oil—Reduced Calorie ☞ Vitamin K = 0.5 mcg; Serving size: 1 tbsp, 15 g

Creamy Dressing—Prepared With Sour Cream—And/or Buttermilk And Oil—Reduced Calorie Cholesterol-Free ☞ Vitamin K = 5.2 mcg; Serving size: 1 tbsp, 15 g

Creamy Dressing—Prepared With Sour Cream—And/or Buttermilk And Oil—Reduced Calorie Fat-Free ☞ Vitamin K = 0.4 mcg; Serving size: 1 tbsp, 17 g

Creamy Poppyseed Salad Dressing ☞ Vitamin K = 16.6 mcg; Serving size: 2 tbsp, 33 g

Dressing Honey Mustard Fat-Free ☞ Vitamin K = 0.1 mcg; Serving size: 2 tbsp, 30 g

Fat Back Cooked ☞ Vitamin K = 0 mcg; Serving size: 1 slice (2-1/4" x 1-3/4" x 1/4"), 26 g

Fat Turkey ☞ Vitamin K = 0 mcg; Serving size: 1 tbsp, 12.8 g

Honey Butter ☞ Vitamin K = 8.1 mcg; Serving size: 1 cup, 288 g

Lard ☞ Vitamin K = 0 mcg; Serving size: 1 tbsp, 12.8 g

Margarine-Like Butter-Margarine—Blend 80% Fat Stick Without Salt ☞ Vitamin K = 9.9 mcg; Serving size: 1 tablespoon, 14 g

Margarine-Like Margarine-Butter Blend Soybean Oil—And Butter ☞ Vitamin K = 12.2 mcg; Serving size: 1 tbsp, 14.1 g

Margarine-Like Shortening—Industrial Soy Cottonseed And Soy Principal Use Flaky Pastries ☞ Vitamin K = 6 mcg; Serving size: 1 tbsp, 14 g

Margarine-Like Spread—Benecol Light Spread ☞ Vitamin K = 7.9 mcg; Serving size: 1 tablespoon, 14 g

Margarine-Like Spread—Liquid Salted ☞ Vitamin K = 230 mcg; Serving size: 1 cup, 227 g

Margarine-Like Spread—Smart Balance Light Buttery Spread ☞ Vitamin K = 6.6 mcg; Serving size: 1 tbsp, 14 g

Margarine-Like Spread—Smart Balance Omega Plus Spread (With Plant Sterols & Fish Oil) ☞ Vitamin K = 7.4 mcg; Serving size: 1 table-spoon, 14 g

Margarine-Like Spread—Smart Balance Regular Buttery Spread With Flax Oil ☞ Vitamin K = 7.8 mcg; Serving size: 1 tablespoon, 14 g

Margarine-Like Spread—Smart Beat Smart Squeeze ☞ Vitamin K = 0.6 mcg; Serving size: 1 tablespoon, 14 g

Margarine-Like Spread—Smart Beat Super Light Without Saturated Fat ☞ Vitamin K = 1.7 mcg; Serving size: 1 tablespoon, 14 g

Margarine-Like Spread—With Yogurt 70% Fat Stick With Salt ☞ Vitamin K = 13 mcg; Serving size: 1 tablespoon, 14 g

Margarine-Like Spread—With Yogurt Approximately 40% Fat Tub With Salt ☞ Vitamin K = 13 mcg; Serving size: 1 tablespoon, 14 g

Margarine-Like Vegetable Oil-Butter Spread Reduced Calorie Tub With Salt ☞ Vitamin K = 8.1 mcg; Serving size: 1 tablespoon, 14 g

Margarine-Like Vegetable Oil-Butter Spread Tub With Salt ☞ Vitamin K = 6.5 mcg; Serving size: 1 tablespoon, 14 g

Margarine-Like Vegetable Oil—Spread 20% Fat With Salt ☞ Vitamin K = 10.6 mcg; Serving size: 1 tbsp, 15 g

Margarine-Like Vegetable Oil—Spread 20% Fat Without Salt ☞ Vitamin K = 11.9 mcg; Serving size: 1 tbsp, 12.8 g

Margarine-Like Vegetable Oil—Spread 60% Fat Stick With Salt ☞ Vitamin K = 14.5 mcg; Serving size: 1 tbsp, 14.3 g

Margarine-Like Vegetable Oil—Spread 60% Fat Stick With Salt With Added Vitamin D ☞ Vitamin K = 14.2 mcg; Serving size: 1 tbsp, 14 g

Margarine-Like Vegetable Oil—Spread 60% Fat Stick/tub/bottle With Salt ☞ Vitamin K = 14.5 mcg; Serving size: 1 tbsp, 14.3 g

Margarine-Like Vegetable Oil—Spread 60% Fat Stick/tub/bottle Without Salt ☞ Vitamin K = 14.2 mcg; Serving size: 1 tbsp, 14 g

Margarine-Like Vegetable Oil—Spread 60% Fat Stick/tub/bottle Without Salt With Added Vitamin D ☞ Vitamin K = 14.2 mcg; Serving size: 1 tbsp, 14 g

Margarine-Like Vegetable Oil—Spread 60% Fat Tub With Salt ☞ Vitamin K = 14.2 mcg; Serving size: 1 tbsp, 14 g

Margarine-Like Vegetable Oil—Spread 60% Fat Tub With Salt With Added Vitamin D ☞ Vitamin K = 14.2 mcg; Serving size: 1 tbsp, 14 g

Margarine-Like Vegetable Oil—Spread Approximately 37% Fat Unspecified Oils With Salt With Added Vitamin D ☞ Vitamin K = 11.1 mcg; Serving size: 1 tbsp, 14.9 g

Margarine-Like Vegetable Oil—Spread Fat-free Liquid With Salt ☞ Vitamin K = 0 mcg; Serving size: 1 tbsp, 15 g

Margarine-Like Vegetable Oil—Spread Fat-Free Tub ☛ Vitamin K = 0 mcg; Serving size: 1 tbsp, 14.6 g

Margarine-Like Vegetable Oil—Spread Stick Or Tub Sweetened ☛ Vitamin K = 13 mcg; Serving size: 1 tablespoon, 14 g

Margarine-Like Vegetable Oil—Spread Unspecified Oils Approximately 37% Fat With Salt ☛ Vitamin K = 11.1 mcg; Serving size: 1 tbsp, 14.9 g

Margarine-Like Vegetable-Oil—Spread Stick/tub/bottle 60% Fat With Added Vitamin D ☛ Vitamin K = 14.2 mcg; Serving size: 1 tbsp, 14 g

Margarine—(Unsalted) ☛ Vitamin K = 13.2 mcg; Serving size: 1 tbsp, 14.2 g

Margarine—80% Fat Stick Includes Regular And Hydrogenated Corn And Soybean Oils ☛ Vitamin K = 10.5 mcg; Serving size: 1 tbsp, 14 g

Margarine—Industrial Non-Dairy Cottonseed Soy Oil—(Partially Hydrogenated) For Flaky Pastries ☛ Vitamin K = 14.9 mcg; Serving size: 1 tbsp, 14 g

Margarine—Industrial Soy And Partially Hydrogenated Soy Oil—Use For Baking Sauces And Candy ☛ Vitamin K = 10.5 mcg; Serving size: 1 tbsp, 14 g

Margarine—Like Spread Whipped Tub Salted ☛ Vitamin K = 10.1 mcg; Serving size: 1 tablespoon, 10 g

Margarine—Regular 80% Fat Composite Stick With Salt ☛ Vitamin K = 13 mcg; Serving size: 1 tbsp, 14 g

Margarine—Regular 80% Fat Composite Stick With Salt With Added Vitamin D ☛ Vitamin K = 13 mcg; Serving size: 1 tablespoon, 14 g

Margarine—Regular 80% Fat Composite Stick Without Salt With Added Vitamin D ☛ Vitamin K = 13 mcg; Serving size: 1 tbsp, 14 g

Margarine—Regular 80% Fat Composite Tub With Salt ☛ Vitamin K = 13 mcg; Serving size: 1 tbsp, 14.2 g

Margarine—Regular 80% Fat Composite Tub With Salt With Added Vitamin D ☛ Vitamin K = 12.8 mcg; Serving size: 1 tbsp, 14 g

Margarine—Regular 80% Fat Composite Tub Without Salt ☛ Vitamin K = 13 mcg; Serving size: 1 tbsp, 14.2 g

Mayonnaise Reduced-Fat With Olive Oil ☛ Vitamin K = 8.1 mcg; Serving size: 1 tbsp, 15 g

Mayonnaise—Low Sodium Reduced Calorie Or Diet ☛ Vitamin K = 3.5 mcg; Serving size: 1 tbsp, 14 g

Mayonnaise—Prepared With Tofu ☛ Vitamin K = 8 mcg; Serving size: 1 tbsp, 15 g

Mayonnaise—Reduced-Calorie Or Diet Cholesterol-Free ☛ Vitamin K = 3.6 mcg; Serving size: 1 tbsp, 14.6 g

Oil—Almond ☛ Vitamin K = 1 mcg; Serving size: 1 tablespoon, 13.6 g

Oil—Canola ☛ Vitamin K = 10 mcg; Serving size: 1 tbsp, 14 g

Oil—Coconut ☛ Vitamin K = 0.1 mcg; Serving size: 1 tbsp, 13.6 g

Oil—Corn ☛ Vitamin K = 0.3 mcg; Serving size: 1 tbsp, 13.6 g

Oil—Corn And Canola ☛ Vitamin K = 5.9 mcg; Serving size: 1 tbsp, 14 g

Oil—Corn Peanut And Olive ☛ Vitamin K = 2.9 mcg; Serving size: 1 tablespoon, 14 g

Oil—Cottonseed ☛ Vitamin K = 3.4 mcg; Serving size: 1 tablespoon, 13.6 g

Oil—Flaxseed ☛ Vitamin K = 1.3 mcg; Serving size: 1 tbsp, 13.6 g

Oil—Flaxseed Contains Added Sliced Flaxseed ☛ Vitamin K = 0.5 mcg; Serving size: 1 tablespoon, 13.7 g

Oil—Industrial Canola For Salads Woks And Light Frying ☛ Vitamin K = 9.7 mcg; Serving size: 1 tablespoon, 13.6 g

Oil—Industrial Canola High Oleic ☛ Vitamin K = 10 mcg; Serving size: 1 tablespoon, 14 g

Oil—Industrial Canola Oil—For Deep Fat Frying ☛ Vitamin K = 9.7 mcg; Serving size: 1 tablespoon, 13.6 g

Oil—Oat ☛ Vitamin K = 3.4 mcg; Serving size: 1 tbsp, 13.6 g

Oil—Olive ☛ Vitamin K = 8.1 mcg; Serving size: 1 tablespoon, 13.5 g

Oil—Palm ☛ Vitamin K = 1.1 mcg; Serving size: 1 tbsp, 13.6 g

Oil—Palm Kernel ☛ Vitamin K = 3.4 mcg; Serving size: 1 tablespoon, 13.6 g

Oil—Pam Cooking Spray Original ☛ Vitamin K = 0 mcg; Serving size: 1 spray , about 1/3 second, 0.3 g

Oil—Peanut ☛ Vitamin K = 0.1 mcg; Serving size: 1 tbsp, 13.5 g

Oil—Rice Bran ☛ Vitamin K = 3.4 mcg; Serving size: 1 tablespoon, 13.6 g

Oil—Safflower Salad Or Cooking High Oleic (Primary Safflower Oil —Of Commerce) ☛ Vitamin K = 1 mcg; Serving size: 1 tablespoon, 13.6 g

Oil—Safflower Salad Or Cooking Linoleic (Over 70%) ☛ Vitamin K = 1 mcg; Serving size: 1 tbsp, 13.6 g

Oil—Sesame ☛ Vitamin K = 1.8 mcg; Serving size: 1 tablespoon, 13.6 g

Oil—Soybean ☛ Vitamin K = 25 mcg; Serving size: 1 tbsp, 13.6 g

Oil—Soybean Salad Or Cooking ☛ Vitamin K = 3.4 mcg; Serving size: 1 tbsp, 13.6 g

Oil—Soybean Salad Or Cooking And Cottonseed ☛ Vitamin K = 3.4 mcg; Serving size: 1 tablespoon, 13.6 g

Oil—Sunflower High Oleic (70% And Over) ☞ Vitamin K = 0.8 mcg; Serving size: 1 tbsp, 14 g

Oil—Sunflower Linoleic ☞ Vitamin K = 0.7 mcg; Serving size: 1 tbsp, 13.6 g

Oil—Sunflower Linoleic (Approx. 65%) ☞ Vitamin K = 0.7 mcg; Serving size: 1 tbsp, 13.6 g

Oil—Sunflower Linoleic (Less Than 60%) ☞ Vitamin K = 0.7 mcg; Serving size: 1 tbsp, 13.6 g

Oil—Walnut ☞ Vitamin K = 2 mcg; Serving size: 1 tbsp, 13.6 g

Oil—Wheat Germ ☞ Vitamin K = 1.1 mcg; Serving size: 1 tsp, 4.5 g

Rendered Chicken Fat ☞ Vitamin K = 0 mcg; Serving size: 1 tbsp, 12.8 g

Salad Dressing—Bacon And Tomato ☞ Vitamin K = 10.4 mcg; Serving size: 1 tbsp, 15 g

Salad Dressing—Blue Or Roquefort Cheese Dressing Commercially Made Regular ☞ Vitamin K = 12.9 mcg; Serving size: 1 tbsp, 15 g

Salad Dressing—Blue Or Roquefort Cheese Dressing Fat-Free ☞ Vitamin K = 0 mcg; Serving size: 1 tbsp, 17 g

Salad Dressing—Blue Or Roquefort Cheese Dressing Light ☞ Vitamin K = 14.6 mcg; Serving size: 1 tbsp, 16 g

Salad Dressing—Blue Or Roquefort Cheese Reduced Calorie ☞ Vitamin K = 0.8 mcg; Serving size: 1 tbsp, 15 g

Salad Dressing—Buttermilk Lite ☞ Vitamin K = 5.2 mcg; Serving size: 1 tablespoon, 15 g

Salad Dressing—Caesar Dressing Regular ☞ Vitamin K = 15.4 mcg; Serving size: 1 tbsp, 14.7 g

Salad Dressing—Caesar Fat-Free ☞ Vitamin K = 0 mcg; Serving size: 2 tbsp, 34 g

Salad Dressing—Caesar Reduced Calorie ☛ Vitamin K = 0.2 mcg; Serving size: 1 tbsp, 15 g

Salad Dressing—Coleslaw ☛ Vitamin K = 159.3 mcg; Serving size: 1 cup, 250 g

Salad Dressing—Coleslaw ☛ Vitamin K = 10.6 mcg; Serving size: 1 tbsp, 16 g

Salad Dressing—Coleslaw Dressing Reduced-Fat ☛ Vitamin K = 6.7 mcg; Serving size: 1 tbsp, 17 g

Salad Dressing—French Dressing Commercially Made Regular ☛ Vitamin K = 19.4 mcg; Serving size: 1 tbsp, 16 g

Salad Dressing—French Dressing Commercially Made Regular Without Salt ☛ Vitamin K = 18.2 mcg; Serving size: 1 tablespoon, 15 g

Salad Dressing—French Dressing Fat-Free ☛ Vitamin K = 0 mcg; Serving size: 1 tablespoon, 16 g

Salad Dressing—French Dressing Reduced Calorie ☛ Vitamin K = 0.8 mcg; Serving size: 1 tbsp, 16 g

Salad Dressing—French Dressing Reduced-Fat ☛ Vitamin K = 2.8 mcg; Serving size: 1 tablespoon, 16 g

Salad Dressing—French Or Catalina Dressing ☛ Vitamin K = 303.5 mcg; Serving size: 1 cup, 250 g

Salad Dressing—Green Goddess Regular ☛ Vitamin K = 14.5 mcg; Serving size: 1 tbsp, 15 g

Salad Dressing—Home Recipe Vinegar And Oil ☛ Vitamin K = 15.8 mcg; Serving size: 1 tablespoon, 16 g

Salad Dressing—Honey Mustard ☛ Vitamin K = 21 mcg; Serving size: 2 tbsp, 30 g

Salad Dressing—Honey Mustard Dressing Reduced Calorie ☛ Vitamin K = 4 mcg; Serving size: 2 tbsp (1 serving), 30 g

Salad Dressing—Italian Dressing Commercially Made Regular ☛ Vitamin K = 8.2 mcg; Serving size: 1 tbsp, 14.7 g

Salad Dressing—Italian Dressing Commercially Made Regular Without Salt ☛ Vitamin K = 8.2 mcg; Serving size: 1 tablespoon, 14.7 g

Salad Dressing—Italian Dressing Fat-Free ☛ Vitamin K = 0.2 mcg; Serving size: 1 tbsp, 14 g

Salad Dressing—Italian Dressing Reduced Calorie ☛ Vitamin K = 1.8 mcg; Serving size: 1 tbsp, 14 g

Salad Dressing—Italian Dressing Reduced-Fat Without Salt ☛ Vitamin K = 1.9 mcg; Serving size: 1 tablespoon, 15 g

Salad Dressing—Italian Salad ☛ Vitamin K = 1.9 mcg; Serving size: 1 tablespoon, 15 g

Salad Dressing—Korean Dressing Or Marinade ☛ Vitamin K = 84.4 mcg; Serving size: 1 cup, 246 g

Salad Dressing—Kraft Mayo Fat-free Mayonnaise Dressing ☛ Vitamin K = 0 mcg; Serving size: 1 tbsp, 16 g

Salad Dressing—Kraft Mayo Light Mayonnaise ☛ Vitamin K = 23.3 mcg; Serving size: 1 tbsp, 15 g

Salad Dressing—Lowfat French ☛ Vitamin K = 0.8 mcg; Serving size: 1 tablespoon, 16 g

Salad Dressing—Mayonnaise ☛ Vitamin K = 3.7 mcg; Serving size: 1 tbsp, 15 g

Salad Dressing—Mayonnaise ☛ Vitamin K = 6.2 mcg; Serving size: 1 tbsp, 14.7 g

Salad Dressing—Mayonnaise And Mayonnaise-Type Reduced Calorie ☛ Vitamin K = 3.6 mcg; Serving size: 1 tbsp, 14.5 g

Salad Dressing—Mayonnaise Imitation Soybean ☛ Vitamin K = 6.3 mcg; Serving size: 1 tbsp, 15 g

Salad Dressing—Mayonnaise Imitation Soybean Without Cholesterol ☛ Vitamin K = 6 mcg; Serving size: 1 tablespoon, 14.1 g

Salad Dressing—Mayonnaise Light ☛ Vitamin K = 8.1 mcg; Serving size: 1 tablespoon, 15 g

Salad Dressing—Mayonnaise Light Smart Balance Omega Plus Light ☛ Vitamin K = 9.2 mcg; Serving size: 1 tbsp, 14 g

Salad Dressing—Mayonnaise Regular ☛ Vitamin K = 22.5 mcg; Serving size: 1 tbsp, 13.8 g

Salad Dressing—Mayonnaise Soybean And Safflower Oil—With Salt ☛ Vitamin K = 3.4 mcg; Serving size: 1 tablespoon, 13.8 g

Salad Dressing—Mayonnaise-Like Fat-Free ☛ Vitamin K = 4 mcg; Serving size: 1 tbsp, 16 g

Salad Dressing—Peppercorn Dressing Commercially Made Regular ☛ Vitamin K = 16.8 mcg; Serving size: 1 tbsp, 13.4 g

Salad Dressing—Ranch Dressing Fat-Free ☛ Vitamin K = 0.3 mcg; Serving size: 1 tablespoon, 14 g

Salad Dressing—Ranch Dressing Reduced-Fat ☛ Vitamin K = 5.2 mcg; Serving size: 1 tablespoon, 15 g

Salad Dressing—Ranch Dressing Regular ☛ Vitamin K = 20.1 mcg; Serving size: 1 tablespoon, 15 g

Salad Dressing—Russian ☛ Vitamin K = 8.1 mcg; Serving size: 1 tbsp, 15 g

Salad Dressing—Russian Dressing Reduced Calorie ☛ Vitamin K = 1.1 mcg; Serving size: 1 tablespoon, 16 g

Salad Dressing—Sesame Seed ☛ Vitamin K = 8.4 mcg; Serving size: 1 tablespoon, 15 g

Salad Dressing—Sweet And Sour ☛ Vitamin K = 6.3 mcg; Serving size: 1 tbsp, 16 g

Salad Dressing—Thousand Island Dressing Fat-Free ☛ Vitamin K = 0.6 mcg; Serving size: 1 tbsp, 16 g

Salad Dressing—Thousand Island Dressing Reduced-Fat ☛ Vitamin K = 4.1 mcg; Serving size: 1 tablespoon, 15 g

Salad Dressing—Yogurt Dressing ☛ Vitamin K = 4.2 mcg; Serving size: 1 cup, 246 g

Sandwich Spread With Chopped Pickle Regular Unspecified Oils ☛ Vitamin K = 3.7 mcg; Serving size: 1 tablespoon, 15 g

Shortening—Cake Mix Soybean (Hydrogenated) And Cottonseed (Hydrogenated) ☛ Vitamin K = 5.5 mcg; Serving size: 1 tbsp, 12.8 g

Shortening—Confectionery Coconut (Hydrogenated) And Or Palm Kernel (Hydrogenated) ☛ Vitamin K = 5.5 mcg; Serving size: 1 tbsp, 12.8 g

Shortening—Frying (Heavy Duty) Soybean (Hydrogenated) Linoleic (Less Than 1%) ☛ Vitamin K = 5.5 mcg; Serving size: 1 tbsp, 12.8 g

Shortening—Household Lard And Vegetable Oil ☛ Vitamin K = 2.8 mcg; Serving size: 1 tablespoon, 12.8 g

Shortening—Household Soybean-Cottonseed ☛ Vitamin K = 5.5 mcg; Serving size: 1 tbsp, 12.8 g

Shortening—Industrial Soy And Corn For Frying ☛ Vitamin K = 5.5 mcg; Serving size: 1 tbsp, 12.8 g

Shortening—Industrial Soy For Baking And Confections ☛ Vitamin K = 5.5 mcg; Serving size: 1 tbsp, 12.8 g

Shortening—Industrial Soy Pourable Liquid Fry Shortening ☛ Vitamin K = 3.4 mcg; Serving size: 1 tbsp, 13.6 g

Shortening—Industrial Soybean (Hydrogenated) And Cottonseed ☛ Vitamin K = 5.5 mcg; Serving size: 1 tbsp, 12.8 g

Shortening—Special Purpose For Baking Soybean (Hydrogenated)

Palm And Cottonseed ☛ Vitamin K = 5.5 mcg; Serving size: 1 tbsp, 12.8 g

Shortening—Special Purpose For Cakes And Frostings Soybean (Hydrogenated) ☛ Vitamin K = 5.5 mcg; Serving size: 1 tbsp, 12.8 g

Soybean Lecithin ☛ Vitamin K = 25 mcg; Serving size: 1 tablespoon, 13.6 g

Table Fat Nfs ☛ Vitamin K = 101.5 mcg; Serving size: 1 cup, 227 g

Tartar Sauce Reduced-Fat/calorie ☛ Vitamin K = 64.3 mcg; Serving size: 1 cup, 224 g

Thousand Island ☛ Vitamin K = 11.1 mcg; Serving size: 1 tbsp, 16 g

USDA Commodity Food Oil—Vegetable Soybean Refined ☛ Vitamin K = 25 mcg; Serving size: 1 tablespoon, 13.6 g

Vegetable Oil-Butter Spread Reduced Calorie ☛ Vitamin K = 7.9 mcg; Serving size: 1 tbsp, 13 g

Vegetable Oil-Butter Spread Stick Salted ☛ Vitamin K = 223.6 mcg; Serving size: 1 cup, 227 g

Vegetable Shortening ☛ Vitamin K = 6.8 mcg; Serving size: 1 tbsp, 12.8 g

19

FINFISH AND SHELLFISH PRODUCTS

Abalone Floured Or Breaded Fried ☛ Vitamin K = 9 mcg; Serving size: 1 oz, cooked, 28 g

Abalone—Steamed Or Poached ☛ Vitamin K = 12.8 mcg; Serving size: 1 oz, cooked, 28 g

Anchovies (Raw) ☛ Vitamin K = 0.1 mcg; Serving size: 3 oz, 85 g

Atlantic Herring ☛ Vitamin K = 0.1 mcg; Serving size: 1 fillet, 143 g

Atlantic Mackerel (Raw) ☛ Vitamin K = 5.6 mcg; Serving size: 1 fillet, 112 g

Baked Conch ☛ Vitamin K = 0.3 mcg; Serving size: 1 cup, sliced, 127 g

Barracuda—Baked Or Broiled (Cooked with Fat) ☛ Vitamin K = 5.1 mcg; Serving size: 1 small fillet, 113 g

Barracuda—Baked Or Broiled (Cooked without Fat) ☛ Vitamin K = 0.1 mcg; Serving size: 1 small fillet, 113 g

Barracuda—Coated Fried ☛ Vitamin K = 12.9 mcg; Serving size: 1 small fillet, 113 g

Barracuda—Coated—Baked Or Broiled (Cooked with Fat) ☛ Vitamin K = 8.2 mcg; Serving size: 1 small fillet, 113 g

Barracuda—Coated—Baked Or Broiled (Cooked without Fat) ☛ Vitamin K = 0.9 mcg; Serving size: 1 small fillet, 113 g

Barracuda—Steamed Or Poached ☛ Vitamin K = 0.1 mcg; Serving size: 1 small fillet, 113 g

Biscayne Codfish (Puerto Rican Style) ☛ Vitamin K = 15.4 mcg; Serving size: 1 cup, 175 g

Blue Crab ☛ Vitamin K = 0.4 mcg; Serving size: 1 cup, flaked and pieces, 118 g

Bluefin Tuna (Raw) ☛ Vitamin K = 0 mcg; Serving size: 3 oz, 85 g

Bouillabaisse ☛ Vitamin K = 21.3 mcg; Serving size: 1 cup, 227 g

Canned Anchovies ☛ Vitamin K = 3.4 mcg; Serving size: 1 oz, boneless, 28.4 g

Canned Atlantic Cod ☛ Vitamin K = 0.1 mcg; Serving size: 3 oz, 85 g

Canned Blue Crab ☛ Vitamin K = 0.4 mcg; Serving size: 1 cup, 135 g

Canned Clams ☛ Vitamin K = 0.3 mcg; Serving size: 3 oz, 85 g

Canned Eastern Oysters ☛ Vitamin K = 0.1 mcg; Serving size: 3 oz, 85 g

Canned Pink Salmon ☛ Vitamin K = 0.1 mcg; Serving size: 3 oz, 85 g

Canned Pink Salmon (With Skin And Bones) ☛ Vitamin K = 0.1 mcg; Serving size: 3 oz, 85 g

Canned Salmon ☛ Vitamin K = 0.1 mcg; Serving size: 3 oz, 85 g

Canned Sardines ☛ Vitamin K = 3.9 mcg; Serving size: 1 cup, drained, 149 g

Canned Shrimp ☛ Vitamin K = 0 mcg; Serving size: 1 cup, 128 g

Canned Sockeye Salmon ☞ Vitamin K = 0.1 mcg; Serving size: 3 oz, 85 g

Canned Sockeye Salmon (With Skin And Bones) ☞ Vitamin K = 0.1 mcg; Serving size: 3 oz, 85 g

Canned White Tuna (Oil Packed) ☞ Vitamin K = 5.9 mcg; Serving size: 3 oz, 85 g

Canned White Tuna (Water Packed) ☞ Vitamin K = 2.1 mcg; Serving size: 3 oz, 85 g

Carp Raw ☞ Vitamin K = 0.1 mcg; Serving size: 3 oz, 85 g

Carp Smoked ☞ Vitamin K = 0.1 mcg; Serving size: 1 oz, 28 g

Carp—Baked Or Broiled (Cooked with Fat) ☞ Vitamin K = 7.7 mcg; Serving size: 1 small fillet, 170 g

Carp—Baked Or Broiled (Cooked without Fat) ☞ Vitamin K = 0.2 mcg; Serving size: 1 small fillet, 170 g

Carp—Coated Fried ☞ Vitamin K = 19.4 mcg; Serving size: 1 small fillet, 170 g

Carp—Coated—Baked Or Broiled (Cooked with Fat) ☞ Vitamin K = 12.4 mcg; Serving size: 1 small fillet, 170 g

Carp—Coated—Baked Or Broiled (Cooked without Fat) ☞ Vitamin K = 1.4 mcg; Serving size: 1 small fillet, 170 g

Carp—Steamed Or Poached ☞ Vitamin K = 0.2 mcg; Serving size: 1 small fillet, 170 g

Cassava Fritter Stuffed With Crab Meat Puerto Rican Style ☞ Vitamin K = 10.3 mcg; Serving size: 1 empanada (5" x 2-1/2" x 1/2"), 126 g

Catfish Channel Farmed Raw ☞ Vitamin K = 1.8 mcg; Serving size: 3 oz, 85 g

Catfish Channel Farmed—Cooked—Dry Heat ☞ Vitamin K = 3.6 mcg; Serving size: 1 fillet, 143 g

Catfish—Baked Or Broiled —Prepared with Butter ☛ Vitamin K = 3.2 mcg; Serving size: 1 small fillet, 113 g

Catfish—Baked Or Broiled —Prepared with Cooking Spray ☛ Vitamin K = 2.9 mcg; Serving size: 1 small fillet, 113 g

Catfish—Baked Or Broiled —Prepared with Margarine ☛ Vitamin K = 7.3 mcg; Serving size: 1 small fillet, 113 g

Catfish—Baked Or Broiled —Prepared with Oil ☛ Vitamin K = 7.8 mcg; Serving size: 1 small fillet, 113 g

Catfish—Baked Or Broiled —Prepared without Fat ☛ Vitamin K = 2.9 mcg; Serving size: 1 small fillet, 113 g

Catfish—Coated Fried—Prepared with Butter ☛ Vitamin K = 3.8 mcg; Serving size: 1 small fillet, 113 g

Catfish—Coated Fried—Prepared with Cooking Spray ☛ Vitamin K = 3.7 mcg; Serving size: 1 small fillet, 113 g

Catfish—Coated Fried—Prepared with Margarine ☛ Vitamin K = 13.1 mcg; Serving size: 1 small fillet, 113 g

Catfish—Coated Fried—Prepared with Oil ☛ Vitamin K = 14.8 mcg; Serving size: 1 small fillet, 113 g

Catfish—Coated Fried—Prepared without Fat ☛ Vitamin K = 3.7 mcg; Serving size: 1 small fillet, 113 g

Catfish—Coated—Baked Or Broiled —Prepared with Butter ☛ Vitamin K = 3.4 mcg; Serving size: 1 small fillet, 113 g

Catfish—Coated—Baked Or Broiled —Prepared with Cooking Spray ☛ Vitamin K = 3.1 mcg; Serving size: 1 small fillet, 113 g

Catfish—Coated—Baked Or Broiled —Prepared with Margarine ☛ Vitamin K = 9.6 mcg; Serving size: 1 small fillet, 113 g

Catfish—Coated—Baked Or Broiled —Prepared with Oil ☛ Vitamin K = 10.4 mcg; Serving size: 1 small fillet, 113 g

Catfish—Coated—Baked Or Broiled —Prepared without Fat ⮞ Vitamin K = 3.1 mcg; Serving size: 1 small fillet, 113 g

Catfish—Steamed Or Poached ⮞ Vitamin K = 2.9 mcg; Serving size: 1 small fillet, 113 g

Caviar Black And Red Granular ⮞ Vitamin K = 0.1 mcg; Serving size: 1 tbsp, 16 g

Ceviche ⮞ Vitamin K = 10.3 mcg; Serving size: 1 cup, 250 g

Cisco Smoked ⮞ Vitamin K = 0 mcg; Serving size: 1 oz, 28.4 g

Clam Cake Or Patty ⮞ Vitamin K = 28.8 mcg; Serving size: 1 cake or patty, 120 g

Clam Sauce White ⮞ Vitamin K = 27.8 mcg; Serving size: 1 cup, 240 g

Clams (Raw) ⮞ Vitamin K = 0.2 mcg; Serving size: 3 oz, 85 g

Clams Casino ⮞ Vitamin K = 2.9 mcg; Serving size: 1 clam, 30 g

Clams Smoked—In Oil ⮞ Vitamin K = 1.7 mcg; Serving size: 1 oz, 28 g

Clams Steamed Or Boiled ⮞ Vitamin K = 0.1 mcg; Serving size: 1 oz (without shell, cooked), 28 g

Clams Stuffed ⮞ Vitamin K = 3.2 mcg; Serving size: 1 small (12 in 11 oz frozen package), 26 g

Clams—Baked Or Broiled (Cooked with Fat) ⮞ Vitamin K = 1.3 mcg; Serving size: 1 oz (without shell, cooked), 28 g

Clams—Baked Or Broiled (Cooked without Fat) ⮞ Vitamin K = 0.1 mcg; Serving size: 1 oz (without shell, cooked), 28 g

Clams—Canned ⮞ Vitamin K = 0.1 mcg; Serving size: 1 oz, 28 g

Clams—Coated Fried ⮞ Vitamin K = 3.3 mcg; Serving size: 1 oz (without shell, cooked), 28 g

Clams—Coated—Baked Or Broiled (Cooked with Fat) ⮞ Vitamin K = 2 mcg; Serving size: 1 oz (without shell, cooked), 28 g

Clams—Coated—Baked Or Broiled (Cooked without Fat) ☛ Vitamin K = 0.2 mcg; Serving size: 1 oz (without shell, cooked), 28 g

Cod Atlantic Raw ☛ Vitamin K = 0.1 mcg; Serving size: 3 oz, 85 g

Cod Pacific Raw (Previously Frozen or Not) ☛ Vitamin K = 0 mcg; Serving size: 1 fillet, 116 g

Cod Smoked ☛ Vitamin K = 0 mcg; Serving size: 1 oz, boneless, 28 g

Cod—Baked Or Broiled —Prepared with Butter ☛ Vitamin K = 0.5 mcg; Serving size: 1 small fillet, 170 g

Cod—Baked Or Broiled —Prepared with Cooking Spray ☛ Vitamin K = 0 mcg; Serving size: 1 small fillet, 170 g

Cod—Baked Or Broiled —Prepared with Margarine ☛ Vitamin K = 6.6 mcg; Serving size: 1 small fillet, 170 g

Cod—Baked Or Broiled —Prepared with Oil ☛ Vitamin K = 7.3 mcg; Serving size: 1 small fillet, 170 g

Cod—Baked Or Broiled —Prepared without Fat ☛ Vitamin K = 0 mcg; Serving size: 1 small fillet, 170 g

Cod—Coated Fried—Prepared with Butter ☛ Vitamin K = 2.7 mcg; Serving size: 1 small fillet, 170 g

Cod—Coated Fried—Prepared with Cooking Spray ☛ Vitamin K = 2 mcg; Serving size: 1 small fillet, 170 g

Cod—Coated Fried—Prepared with Margarine ☛ Vitamin K = 16.7 mcg; Serving size: 1 small fillet, 170 g

Cod—Coated Fried—Prepared with Oil ☛ Vitamin K = 19.2 mcg; Serving size: 1 small fillet, 170 g

Cod—Coated Fried—Prepared without Fat ☛ Vitamin K = 2 mcg; Serving size: 1 small fillet, 170 g

Cod—Coated—Baked Or Broiled —Prepared with Butter ☛ Vitamin K = 1.7 mcg; Serving size: 1 small fillet, 170 g

Cod—Coated—Baked Or Broiled —Prepared with Cooking Spray ☞ Vitamin K = 1.2 mcg; Serving size: 1 small fillet, 170 g

Cod—Coated—Baked Or Broiled —Prepared with Margarine ☞ Vitamin K = 11.2 mcg; Serving size: 1 small fillet, 170 g

Cod—Coated—Baked Or Broiled —Prepared with Oil ☞ Vitamin K = 12.2 mcg; Serving size: 1 small fillet, 170 g

Cod—Coated—Baked Or Broiled —Prepared without Fat ☞ Vitamin K = 1.2 mcg; Serving size: 1 small fillet, 170 g

Cod—Steamed Or Poached ☞ Vitamin K = 0 mcg; Serving size: 1 small fillet, 170 g

Codfish Ball Or Cake ☞ Vitamin K = 5.1 mcg; Serving size: 1 ball, 63 g

Codfish Fritter Puerto Rican Style ☞ Vitamin K = 2.8 mcg; Serving size: 1 fritter (3-1/2" x 3-1/2"), 34 g

Codfish Salad Puerto Rican Style Serenata ☞ Vitamin K = 16.7 mcg; Serving size: 1 cup, 145 g

Codfish With Starchy Vegetables ☞ Vitamin K = 8 mcg; Serving size: 1 cup, 173 g

Codfish—Stewed (Puerto Rican Style) ☞ Vitamin K = 9.2 mcg; Serving size: 1 cup, 200 g

Crab Deviled ☞ Vitamin K = 41 mcg; Serving size: 1 cup, 175 g

Crab Hard Shell Steamed ☞ Vitamin K = 0.4 mcg; Serving size: 1 cup (cooked, flaked and pieces), 118 g

Crab Imperial ☞ Vitamin K = 15.5 mcg; Serving size: 1 cup, 259 g

Crab Salad ☞ Vitamin K = 84 mcg; Serving size: 1 cup, 208 g

Crab Salad—Prepared with—Imitation—Crab ☞ Vitamin K = 87.2 mcg; Serving size: 1 cup, 208 g

Crab Soft Shell—Coated Fried ☞ Vitamin K = 3.4 mcg; Serving size: 1

oz, cooked, 28 g

Crab—Baked Or Broiled (Cooked with Fat) ☛ Vitamin K = 5.4 mcg; Serving size: 1 cup (cooked, flaked and pieces), 118 g

Crab—Baked Or Broiled (Cooked without Fat) ☛ Vitamin K = 0.5 mcg; Serving size: 1 cup (cooked, flaked and pieces), 118 g

Crab—Coated—Baked Or Broiled (Cooked with Fat) ☛ Vitamin K = 8.6 mcg; Serving size: 1 cup (cooked, flaked and pieces), 118 g

Crab—Coated—Baked Or Broiled (Cooked without Fat) ☛ Vitamin K = 1.1 mcg; Serving size: 1 cup (cooked, flaked and pieces), 118 g

Crabs In Tomato-Based Sauce Puerto Rican Style ☛ Vitamin K = 16.7 mcg; Serving size: 1 cup, 170 g

Crayfish ☛ Vitamin K = 0.1 mcg; Serving size: 3 oz, 85 g

Crayfish Boiled Or Steamed ☛ Vitamin K = 0 mcg; Serving size: 1 oz (without shell, cooked), 28 g

Crayfish Mixed Species Wild Raw ☛ Vitamin K = 0.1 mcg; Serving size: 3 oz, 85 g

Crayfish—Coated Fried ☛ Vitamin K = 3.3 mcg; Serving size: 1 oz (without shell, cooked), 28 g

Croaker Atlantic Raw ☛ Vitamin K = 0.1 mcg; Serving size: 1 fillet, 79 g

Croaker—Baked Or Broiled (Cooked with Fat) ☛ Vitamin K = 5.1 mcg; Serving size: 1 small fillet, 113 g

Croaker—Baked Or Broiled (Cooked without Fat) ☛ Vitamin K = 0.1 mcg; Serving size: 1 small fillet, 113 g

Croaker—Coated Fried ☛ Vitamin K = 12.9 mcg; Serving size: 1 small fillet, 113 g

Croaker—Coated—Baked Or Broiled (Cooked with Fat) ☛ Vitamin K = 8.2 mcg; Serving size: 1 small fillet, 113 g

Croaker—Coated—Baked Or Broiled (Cooked without Fat) ☛ Vitamin K = 0.9 mcg; Serving size: 1 small fillet, 113 g

Croaker—Steamed Or Poached ☛ Vitamin K = 0.1 mcg; Serving size: 1 small fillet, 113 g

Dried Salted Atlantic Cod ☛ Vitamin K = 0.1 mcg; Serving size: 1 oz, 28.4 g

Eel Mixed Species Raw ☛ Vitamin K = 0 mcg; Serving size: 3 oz, 85 g

Eel Smoked ☛ Vitamin K = 0 mcg; Serving size: 1 oz, boneless, 28 g

Eel—Steamed Or Poached ☛ Vitamin K = 0 mcg; Serving size: 1 oz, boneless, raw, 23 g

Farmed Atlantic Salmon ☛ Vitamin K = 0.1 mcg; Serving size: 3 oz, 85 g

Farmed Atlantic Salmon (Raw) ☛ Vitamin K = 0.4 mcg; Serving size: 3 oz, 85 g

Fish And Noodles—With Mushroom Sauce ☛ Vitamin K = 18.8 mcg; Serving size: 1 cup, 224 g

Fish And Rice With Cream Sauce ☛ Vitamin K = 6.2 mcg; Serving size: 1 cup, 248 g

Fish And Rice With Mushroom Sauce ☛ Vitamin K = 23.6 mcg; Serving size: 1 cup, 248 g

Fish And Rice With Tomato-Based Sauce ☛ Vitamin K = 16.1 mcg; Serving size: 1 cup, 248 g

Fish And Vegetables Excluding Carrots Broccoli And Dark- Green Leafy; No Potatoes Tomato-Based Sauce ☛ Vitamin K = 33.8 mcg; Serving size: 1 cup, 224 g

Fish And Vegetables Including Carrots Broccoli And/or Dark-Green Leafy; No Potatoes Tomato-Based Sauce ☛ Vitamin K = 55.3 mcg; Serving size: 1 cup, 224 g

Fish Curry ☛ Vitamin K = 115.9 mcg; Serving size: 1 cup, 236 g

Fish In Lemon-Butter Sauce With Starch Item Vegetable Frozen Meal ☛ Vitamin K = 17.3 mcg; Serving size: 1 meal (10 oz), 284 g

Fish Moochim ☛ Vitamin K = 0.2 mcg; Serving size: 1 tablespoon, 5 g

Fish Noodles—And Vegetables Excluding Carrots Broccoli And Dark-Green Leafy; Cheese Sauce ☛ Vitamin K = 9.3 mcg; Serving size: 1 cup, 244 g

Fish Noodles—And Vegetables Including Carrots Broccoli And/or Dark Green Leafy; Cheese Sauce ☛ Vitamin K = 23.2 mcg; Serving size: 1 cup, 244 g

Fish Shish Kabob With Vegetables Excluding Potatoes ☛ Vitamin K = 10.1 mcg; Serving size: 1 shishkabob, 202 g

Fish Timbale Or Mousse ☛ Vitamin K = 1.6 mcg; Serving size: 1 cup, 175 g

Fish Tofu And Vegetables Tempura ☛ Vitamin K = 18.6 mcg; Serving size: 1 cup, 63 g

Fish With Tomato-Based Sauce ☛ Vitamin K = 2 mcg; Serving size: 1 cup, 222 g

Flat Fish (Flounder Or Sole) ☛ Vitamin K = 0.1 mcg; Serving size: 1 fillet, 127 g

Flatfish (Flounder And Sole Species) Raw ☛ Vitamin K = 0 mcg; Serving size: 1 oz, boneless, 28.4 g

Flounder Smoked ☛ Vitamin K = 0.1 mcg; Serving size: 1 oz, boneless, 28 g

Flounder With Chopped Broccoli Diet Frozen Meal ☛ Vitamin K = 119 mcg; Serving size: 1 meal (12.4 oz), 351 g

Flounder With Crab Stuffing ☛ Vitamin K = 30.5 mcg; Serving size: 1 piece, 210 g

Flounder—Baked Or Broiled —Prepared with Butter ☛ Vitamin K = 0.5 mcg; Serving size: 1 small fillet, 113 g

Flounder—Baked Or Broiled —Prepared with Cooking Spray ☛ Vitamin K = 0.1 mcg; Serving size: 1 small fillet, 113 g

Flounder—Baked Or Broiled —Prepared with Margarine ☛ Vitamin K = 4.5 mcg; Serving size: 1 small fillet, 113 g

Flounder—Baked Or Broiled —Prepared with Oil ☛ Vitamin K = 5.1 mcg; Serving size: 1 small fillet, 113 g

Flounder—Baked Or Broiled —Prepared without Fat ☛ Vitamin K = 0.1 mcg; Serving size: 1 small fillet, 113 g

Flounder—Coated Fried—Prepared with Butter ☛ Vitamin K = 1.9 mcg; Serving size: 1 small fillet, 113 g

Flounder—Coated Fried—Prepared with Cooking Spray ☛ Vitamin K = 1.5 mcg; Serving size: 1 small fillet, 113 g

Flounder—Coated Fried—Prepared with Margarine ☛ Vitamin K = 11.2 mcg; Serving size: 1 small fillet, 113 g

Flounder—Coated Fried—Prepared with Oil ☛ Vitamin K = 12.9 mcg; Serving size: 1 small fillet, 113 g

Flounder—Coated Fried—Prepared without Fat ☛ Vitamin K = 1.5 mcg; Serving size: 1 small fillet, 113 g

Flounder—Coated—Baked Or Broiled —Prepared with Butter ☛ Vitamin K = 1.2 mcg; Serving size: 1 small fillet, 113 g

Flounder—Coated—Baked Or Broiled —Prepared with Cooking Spray ☛ Vitamin K = 0.9 mcg; Serving size: 1 small fillet, 113 g

Flounder—Coated—Baked Or Broiled —Prepared with Margarine ☛ Vitamin K = 7.6 mcg; Serving size: 1 small fillet, 113 g

Flounder—Coated—Baked Or Broiled —Prepared with Oil ☛ Vitamin K = 8.2 mcg; Serving size: 1 small fillet, 113 g

Flounder—Coated—Baked Or Broiled —Prepared without Fat ☞ Vitamin K = 0.9 mcg; Serving size: 1 small fillet, 113 g

Flounder—Steamed Or Poached ☞ Vitamin K = 0.1 mcg; Serving size: 1 small fillet, 113 g

Fried Fish With Sauce Puerto Rican Style ☞ Vitamin K = 12.4 mcg; Serving size: 1 slice (4" x 3-1/2" x 1/2") with sauce, 213 g

Frog Legs Raw ☞ Vitamin K = 0 mcg; Serving size: 1 leg, 45 g

Frog Legs Steamed ☞ Vitamin K = 0 mcg; Serving size: 1 oz, boneless, cooked, 28 g

Gefilte Fish ☞ Vitamin K = 0.5 mcg; Serving size: 1 cup, 227 g

Gumbo No Rice ☞ Vitamin K = 12.9 mcg; Serving size: 1 cup, 244 g

Gumbo With Rice ☞ Vitamin K = 12 mcg; Serving size: 1 cup, 244 g

Haddock Cake Or Patty ☞ Vitamin K = 7.2 mcg; Serving size: 1 cake or patty, 120 g

Haddock Raw ☞ Vitamin K = 0.1 mcg; Serving size: 3 oz, 85 g

Haddock With Chopped Spinach Diet Frozen Meal ☞ Vitamin K = 104 mcg; Serving size: 1 meal (9 oz), 255 g

Haddock—Baked Or Broiled (Cooked with Fat) ☞ Vitamin K = 7.7 mcg; Serving size: 1 small fillet, 170 g

Haddock—Baked Or Broiled (Cooked without Fat) ☞ Vitamin K = 0.2 mcg; Serving size: 1 small fillet, 170 g

Haddock—Coated Fried ☞ Vitamin K = 19.4 mcg; Serving size: 1 small fillet, 170 g

Haddock—Coated—Baked Or Broiled (Cooked with Fat) ☞ Vitamin K = 12.4 mcg; Serving size: 1 small fillet, 170 g

Haddock—Coated—Baked Or Broiled (Cooked without Fat) ☞ Vitamin K = 1.4 mcg; Serving size: 1 small fillet, 170 g

Haddock—Steamed Or Poached ☞ Vitamin K = 0.2 mcg; Serving size: 1 small fillet, 170 g

Halibut Atlantic And Pacific Raw ☞ Vitamin K = 0 mcg; Serving size: 3 oz, 85 g

Halibut Greenland Raw ☞ Vitamin K = 0.1 mcg; Serving size: 3 oz, 85 g

Halibut Smoked ☞ Vitamin K = 0 mcg; Serving size: 1 oz, boneless, 28 g

Halibut—Baked Or Broiled —Prepared with Butter ☞ Vitamin K = 0.5 mcg; Serving size: 1 small fillet, 170 g

Halibut—Baked Or Broiled —Prepared with Cooking Spray ☞ Vitamin K = 0 mcg; Serving size: 1 small fillet, 170 g

Halibut—Baked Or Broiled —Prepared with Margarine ☞ Vitamin K = 6.6 mcg; Serving size: 1 small fillet, 170 g

Halibut—Baked Or Broiled —Prepared with Oil ☞ Vitamin K = 7.3 mcg; Serving size: 1 small fillet, 170 g

Halibut—Baked Or Broiled —Prepared without Fat ☞ Vitamin K = 0 mcg; Serving size: 1 small fillet, 170 g

Halibut—Coated Fried—Prepared with Butter ☞ Vitamin K = 2.7 mcg; Serving size: 1 small fillet, 170 g

Halibut—Coated Fried—Prepared with Cooking Spray ☞ Vitamin K = 2 mcg; Serving size: 1 small fillet, 170 g

Halibut—Coated Fried—Prepared with Margarine ☞ Vitamin K = 16.7 mcg; Serving size: 1 small fillet, 170 g

Halibut—Coated Fried—Prepared with Oil ☞ Vitamin K = 19.2 mcg; Serving size: 1 small fillet, 170 g

Halibut—Coated Fried—Prepared without Fat ☞ Vitamin K = 2 mcg; Serving size: 1 small fillet, 170 g

Halibut—Coated—Baked Or Broiled —Prepared with Butter ☛ Vitamin K = 1.7 mcg; Serving size: 1 small fillet, 170 g

Halibut—Coated—Baked Or Broiled —Prepared with Cooking Spray ☛ Vitamin K = 1.2 mcg; Serving size: 1 small fillet, 170 g

Halibut—Coated—Baked Or Broiled —Prepared with Margarine ☛ Vitamin K = 11.2 mcg; Serving size: 1 small fillet, 170 g

Halibut—Coated—Baked Or Broiled —Prepared with Oil ☛ Vitamin K = 12.2 mcg; Serving size: 1 small fillet, 170 g

Halibut—Coated—Baked Or Broiled —Prepared without Fat ☛ Vitamin K = 1.2 mcg; Serving size: 1 small fillet, 170 g

Halibut—Steamed Or Poached ☛ Vitamin K = 0 mcg; Serving size: 1 small fillet, 170 g

Herring Atlantic Raw ☛ Vitamin K = 0 mcg; Serving size: 1 oz, boneless, 28.4 g

Herring—Baked Or Broiled (Cooked with Fat) ☛ Vitamin K = 1 mcg; Serving size: 1 oz, boneless, raw, 23 g

Herring—Baked Or Broiled (Cooked without Fat) ☛ Vitamin K = 0 mcg; Serving size: 1 oz, boneless, raw, 23 g

Herring—Coated Fried ☛ Vitamin K = 3.1 mcg; Serving size: 1 oz, boneless, raw, 27 g

Herring—Coated—Baked Or Broiled (Cooked with Fat) ☛ Vitamin K = 2 mcg; Serving size: 1 oz, boneless, raw, 27 g

Herring—Coated—Baked Or Broiled (Cooked without Fat) ☛ Vitamin K = 0.2 mcg; Serving size: 1 oz, boneless, raw, 27 g

Herring—Dried Salted ☛ Vitamin K = 0.1 mcg; Serving size: 1 oz, boneless, 28 g

Herring—Pickled In Cream Sauce ☛ Vitamin K = 0.1 mcg; Serving size: 1 oz, boneless, 28 g

Imitation Crab Meat ☛ Vitamin K = 0.3 mcg; Serving size: 3 oz, 85 g

Jellyfish—Dried Salted ☛ Vitamin K = 0.1 mcg; Serving size: 1 cup, 58 g

Kippered Herring ☛ Vitamin K = 0 mcg; Serving size: 1 oz, boneless, 28.4 g

Lau Lau ☛ Vitamin K = 0 mcg; Serving size: 1 lau lau, 214 g

Lobster (Cooked) ☛ Vitamin K = 0 mcg; Serving size: 1 cup, 145 g

Lobster Gumbo ☛ Vitamin K = 21.7 mcg; Serving size: 1 cup, 244 g

Lobster Newburg ☛ Vitamin K = 4.1 mcg; Serving size: 1 cup, 244 g

Lobster Northern Raw ☛ Vitamin K = 0 mcg; Serving size: 1 lobster, 150 g

Lobster Salad ☛ Vitamin K = 70.6 mcg; Serving size: 1 cup, 182 g

Lobster Steamed Or Boiled ☛ Vitamin K = 0 mcg; Serving size: 1 small lobster (1 lb live weight), 118 g

Lobster With Bread Stuffing Baked ☛ Vitamin K = 2.8 mcg; Serving size: 1 lobster, 400 g

Lobster With Butter Sauce ☛ Vitamin K = 1.5 mcg; Serving size: 1 cup, 188 g

Lobster With Sauce Puerto Rican Style ☛ Vitamin K = 19.6 mcg; Serving size: 1 cup, 242 g

Lobster—Baked Or Broiled (Cooked with Fat) ☛ Vitamin K = 5 mcg; Serving size: 1 small lobster (1 lb live weight), 118 g

Lobster—Baked Or Broiled (Cooked without Fat) ☛ Vitamin K = 0 mcg; Serving size: 1 small lobster (1 lb live weight), 118 g

Lobster—Coated Fried ☛ Vitamin K = 3.3 mcg; Serving size: 1 oz (without shell, cooked), 28 g

Lobster—Coated—Baked Or Broiled (Cooked with Fat) ☛ Vitamin K

= 8.4 mcg; Serving size: 1 small lobster (1 lb live weight), 118 g

Lobster—Coated—Baked Or Broiled (Cooked without Fat) ☞ Vitamin K = 0.7 mcg; Serving size: 1 small lobster (1 lb live weight), 118 g

Lomi Salmon ☞ Vitamin K = 54.1 mcg; Serving size: 1 cup, 234 g

Mackerel Cake Or Patty ☞ Vitamin K = 7.9 mcg; Serving size: 1 cake or patty, 120 g

Mackerel Jack—Canned Drained Solids ☞ Vitamin K = 0 mcg; Serving size: 1 oz, boneless, 28.4 g

Mackerel Pacific And Jack Mixed Species Raw ☞ Vitamin K = 0.1 mcg; Serving size: 3 oz, 85 g

Mackerel Pacific And Jack Mixed Species—Cooked—Dry Heat ☞ Vitamin K = 0 mcg; Serving size: 1 oz, boneless, 28.4 g

Mackerel Raw ☞ Vitamin K = 1 mcg; Serving size: 1 oz, boneless, raw, 28 g

Mackerel Salted ☞ Vitamin K = 6.2 mcg; Serving size: 1 piece (5-1/2 inch x 1-1/2 inch x 1/2 inch), 80 g

Mackerel Smoked ☞ Vitamin K = 0 mcg; Serving size: 1 oz, boneless, 28 g

Mackerel Spanish Raw ☞ Vitamin K = 0.1 mcg; Serving size: 3 oz, 85 g

Mackerel—Baked Or Broiled (Cooked with Fat) ☞ Vitamin K = 14.3 mcg; Serving size: 1 small fillet, 170 g

Mackerel—Baked Or Broiled (Cooked without Fat) ☞ Vitamin K = 7.1 mcg; Serving size: 1 small fillet, 170 g

Mackerel—Coated Fried ☞ Vitamin K = 24 mcg; Serving size: 1 small fillet, 170 g

Mackerel—Coated—Baked Or Broiled (Cooked with Fat) ☞ Vitamin K = 17.7 mcg; Serving size: 1 small fillet, 170 g

Mackerel—Coated—Baked Or Broiled (Cooked without Fat) ☛ Vitamin K = 6.6 mcg; Serving size: 1 small fillet, 170 g

Mackerel—Pickled ☛ Vitamin K = 2.4 mcg; Serving size: 1 oz, boneless, 28 g

Mollusks Abalone Mixed Species Raw ☛ Vitamin K = 19.6 mcg; Serving size: 3 oz, 85 g

Mollusks Clam Mixed Species—Canned Liquid ☛ Vitamin K = 0.2 mcg; Serving size: 3 oz, 85 g

Mollusks Mussel Blue Raw ☛ Vitamin K = 0.2 mcg; Serving size: 1 cup, 150 g

Mollusks Octopus Common Raw ☛ Vitamin K = 0.1 mcg; Serving size: 3 oz, 85 g

Mollusks Oyster Eastern Wild Raw ☛ Vitamin K = 0.8 mcg; Serving size: 6 medium, 84 g

Mollusks Snail Raw ☛ Vitamin K = 0.1 mcg; Serving size: 3 oz, 85 g

Mollusks Whelk Unspecified Raw ☛ Vitamin K = 0.1 mcg; Serving size: 3 oz, 85 g

Mullet Striped Raw ☛ Vitamin K = 0 mcg; Serving size: 1 oz, 28.4 g

Mullet—Baked Or Broiled (Cooked with Fat) ☛ Vitamin K = 5.1 mcg; Serving size: 1 small fillet, 113 g

Mullet—Baked Or Broiled (Cooked without Fat) ☛ Vitamin K = 0.1 mcg; Serving size: 1 small fillet, 113 g

Mullet—Coated Fried ☛ Vitamin K = 12.9 mcg; Serving size: 1 small fillet, 113 g

Mullet—Coated—Baked Or Broiled (Cooked with Fat) ☛ Vitamin K = 8.2 mcg; Serving size: 1 small fillet, 113 g

Mullet—Coated—Baked Or Broiled (Cooked without Fat) ☛ Vitamin K = 0.9 mcg; Serving size: 1 small fillet, 113 g

Mullet—Steamed Or Poached ☛ Vitamin K = 0.1 mcg; Serving size: 1 small fillet, 113 g

Mussels With Tomato-Based Sauce ☛ Vitamin K = 1.9 mcg; Serving size: 1 cup, 240 g

Mussels—Steamed Or Poached ☛ Vitamin K = 0.1 mcg; Serving size: 1 oz, cooked, 28 g

Ocean Perch Atlantic Raw ☛ Vitamin K = 0 mcg; Serving size: 1 oz, boneless, 28.4 g

Ocean Perch—Baked Or Broiled (Cooked with Fat) ☛ Vitamin K = 5.1 mcg; Serving size: 1 small fillet, 113 g

Ocean Perch—Baked Or Broiled (Cooked without Fat) ☛ Vitamin K = 0.1 mcg; Serving size: 1 small fillet, 113 g

Ocean Perch—Coated Fried ☛ Vitamin K = 12.9 mcg; Serving size: 1 small fillet, 113 g

Ocean Perch—Coated—Baked Or Broiled (Cooked with Fat) ☛ Vitamin K = 8.2 mcg; Serving size: 1 small fillet, 113 g

Ocean Perch—Coated—Baked Or Broiled (Cooked without Fat) ☛ Vitamin K = 0.9 mcg; Serving size: 1 small fillet, 113 g

Ocean Perch—Steamed Or Poached ☛ Vitamin K = 0.1 mcg; Serving size: 1 small fillet, 113 g

Octopus (Cooked) ☛ Vitamin K = 0.1 mcg; Serving size: 3 oz, 85 g

Octopus Salad Puerto Rican Style ☛ Vitamin K = 17.6 mcg; Serving size: 1 cup, 180 g

Octopus Smoked ☛ Vitamin K = 0.1 mcg; Serving size: 1 oz, boneless, cooked, 28 g

Octopus Steamed ☛ Vitamin K = 0 mcg; Serving size: 1 oz, boneless, cooked, 28 g

Octopus—Dried ☛ Vitamin K = 0.1 mcg; Serving size: 1 oz, 28 g

Octopus—Dried Boiled ☞ Vitamin K = 0.1 mcg; Serving size: 1 cup, cooked, 106 g

Oyster Fritter ☞ Vitamin K = 9.7 mcg; Serving size: 1 fritter, 40 g

Oyster Pie ☞ Vitamin K = 77.4 mcg; Serving size: 1 pie, 656 g

Oysters Rockefeller ☞ Vitamin K = 37.7 mcg; Serving size: 1 oyster, no shell, 24 g

Oysters Smoked ☞ Vitamin K = 0.4 mcg; Serving size: 1 oz, 28 g

Oysters Steamed ☞ Vitamin K = 0.6 mcg; Serving size: 1 oz (without shell, cooked), 28 g

Oysters—Baked Or Broiled (Cooked with Fat) ☞ Vitamin K = 1.5 mcg; Serving size: 1 oz (without shell, cooked), 28 g

Oysters—Baked Or Broiled (Cooked without Fat) ☞ Vitamin K = 0.3 mcg; Serving size: 1 oz (without shell, cooked), 28 g

Oysters—Canned ☞ Vitamin K = 0 mcg; Serving size: 1 oz, cooked, 28 g

Oysters—Coated Fried ☞ Vitamin K = 3.5 mcg; Serving size: 1 oz (without shell, cooked), 28 g

Oysters—Coated—Baked Or Broiled (Cooked with Fat) ☞ Vitamin K = 2.2 mcg; Serving size: 1 oz (without shell, cooked), 28 g

Oysters—Coated—Baked Or Broiled (Cooked without Fat) ☞ Vitamin K = 0.4 mcg; Serving size: 1 oz (without shell, cooked), 28 g

Perch Mixed Species Raw ☞ Vitamin K = 0.1 mcg; Serving size: 1 fillet, 60 g

Perch—Baked Or Broiled —Prepared with Butter ☞ Vitamin K = 0.5 mcg; Serving size: 1 small fillet, 113 g

Perch—Baked Or Broiled —Prepared with Cooking Spray ☞ Vitamin K = 0.1 mcg; Serving size: 1 small fillet, 113 g

Perch—Baked Or Broiled —Prepared with Margarine ☞ Vitamin K = 4.5 mcg; Serving size: 1 small fillet, 113 g

Perch—Baked Or Broiled —Prepared with Oil ☞ Vitamin K = 5.1 mcg; Serving size: 1 small fillet, 113 g

Perch—Baked Or Broiled —Prepared without Fat ☞ Vitamin K = 0.1 mcg; Serving size: 1 small fillet, 113 g

Perch—Coated Fried—Prepared with Butter ☞ Vitamin K = 1.9 mcg; Serving size: 1 small fillet, 113 g

Perch—Coated Fried—Prepared with Cooking Spray ☞ Vitamin K = 1.5 mcg; Serving size: 1 small fillet, 113 g

Perch—Coated Fried—Prepared with Margarine ☞ Vitamin K = 11.2 mcg; Serving size: 1 small fillet, 113 g

Perch—Coated Fried—Prepared with Oil ☞ Vitamin K = 12.9 mcg; Serving size: 1 small fillet, 113 g

Perch—Coated Fried—Prepared without Fat ☞ Vitamin K = 1.5 mcg; Serving size: 1 small fillet, 113 g

Perch—Coated—Baked Or Broiled —Prepared with Butter ☞ Vitamin K = 1.2 mcg; Serving size: 1 small fillet, 113 g

Perch—Coated—Baked Or Broiled —Prepared with Cooking Spray ☞ Vitamin K = 0.9 mcg; Serving size: 1 small fillet, 113 g

Perch—Coated—Baked Or Broiled —Prepared with Margarine ☞ Vitamin K = 7.6 mcg; Serving size: 1 small fillet, 113 g

Perch—Coated—Baked Or Broiled —Prepared with Oil ☞ Vitamin K = 8.2 mcg; Serving size: 1 small fillet, 113 g

Perch—Coated—Baked Or Broiled —Prepared without Fat ☞ Vitamin K = 0.9 mcg; Serving size: 1 small fillet, 113 g

Perch—Steamed Or Poached ☞ Vitamin K = 0.1 mcg; Serving size: 1 small fillet, 113 g

Pickled Herring ☛ Vitamin K = 0.3 mcg; Serving size: 1 cup, 140 g

Pike Northern Raw ☛ Vitamin K = 0.1 mcg; Serving size: 3 oz, 85 g

Pike—Baked Or Broiled (Cooked with Fat) ☛ Vitamin K = 7.7 mcg; Serving size: 1 small fillet, 170 g

Pike—Baked Or Broiled (Cooked without Fat) ☛ Vitamin K = 0.2 mcg; Serving size: 1 small fillet, 170 g

Pike—Coated Fried ☛ Vitamin K = 19.4 mcg; Serving size: 1 small fillet, 170 g

Pike—Coated—Baked Or Broiled (Cooked with Fat) ☛ Vitamin K = 12.4 mcg; Serving size: 1 small fillet, 170 g

Pike—Coated—Baked Or Broiled (Cooked without Fat) ☛ Vitamin K = 1.4 mcg; Serving size: 1 small fillet, 170 g

Pike—Steamed Or Poached ☛ Vitamin K = 0.2 mcg; Serving size: 1 small fillet, 170 g

Pink Salmon (Raw) ☛ Vitamin K = 0.3 mcg; Serving size: 3 oz, 85 g

Pollock Alaska Raw (Previously Frozen or Not) ☛ Vitamin K = 0 mcg; Serving size: 1 fillet, 77 g

Pollock Atlantic Raw ☛ Vitamin K = 0.1 mcg; Serving size: 3 oz, 85 g

Pompano Florida Raw ☛ Vitamin K = 0 mcg; Serving size: 1 oz, boneless, 28.4 g

Pompano Smoked ☛ Vitamin K = 0 mcg; Serving size: 1 oz, boneless, 28 g

Pompano—Baked Or Broiled (Cooked with Fat) ☛ Vitamin K = 5.1 mcg; Serving size: 1 small fillet, 113 g

Pompano—Baked Or Broiled (Cooked without Fat) ☛ Vitamin K = 0.1 mcg; Serving size: 1 small fillet, 113 g

Pompano—Coated Fried ☞ Vitamin K = 12.9 mcg; Serving size: 1 small fillet, 113 g

Pompano—Coated—Baked Or Broiled (Cooked with Fat) ☞ Vitamin K = 8.2 mcg; Serving size: 1 small fillet, 113 g

Pompano—Coated—Baked Or Broiled (Cooked without Fat) ☞ Vitamin K = 0.9 mcg; Serving size: 1 small fillet, 113 g

Pompano—Steamed Or Poached ☞ Vitamin K = 0.1 mcg; Serving size: 1 small fillet, 113 g

Porgy—Baked Or Broiled (Cooked with Fat) ☞ Vitamin K = 5.1 mcg; Serving size: 1 small fillet, 113 g

Porgy—Baked Or Broiled (Cooked without Fat) ☞ Vitamin K = 0.1 mcg; Serving size: 1 small fillet, 113 g

Porgy—Coated Fried ☞ Vitamin K = 12.9 mcg; Serving size: 1 small fillet, 113 g

Porgy—Coated—Baked Or Broiled (Cooked with Fat) ☞ Vitamin K = 8.2 mcg; Serving size: 1 small fillet, 113 g

Porgy—Coated—Baked Or Broiled (Cooked without Fat) ☞ Vitamin K = 0.9 mcg; Serving size: 1 small fillet, 113 g

Porgy—Steamed Or Poached ☞ Vitamin K = 0.1 mcg; Serving size: 1 small fillet, 113 g

Rainbow Trout (Raw) ☞ Vitamin K = 0.1 mcg; Serving size: 1 fillet, 79 g

Ray—Baked Or Broiled (Cooked with Fat) ☞ Vitamin K = 1 mcg; Serving size: 1 oz, boneless, raw, 23 g

Ray—Baked Or Broiled (Cooked without Fat) ☞ Vitamin K = 0 mcg; Serving size: 1 oz, boneless, raw, 23 g

Ray—Coated Fried ☞ Vitamin K = 3.1 mcg; Serving size: 1 oz, boneless, raw, 27 g

Ray—Coated—Baked Or Broiled (Cooked with Fat) ☞ Vitamin K = 2 mcg; Serving size: 1 oz, boneless, raw, 27 g

Ray—Coated—Baked Or Broiled (Cooked without Fat) ☞ Vitamin K = 0.2 mcg; Serving size: 1 oz, boneless, raw, 27 g

Ray—Steamed Or Poached ☞ Vitamin K = 0 mcg; Serving size: 1 oz, boneless, raw, 23 g

Rockfish Pacific Mixed Species Raw ☞ Vitamin K = 0 mcg; Serving size: 3 oz, 85 g

Rockfish Pacific Mixed Species—Cooked—Dry Heat ☞ Vitamin K = 0 mcg; Serving size: 1 fillet, 149 g

Roe ☞ Vitamin K = 0 mcg; Serving size: 1 tbsp, 14 g

Roe Shad Cooked ☞ Vitamin K = 1.3 mcg; Serving size: 1 oz, 28 g

Roughy Orange Raw ☞ Vitamin K = 0.6 mcg; Serving size: 3 oz, 85 g

Salmon Cake Or Patty ☞ Vitamin K = 15.1 mcg; Serving size: 1 ball, 63 g

Salmon Chum—Canned Drained Solids With Bone ☞ Vitamin K = 0.1 mcg; Serving size: 3 oz, 85 g

Salmon Coho Wild Raw ☞ Vitamin K = 0.1 mcg; Serving size: 3 oz, 85 g

Salmon Loaf ☞ Vitamin K = 18 mcg; Serving size: 1 slice, 105 g

Salmon Pink—Canned Total Can Contents ☞ Vitamin K = 0.4 mcg; Serving size: 3 oz, 85 g

Salmon Pink—Cooked—Dry Heat ☞ Vitamin K = 0.4 mcg; Serving size: 3 oz, 85 g

Salmon Salad ☞ Vitamin K = 89.4 mcg; Serving size: 1 cup, 208 g

Salmon Sockeye Raw ☞ Vitamin K = 0 mcg; Serving size: 1 oz, boneless, 28.4 g

Salmon—Baked Or Broiled —Prepared with Butter ☞ Vitamin K =

1.4 mcg; Serving size: 1 small fillet, 170 g

Salmon—Baked Or Broiled —Prepared with Cooking Spray ☞ Vitamin K = 0.9 mcg; Serving size: 1 small fillet, 170 g

Salmon—Baked Or Broiled —Prepared with Margarine ☞ Vitamin K = 7.5 mcg; Serving size: 1 small fillet, 170 g

Salmon—Baked Or Broiled —Prepared with Oil ☞ Vitamin K = 8.2 mcg; Serving size: 1 small fillet, 170 g

Salmon—Baked Or Broiled —Prepared without Fat ☞ Vitamin K = 0.9 mcg; Serving size: 1 small fillet, 170 g

Salmon—Canned ☞ Vitamin K = 0.1 mcg; Serving size: 1 oz, 28 g

Salmon—Coated Fried—Prepared with Butter ☞ Vitamin K = 3.4 mcg; Serving size: 1 small fillet, 170 g

Salmon—Coated Fried—Prepared with Cooking Spray ☞ Vitamin K = 2.7 mcg; Serving size: 1 small fillet, 170 g

Salmon—Coated Fried—Prepared with Margarine ☞ Vitamin K = 17.3 mcg; Serving size: 1 small fillet, 170 g

Salmon—Coated Fried—Prepared with Oil ☞ Vitamin K = 19.7 mcg; Serving size: 1 small fillet, 170 g

Salmon—Coated Fried—Prepared without Fat ☞ Vitamin K = 2.7 mcg; Serving size: 1 small fillet, 170 g

Salmon—Coated—Baked Or Broiled —Prepared with Butter ☞ Vitamin K = 2.4 mcg; Serving size: 1 small fillet, 170 g

Salmon—Coated—Baked Or Broiled —Prepared with Cooking Spray ☞ Vitamin K = 1.7 mcg; Serving size: 1 small fillet, 170 g

Salmon—Coated—Baked Or Broiled —Prepared with Margarine ☞ Vitamin K = 11.9 mcg; Serving size: 1 small fillet, 170 g

Salmon—Coated—Baked Or Broiled —Prepared with Oil ☞ Vitamin K = 12.9 mcg; Serving size: 1 small fillet, 170 g

Salmon—Coated—Baked Or Broiled —Prepared without Fat ☛ Vitamin K = 1.7 mcg; Serving size: 1 small fillet, 170 g

Salmon—Dried ☛ Vitamin K = 0.3 mcg; Serving size: 1 oz, boneless, 28 g

Salmon—Steamed Or Poached ☛ Vitamin K = 0.9 mcg; Serving size: 1 small fillet, 170 g

Sardine Pacific—Canned In Tomato Sauce Drained Solids With Bone ☛ Vitamin K = 0.4 mcg; Serving size: 1 cup, 89 g

Sardines—Dried ☛ Vitamin K = 0.1 mcg; Serving size: 1 oz, 28 g

Scallops ☛ Vitamin K = 0 mcg; Serving size: 3 oz, 85 g

Scallops (Raw) ☛ Vitamin K = 0 mcg; Serving size: 1 unit 2 large or 5 small, 30 g

Scallops And Noodles—With Cheese Sauce ☛ Vitamin K = 0.7 mcg; Serving size: 1 cup, 224 g

Scallops Steamed Or Boiled ☛ Vitamin K = 0 mcg; Serving size: 1 cup, raw, yield cooked, 120 g

Scallops With Cheese Sauce ☛ Vitamin K = 0.7 mcg; Serving size: 1 cup, 244 g

Scallops—Baked Or Broiled (Cooked with Fat) ☛ Vitamin K = 6 mcg; Serving size: 1 cup, raw, yield cooked, 144 g

Scallops—Baked Or Broiled (Cooked without Fat) ☛ Vitamin K = 0 mcg; Serving size: 1 cup, raw, yield cooked, 144 g

Scallops—Coated Fried ☛ Vitamin K = 3.3 mcg; Serving size: 1 oz, cooked, 28 g

Scallops—Coated—Baked Or Broiled (Cooked with Fat) ☛ Vitamin K = 2 mcg; Serving size: 1 oz, cooked, 28 g

Scallops—Coated—Baked Or Broiled (Cooked without Fat) ☛ Vitamin K = 0.2 mcg; Serving size: 1 oz, cooked, 28 g

Scup Raw ☞ Vitamin K = 0.1 mcg; Serving size: 3 oz, 85 g

Sea Bass Mixed Species Raw ☞ Vitamin K = 0.1 mcg; Serving size: 1 fillet, 129 g

Sea Bass—Baked Or Broiled (Cooked with Fat) ☞ Vitamin K = 5.1 mcg; Serving size: 1 small fillet, 113 g

Sea Bass—Baked Or Broiled (Cooked without Fat) ☞ Vitamin K = 0.1 mcg; Serving size: 1 small fillet, 113 g

Sea Bass—Coated Fried ☞ Vitamin K = 12.9 mcg; Serving size: 1 small fillet, 113 g

Sea Bass—Coated—Baked Or Broiled (Cooked with Fat) ☞ Vitamin K = 8.2 mcg; Serving size: 1 small fillet, 113 g

Sea Bass—Coated—Baked Or Broiled (Cooked without Fat) ☞ Vitamin K = 0.9 mcg; Serving size: 1 small fillet, 113 g

Sea Bass—Pickled ☞ Vitamin K = 1.6 mcg; Serving size: 1 oz, boneless, 28 g

Sea Bass—Steamed Or Poached ☞ Vitamin K = 0.1 mcg; Serving size: 1 small fillet, 113 g

Seafood Garden Salad With Seafood Lettuce Eggs Tomato And/or Carrots Other Vegetables No Dressing ☞ Vitamin K = 58.4 mcg; Serving size: 1 cup, 95 g

Seafood Garden Salad With Seafood Lettuce Eggs Vegetables Excluding Tomato And Carrots No Dressing ☞ Vitamin K = 61.2 mcg; Serving size: 1 cup, 95 g

Seafood Garden Salad With Seafood Lettuce Tomato And/or Carrots Other Vegetables No Dressing ☞ Vitamin K = 68.3 mcg; Serving size: 1 cup, 95 g

Seafood Garden Salad With Seafood Lettuce Vegetables Excluding Tomato And Carrots No Dressing ☞ Vitamin K = 72.3 mcg; Serving size: 1 cup, 95 g

Seafood Newburg ☛ Vitamin K = 4.4 mcg; Serving size: 1 cup, 244 g

Seafood Salad ☛ Vitamin K = 83.6 mcg; Serving size: 1 cup, 208 g

Shad American Raw ☛ Vitamin K = 0.1 mcg; Serving size: 3 oz, 85 g

Shark Mixed Species Raw ☛ Vitamin K = 0.1 mcg; Serving size: 3 oz, 85 g

Shark—Baked Or Broiled (Cooked with Fat) ☛ Vitamin K = 7.7 mcg; Serving size: 1 small fillet, 170 g

Shark—Baked Or Broiled (Cooked without Fat) ☛ Vitamin K = 0.2 mcg; Serving size: 1 small fillet, 170 g

Shark—Coated Fried ☛ Vitamin K = 19.4 mcg; Serving size: 1 small fillet, 170 g

Shark—Coated—Baked Or Broiled (Cooked with Fat) ☛ Vitamin K = 12.4 mcg; Serving size: 1 small fillet, 170 g

Shark—Coated—Baked Or Broiled (Cooked without Fat) ☛ Vitamin K = 1.4 mcg; Serving size: 1 small fillet, 170 g

Shark—Steamed Or Poached ☛ Vitamin K = 0.2 mcg; Serving size: 1 small fillet, 170 g

Shellfish And Noodles—With Tomato-Based Sauce ☛ Vitamin K = 11.6 mcg; Serving size: 1 cup, 224 g

Shellfish Mixture And Vegetables Excluding Carrots Broccoli And Dark-Green Leafy; No Potatoes Mushroom Sauce ☛ Vitamin K = 40.3 mcg; Serving size: 1 cup, 224 g

Shellfish Mixture And Vegetables Including Carrots Broccoli And/or Dark-Green Leafy; No Potatoes Mushroom Sauce ☛ Vitamin K = 59.4 mcg; Serving size: 1 cup, 224 g

Shrimp And Clams In Tomato-Based Sauce With Noodles— Frozen Meal ☛ Vitamin K = 102.5 mcg; Serving size: 1 meal (10 oz), 284 g

Shrimp And Noodles—No Sauce ☞ Vitamin K = 7.2 mcg; Serving size: 1 cup, 157 g

Shrimp And Noodles—With Cheese Sauce ☞ Vitamin K = 0.7 mcg; Serving size: 1 cup, 224 g

Shrimp And Noodles—With Cream Or White Sauce ☞ Vitamin K = 2.9 mcg; Serving size: 1 cup, 224 g

Shrimp And Noodles—With Gravy ☞ Vitamin K = 8.7 mcg; Serving size: 1 cup, 224 g

Shrimp And Noodles—With Mushroom Sauce ☞ Vitamin K = 19 mcg; Serving size: 1 cup, 224 g

Shrimp And Noodles—With Tomato Sauce ☞ Vitamin K = 12.1 mcg; Serving size: 1 cup, 224 g

Shrimp And Vegetables Excluding Carrots Broccoli And Dark-Green Leafy; No Potatoes No Sauce ☞ Vitamin K = 26.9 mcg; Serving size: 1 cup, 162 g

Shrimp And Vegetables In Sauce With Noodles—Diet Frozen Meal ☞ Vitamin K = 25 mcg; Serving size: 1 meal (11 oz), 312 g

Shrimp And Vegetables Including Carrots Broccoli And/or Dark-Green Leafy; No Potatoes No Sauce ☞ Vitamin K = 53.3 mcg; Serving size: 1 cup, 162 g

Shrimp Cake Or Patty ☞ Vitamin K = 28.9 mcg; Serving size: 1 cake or patty, 120 g

Shrimp Cocktail ☞ Vitamin K – 4.1 mcg; Serving size: 1 cup, 230 g

Shrimp Creole No Rice ☞ Vitamin K = 15.5 mcg; Serving size: 1 cup, 246 g

Shrimp Creole With Rice ☞ Vitamin K = 10.4 mcg; Serving size: 1 cup, 243 g

Shrimp Curry ☞ Vitamin K = 117.5 mcg; Serving size: 1 cup, 236 g

Shrimp Garden Salad Shrimp Lettuce Eggs Tomato And/or Carrots Other Vegetables No Dressing ☛ Vitamin K = 58.8 mcg; Serving size: 1 cup, 95 g

Shrimp Garden Salad Shrimp Lettuce Eggs Vegetables Excluding Tomato And Carrots No Dressing ☛ Vitamin K = 61.6 mcg; Serving size: 1 cup, 95 g

Shrimp Gumbo ☛ Vitamin K = 21.7 mcg; Serving size: 1 cup, 244 g

Shrimp In Garlic Sauce Puerto Rican Style ☛ Vitamin K = 94.1 mcg; Serving size: 1 cup, 212 g

Shrimp Mixed Species Raw (Previously Frozen or Not) ☛ Vitamin K = 0 mcg; Serving size: 1 medium, 6 g

Shrimp Mixed Species—Cooked—Breaded And Fried ☛ Vitamin K = 0.9 mcg; Serving size: 3 oz, 85 g

Shrimp Salad ☛ Vitamin K = 75.3 mcg; Serving size: 1 cup, 182 g

Shrimp Scampi ☛ Vitamin K = 40.7 mcg; Serving size: 1 cup, 136 g

Shrimp Shish Kabob With Vegetables Excluding Potatoes ☛ Vitamin K = 10.5 mcg; Serving size: 1 shishkabob, 202 g

Shrimp Steamed Or Boiled ☛ Vitamin K = 0.1 mcg; Serving size: 1 oz (without shell, cooked), 28 g

Shrimp Toast Fried ☛ Vitamin K = 14.8 mcg; Serving size: 1/2 slice, 48 g

Shrimp With Crab Stuffing ☛ Vitamin K = 7.8 mcg; Serving size: 1 cup, 140 g

Shrimp With Lobster Sauce ☛ Vitamin K = 8.1 mcg; Serving size: 1 cup, 185 g

Shrimp—Baked Or Broiled —Prepared with Butter ☛ Vitamin K = 0 mcg; Serving size: 1 tiny shrimp ("popcorn"), 1 g

Shrimp—Baked Or Broiled —Prepared with Cooking Spray ☛

Vitamin K = 0 mcg; Serving size: 1 tiny shrimp ("popcorn"), 1 g

Shrimp—Baked Or Broiled —Prepared with Margarine ☞ Vitamin K = 0 mcg; Serving size: 1 tiny shrimp ("popcorn"), 1 g

Shrimp—Baked Or Broiled —Prepared with Oil ☞ Vitamin K = 0 mcg; Serving size: 1 tiny shrimp ("popcorn"), 1 g

Shrimp—Baked Or Broiled —Prepared without Fat ☞ Vitamin K = 0 mcg; Serving size: 1 tiny shrimp ("popcorn"), 1 g

Shrimp—Coated Fried—Prepared with Butter ☞ Vitamin K = 0.5 mcg; Serving size: 1 oz (without shell, cooked), 28 g

Shrimp—Coated Fried—Prepared with Cooking Spray ☞ Vitamin K = 0.4 mcg; Serving size: 1 oz (without shell, cooked), 28 g

Shrimp—Coated Fried—Prepared with Margarine ☞ Vitamin K = 2.9 mcg; Serving size: 1 oz (without shell, cooked), 28 g

Shrimp—Coated Fried—Prepared with Oil ☞ Vitamin K = 3.4 mcg; Serving size: 1 oz (without shell, cooked), 28 g

Shrimp—Coated Fried—Prepared without Fat ☞ Vitamin K = 0.4 mcg; Serving size: 1 oz (without shell, cooked), 28 g

Shrimp—Coated—Baked Or Broiled —Prepared with Butter ☞ Vitamin K = 0.4 mcg; Serving size: 1 oz (without shell, cooked), 28 g

Shrimp—Coated—Baked Or Broiled —Prepared with Cooking Spray ☞ Vitamin K = 0.3 mcg; Serving size: 1 oz (without shell, cooked), 28 g

Shrimp—Coated—Baked Or Broiled —Prepared with Margarine ☞ Vitamin K = 1.9 mcg; Serving size: 1 oz (without shell, cooked), 28 g

Shrimp—Coated—Baked Or Broiled —Prepared with Oil ☞ Vitamin K = 2 mcg; Serving size: 1 oz (without shell, cooked), 28 g

Shrimp—Coated—Baked Or Broiled —Prepared without Fat ☞ Vitamin K = 0.3 mcg; Serving size: 1 oz (without shell, cooked), 28 g

Shrimp—Dried ☞ Vitamin K = 0 mcg; Serving size: 1 oz, 28 g

Smelt Rainbow Raw ☛ Vitamin K = 0.1 mcg; Serving size: 3 oz, 85 g

Smoked—Haddock ☛ Vitamin K = 0 mcg; Serving size: 1 oz, boneless, 28.4 g

Smoked—Salmon ☛ Vitamin K = 0 mcg; Serving size: 1 oz, boneless, 28.4 g

Smoked—Sturgeon ☛ Vitamin K = 0 mcg; Serving size: 1 oz, 28.4 g

Smoked—Whitefish ☛ Vitamin K = 0.1 mcg; Serving size: 1 cup, cooked, 136 g

Snapper Mixed Species Raw ☛ Vitamin K = 0.1 mcg; Serving size: 3 oz, 85 g

Squid (Raw) ☛ Vitamin K = 0 mcg; Serving size: 1 oz, boneless, 28.4 g

Squid Steamed Or Boiled ☛ Vitamin K = 0 mcg; Serving size: 1 oz, boneless, cooked, 28 g

Squid—Baked Or Broiled (Cooked with Fat) ☛ Vitamin K = 11.4 mcg; Serving size: 1 squid, 272 g

Squid—Baked Or Broiled (Cooked without Fat) ☛ Vitamin K = 0 mcg; Serving size: 1 squid, 272 g

Squid—Canned ☛ Vitamin K = 0 mcg; Serving size: 1 cup, 187 g

Squid—Coated Fried ☛ Vitamin K = 3.3 mcg; Serving size: 1 oz, cooked, 28 g

Squid—Coated—Baked Or Broiled (Cooked with Fat) ☛ Vitamin K = 2 mcg; Serving size: 1 oz, cooked, 28 g

Squid—Coated—Baked Or Broiled (Cooked without Fat) ☛ Vitamin K = 0.2 mcg; Serving size: 1 oz, cooked, 28 g

Squid—Dried ☛ Vitamin K = 0 mcg; Serving size: 1 oz, boneless, 28 g

Squid—Pickled ☛ Vitamin K = 0 mcg; Serving size: 1 oz, boneless, 28 g

Stewed Codfish No Potatoes Puerto Rican Style ➤ Vitamin K = 11.8 mcg; Serving size: 1 cup, 227 g

Stewed Salmon Puerto Rican Style ➤ Vitamin K = 11.2 mcg; Serving size: 1 cup, 212 g

Sticks Frozen Prepared ➤ Vitamin K = 2.7 mcg; Serving size: 1 piece (4 inch x 2 inch x 1/2 inch), 57 g

Sturgeon Mixed Species Raw ➤ Vitamin K = 0.1 mcg; Serving size: 3 oz, 85 g

Sturgeon Steamed ➤ Vitamin K = 0 mcg; Serving size: 1 oz, boneless, raw, 23 g

Sturgeon—Baked Or Broiled (Cooked with Fat) ➤ Vitamin K = 1 mcg; Serving size: 1 oz, boneless, raw, 23 g

Sturgeon—Coated Fried ➤ Vitamin K = 3.1 mcg; Serving size: 1 oz, boneless, raw, 27 g

Surimi ➤ Vitamin K = 0 mcg; Serving size: 1 oz, 28.4 g

Swordfish—Baked Or Broiled (Cooked with Fat) ➤ Vitamin K = 7.7 mcg; Serving size: 1 small fillet, 170 g

Swordfish—Baked Or Broiled (Cooked without Fat) ➤ Vitamin K = 0.2 mcg; Serving size: 1 small fillet, 170 g

Swordfish—Coated Fried ➤ Vitamin K = 19.4 mcg; Serving size: 1 small fillet, 170 g

Swordfish—Coated—Baked Or Broiled (Cooked with Fat) ➤ Vitamin K = 12.4 mcg; Serving size: 1 small fillet, 170 g

Swordfish—Coated—Baked Or Broiled (Cooked without Fat) ➤ Vitamin K = 1.4 mcg; Serving size: 1 small fillet, 170 g

Swordfish—Steamed Or Poached ➤ Vitamin K = 0.2 mcg; Serving size: 1 small fillet, 170 g

SwordRaw ➤ Vitamin K = 0.1 mcg; Serving size: 3 oz, 85 g

Tilapia (Raw) ☞ Vitamin K = 1.6 mcg; Serving size: 1 fillet, 116 g

Tilapia—Baked Or Broiled —Prepared with Butter ☞ Vitamin K = 2.3 mcg; Serving size: 1 small fillet, 113 g

Tilapia—Baked Or Broiled —Prepared with Cooking Spray ☞ Vitamin K = 2 mcg; Serving size: 1 small fillet, 113 g

Tilapia—Baked Or Broiled —Prepared with Margarine ☞ Vitamin K = 6.3 mcg; Serving size: 1 small fillet, 113 g

Tilapia—Baked Or Broiled —Prepared with Oil ☞ Vitamin K = 6.8 mcg; Serving size: 1 small fillet, 113 g

Tilapia—Baked Or Broiled —Prepared without Fat ☞ Vitamin K = 2 mcg; Serving size: 1 small fillet, 113 g

Tilapia—Coated Fried—Prepared with Butter ☞ Vitamin K = 3.2 mcg; Serving size: 1 small fillet, 113 g

Tilapia—Coated Fried—Prepared with Cooking Spray ☞ Vitamin K = 2.9 mcg; Serving size: 1 small fillet, 113 g

Tilapia—Coated Fried—Prepared with Margarine ☞ Vitamin K = 12.4 mcg; Serving size: 1 small fillet, 113 g

Tilapia—Coated Fried—Prepared with Oil ☞ Vitamin K = 14.1 mcg; Serving size: 1 small fillet, 113 g

Tilapia—Coated Fried—Prepared without Fat ☞ Vitamin K = 2.9 mcg; Serving size: 1 small fillet, 113 g

Tilapia—Coated—Baked Or Broiled Made With Oil ☞ Vitamin K = 9.7 mcg; Serving size: 1 small fillet, 113 g

Tilapia—Coated—Baked Or Broiled —Prepared with Butter ☞ Vitamin K = 2.6 mcg; Serving size: 1 small fillet, 113 g

Tilapia—Coated—Baked Or Broiled —Prepared with Cooking Spray ☞ Vitamin K = 2.3 mcg; Serving size: 1 small fillet, 113 g

Tilapia—Coated—Baked Or Broiled —Prepared with Margarine ☞

Vitamin K = 8.9 mcg; Serving size: 1 small fillet, 113 g

Tilapia—Coated—Baked Or Broiled —Prepared without Fat ☛ Vitamin K = 2.3 mcg; Serving size: 1 small fillet, 113 g

Tilapia—Steamed Or Poached ☛ Vitamin K = 2 mcg; Serving size: 1 small fillet, 113 g

Trout Mixed Species Raw ☛ Vitamin K = 0.1 mcg; Serving size: 1 fillet, 79 g

Trout Smoked ☛ Vitamin K = 0.1 mcg; Serving size: 1 oz, boneless, 28 g

Trout—Baked Or Broiled —Prepared with Butter ☛ Vitamin K = 0.5 mcg; Serving size: 1 small fillet, 113 g

Trout—Baked Or Broiled —Prepared with Cooking Spray ☛ Vitamin K = 0.1 mcg; Serving size: 1 small fillet, 113 g

Trout—Baked Or Broiled —Prepared with Margarine ☛ Vitamin K = 4.5 mcg; Serving size: 1 small fillet, 113 g

Trout—Baked Or Broiled —Prepared with Oil ☛ Vitamin K = 5.1 mcg; Serving size: 1 small fillet, 113 g

Trout—Baked Or Broiled —Prepared without Fat ☛ Vitamin K = 0.1 mcg; Serving size: 1 small fillet, 113 g

Trout—Coated Fried—Prepared with Butter ☛ Vitamin K = 1.9 mcg; Serving size: 1 small fillet, 113 g

Trout—Coated Fried—Prepared with Cooking Spray ☛ Vitamin K – 1.5 mcg; Serving size: 1 small fillet, 113 g

Trout—Coated Fried—Prepared with Margarine ☛ Vitamin K = 11.2 mcg; Serving size: 1 small fillet, 113 g

Trout—Coated Fried—Prepared with Oil ☛ Vitamin K = 12.9 mcg; Serving size: 1 small fillet, 113 g

Trout—Coated Fried—Prepared without Fat ☛ Vitamin K = 1.5 mcg;

Serving size: 1 small fillet, 113 g

Trout—Coated—Baked Or Broiled —Prepared with Butter ☛ Vitamin K = 1.2 mcg; Serving size: 1 small fillet, 113 g

Trout—Coated—Baked Or Broiled —Prepared with Cooking Spray ☛ Vitamin K = 0.9 mcg; Serving size: 1 small fillet, 113 g

Trout—Coated—Baked Or Broiled —Prepared with Margarine ☛ Vitamin K = 7.6 mcg; Serving size: 1 small fillet, 113 g

Trout—Coated—Baked Or Broiled —Prepared with Oil ☛ Vitamin K = 8.2 mcg; Serving size: 1 small fillet, 113 g

Trout—Coated—Baked Or Broiled —Prepared without Fat ☛ Vitamin K = 0.9 mcg; Serving size: 1 small fillet, 113 g

Trout—Steamed Or Poached ☛ Vitamin K = 0.1 mcg; Serving size: 1 small fillet, 113 g

Tuna And Rice With Mushroom Sauce ☛ Vitamin K = 23.1 mcg; Serving size: 1 cup, 248 g

Tuna Cake Or Patty ☛ Vitamin K = 28.7 mcg; Serving size: 1 cake or patty, 120 g

Tuna Casserole—With Vegetables And Mushroom Sauce No Noodles ☛ Vitamin K = 16.4 mcg; Serving size: 1 cup, 224 g

Tuna Fresh Smoked ☛ Vitamin K = 0 mcg; Serving size: 1 oz, boneless, 28 g

Tuna Fresh—Baked Or Broiled (Cooked with Fat) ☛ Vitamin K = 7.7 mcg; Serving size: 1 small fillet, 170 g

Tuna Fresh—Baked Or Broiled (Cooked without Fat) ☛ Vitamin K = 0.2 mcg; Serving size: 1 small fillet, 170 g

Tuna Fresh—Coated Fried ☛ Vitamin K = 19.4 mcg; Serving size: 1 small fillet, 170 g

Tuna Fresh—Coated—Baked Or Broiled (Cooked with Fat) ☛

Vitamin K = 12.4 mcg; Serving size: 1 small fillet, 170 g

Tuna Fresh—Coated—Baked Or Broiled Fat Not Added ☞ Vitamin K = 1.4 mcg; Serving size: 1 small fillet, 170 g

Tuna Fresh—Dried ☞ Vitamin K = 0.1 mcg; Serving size: 1 cup, 42 g

Tuna Fresh—Steamed Or Poached ☞ Vitamin K = 0.2 mcg; Serving size: 1 small fillet, 170 g

Tuna Light—Canned In Oil Drained Solids ☞ Vitamin K = 64.2 mcg; Serving size: 1 cup, solid or chunks, 146 g

Tuna Light—Canned In Water Drained Solids ☞ Vitamin K = 0.1 mcg; Serving size: 1 oz, 28.4 g

Tuna Loaf ☞ Vitamin K = 44 mcg; Serving size: 1 slice, 105 g

Tuna Noodle Casserole—With Cream Or White Sauce ☞ Vitamin K = 2.2 mcg; Serving size: 1 cup, 224 g

Tuna Noodle Casserole—With Mushroom Sauce ☞ Vitamin K = 14.1 mcg; Serving size: 1 cup, 224 g

Tuna Noodle Casserole—With Vegetables And Mushroom Sauce ☞ Vitamin K = 12.5 mcg; Serving size: 1 cup, 224 g

Tuna Noodle Casserole—With Vegetables Cream Or White Sauce ☞ Vitamin K = 2.5 mcg; Serving size: 1 cup, 224 g

Tuna Pot Pie ☞ Vitamin K = 160 mcg; Serving size: 1 pie, 769 g

Tuna Salad With Cheese ☞ Vitamin K = 96.9 mcg; Serving size: 1 cup, 238 g

Tuna Salad With Egg ☞ Vitamin K = 97.3 mcg; Serving size: 1 cup, 238 g

Tuna Salad—Prepared with Any Type Of Fat-free Dressing ☞ Vitamin K = 39.7 mcg; Serving size: 1 cup, 238 g

Tuna Salad—Prepared with Creamy Dressing ☞ Vitamin K = 96.6

mcg; Serving size: 1 cup, 238 g

Tuna Salad—Prepared with Italian Dressing ☞ Vitamin K = 55.5 mcg; Serving size: 1 cup, 238 g

Tuna Salad—Prepared with Light Creamy Dressing ☞ Vitamin K = 27.4 mcg; Serving size: 1 cup, 238 g

Tuna Salad—Prepared with Light Italian Dressing ☞ Vitamin K = 33.1 mcg; Serving size: 1 cup, 238 g

Tuna Salad—Prepared with Light Mayonnaise ☞ Vitamin K = 54.7 mcg; Serving size: 1 cup, 238 g

Tuna Salad—Prepared with Light Mayonnaise-Type Salad Dressing ☞ Vitamin K = 54.7 mcg; Serving size: 1 cup, 238 g

Tuna Salad—Prepared with Mayonnaise ☞ Vitamin K = 106.4 mcg; Serving size: 1 cup, 238 g

Tuna Salad—Prepared with Mayonnaise-Type Salad Dressing ☞ Vitamin K = 48.3 mcg; Serving size: 1 cup, 238 g

Tuna With Cream Or White Sauce ☞ Vitamin K = 0.9 mcg; Serving size: 1 cup, 237 g

Turtle Green Raw ☞ Vitamin K = 0.1 mcg; Serving size: 3 oz, 85 g

Whitefish (Raw) ☞ Vitamin K = 0.1 mcg; Serving size: 3 oz, 85 g

Whiting (Raw) ☞ Vitamin K = 0.1 mcg; Serving size: 1 fillet, 92 g

Whiting—Baked Or Broiled —Prepared with Butter ☞ Vitamin K = 0.5 mcg; Serving size: 1 small fillet, 113 g

Whiting—Baked Or Broiled —Prepared with Cooking Spray ☞ Vitamin K = 0.1 mcg; Serving size: 1 small fillet, 113 g

Whiting—Baked Or Broiled —Prepared with Margarine ☞ Vitamin K = 4.5 mcg; Serving size: 1 small fillet, 113 g

Whiting—Baked Or Broiled —Prepared with Oil ☞ Vitamin K = 5.1

mcg; Serving size: 1 small fillet, 113 g

Whiting—Baked Or Broiled —Prepared without Fat ☛ Vitamin K = 0.1 mcg; Serving size: 1 small fillet, 113 g

Whiting—Coated Fried—Prepared with Butter ☛ Vitamin K = 0.5 mcg; Serving size: 1 oz, boneless, raw, 27 g

Whiting—Coated Fried—Prepared with Cooking Spray ☛ Vitamin K = 0.4 mcg; Serving size: 1 oz, boneless, raw, 27 g

Whiting—Coated Fried—Prepared with Margarine ☛ Vitamin K = 2.7 mcg; Serving size: 1 oz, boneless, raw, 27 g

Whiting—Coated Fried—Prepared with Oil ☛ Vitamin K = 12.9 mcg; Serving size: 1 small fillet, 113 g

Whiting—Coated Fried—Prepared without Fat ☛ Vitamin K = 0.4 mcg; Serving size: 1 oz, boneless, raw, 27 g

Whiting—Coated—Baked Or Broiled —Prepared with Butter ☛ Vitamin K = 1.2 mcg; Serving size: 1 small fillet, 113 g

Whiting—Coated—Baked Or Broiled —Prepared with Cooking Spray ☛ Vitamin K = 0.9 mcg; Serving size: 1 small fillet, 113 g

Whiting—Coated—Baked Or Broiled —Prepared with Margarine ☛ Vitamin K = 7.6 mcg; Serving size: 1 small fillet, 113 g

Whiting—Coated—Baked Or Broiled —Prepared with Oil ☛ Vitamin K = 8.2 mcg; Serving size: 1 small fillet, 113 g

Whiting—Coated—Baked Or Broiled —Prepared without Fat ☛ Vitamin K = 0.2 mcg; Serving size: 1 oz, boneless, raw, 27 g

Whiting—Steamed Or Poached ☛ Vitamin K = 0 mcg; Serving size: 1 oz, boneless, raw, 23 g

Yellowfin Tuna (Raw) ☛ Vitamin K = 0 mcg; Serving size: 1 oz, boneless, 28.4 g

Yellowtail (Raw) ☛ Vitamin K = 0.1 mcg; Serving size: 3 oz, 85 g

20

FRUITS AND FRUITS PRODUCTS

Acerola Juice—Raw ☛ Vitamin K = 3.4 mcg; Serving size: 1 cup, 242 g

Ambrosia ☛ Vitamin K = 0.6 mcg; Serving size: 1 cup, 193 g

Apple Baked Unsweetened ☛ Vitamin K = 3.9 mcg; Serving size: 1 apple with liquid, 161 g

Apple Baked With Sugar ☛ Vitamin K = 3.6 mcg; Serving size: 1 apple with liquid, 171 g

Apple Candied ☛ Vitamin K = 4.2 mcg; Serving size: 1 small apple, 198 g

Apple Chips ☛ Vitamin K = 5.2 mcg; Serving size: 1 cup, 28 g

Apple Dried Cooked With Sugar ☛ Vitamin K = 1.7 mcg; Serving size: 1 cup, 280 g

Apple Fried ☛ Vitamin K = 9.3 mcg; Serving size: 1 cup, 179 g

Apple Juice ☛ Vitamin K = 0 mcg; Serving size: 1 cup, 248 g

Apple Juice—Canned—Or Bottled—Unsweetened—With Added Ascorbic Acid ☛ Vitamin K = 0 mcg; Serving size: 1 cup, 248 g

Apple Juice—Canned—Or Bottled—Unsweetened—With Added Ascorbic Acid Calcium And Potassium ☞ Vitamin K = 0 mcg; Serving size: 6 fl oz, 177 g

Apple Juice—Frozen—Concentrate—Unsweetened—Diluted With 3 Volume Water Without Added Ascorbic Acid ☞ Vitamin K = 0 mcg; Serving size: 1 cup, 239 g

Apple Juice—Frozen—Concentrate—Unsweetened—Undiluted Without Added Ascorbic Acid ☞ Vitamin K = 0 mcg; Serving size: 1 can (6 fl oz), 211 g

Apple Pickled ☞ Vitamin K = 0.4 mcg; Serving size: 1 apple, 29 g

Apple Rings Fried ☞ Vitamin K = 1.5 mcg; Serving size: 1 ring, 19 g

Apple Salad With Dressing ☞ Vitamin K = 36 mcg; Serving size: 1 cup, 137 g

Apples ☞ Vitamin K = 2.8 mcg; Serving size: 1 cup, quartered or chopped, 125 g

Apples (Without Skin) ☞ Vitamin K = 0.7 mcg; Serving size: 1 cup slices, 110 g

Apples Dehydrated (Low Moisture) Sulfured Uncooked ☞ Vitamin K = 2.6 mcg; Serving size: 1 cup, 60 g

Apples Dried Sulfured Stewed Without Added Sugar ☞ Vitamin K = 1.8 mcg; Serving size: 1 cup, 255 g

Apples Raw Without Skin Cooked Boiled ☞ Vitamin K = 1 mcg; Serving size: 1 cup slices, 171 g

Apples Raw Without Skin Cooked Microwave ☞ Vitamin K = 1.2 mcg; Serving size: 1 cup slices, 170 g

Apples—Canned—Sweetened Sliced Drained Heated ☞ Vitamin K = 1.2 mcg; Serving size: 1 cup slices, 204 g

Applesauce—Canned—Sweetened Without Salt (Includes USDA Commodity) ☛ Vitamin K = 1.5 mcg; Serving size: 1 cup, 246 g

Applesauce—Canned—Unsweetened Without Added Ascorbic Acid (Includes USDA Commodity) ☛ Vitamin K = 1.2 mcg; Serving size: 1 cup, 244 g

Applesauce—Canned—Unsweetened—With Added Ascorbic Acid ☛ Vitamin K = 1.2 mcg; Serving size: 1 cup, 244 g

Apricot Dried Cooked With Sugar ☛ Vitamin K = 2.7 mcg; Serving size: 1 cup, 270 g

Apricot Nectar—Canned—Without Added Ascorbic Acid ☛ Vitamin K = 3 mcg; Serving size: 1 cup, 251 g

Apricots ☛ Vitamin K = 5.1 mcg; Serving size: 1 cup, halves, 155 g

Apricots Dried Sulfured Stewed Without Added Sugar ☛ Vitamin K = 2.8 mcg; Serving size: 1 cup, halves, 250 g

Apricots—Canned—Heavy Syrup Drained ☛ Vitamin K = 7.2 mcg; Serving size: 1 cup, halves, 219 g

Apricots—Canned—Heavy Syrup Pack—With Skin Solids And Liquids ☛ Vitamin K = 5.7 mcg; Serving size: 1 cup, halves, 258 g

Apricots—Canned—Juice—Pack—With Skin Solids And Liquids ☛ Vitamin K = 5.4 mcg; Serving size: 1 cup, halves, 244 g

Apricots—Canned—Light Syrup Pack—With Skin Solids And Liquids ☛ Vitamin K = 5.6 mcg; Serving size: 1 cup, halves, 253 g

Apricots—Canned—Water Pack—With Skin Solids And Liquids ☛ Vitamin K = 5.3 mcg; Serving size: 1 cup, halves, 243 g

Asian Pears ☛ Vitamin K = 5.5 mcg; Serving size: 1 fruit 2-1/4 inch high x 2-1/2 inch dia, 122 g

Avocados ☛ Vitamin K = 31.5 mcg; Serving size: 1 cup, cubes, 150 g

Banana Baked ☛ Vitamin K = 0.8 mcg; Serving size: 1 banana (7-1/4" long), 128 g

Banana Batter-Dipped Fried ☞ Vitamin K = 17.7 mcg; Serving size: 1 small, 108 g

Banana Red Fried ☞ Vitamin K = 7.2 mcg; Serving size: 1 fruit (7-1/4" long), 94 g

Banana Ripe Fried ☞ Vitamin K = 5.6 mcg; Serving size: 1 small, 73 g

Banana Whip ☞ Vitamin K = 0.4 mcg; Serving size: 1 cup, 130 g

Bananas ☞ Vitamin K = 1.1 mcg; Serving size: 1 cup, mashed, 225 g

Bartlett Pears ☞ Vitamin K = 5.3 mcg; Serving size: 1 cup, sliced, 140 g

Beans String Green Pickled ☞ Vitamin K = 50.2 mcg; Serving size: 1 cup, 135 g

Blackberries ☞ Vitamin K = 28.5 mcg; Serving size: 1 cup, 144 g

Blackberries—Canned—Heavy Syrup Solids And Liquids ☞ Vitamin K = 34 mcg; Serving size: 1 cup, 256 g

Blackberries—Frozen—Unsweetened ☞ Vitamin K = 29.9 mcg; Serving size: 1 cup, unthawed, 151 g

Blackberry Juice—Canned ☞ Vitamin K = 38 mcg; Serving size: 1 cup, 250 g

Blueberries ☞ Vitamin K = 28.6 mcg; Serving size: 1 cup, 148 g

Blueberries (Frozen) ☞ Vitamin K = 25.4 mcg; Serving size: 1 cup, unthawed, 155 g

Blueberries Cooked Or—Canned—Unsweetened Water Pack ☞ Vitamin K = 31.5 mcg; Serving size: 1 cup, 244 g

Blueberries Wild—Canned—Heavy Syrup Drained ☞ Vitamin K = 47.2 mcg; Serving size: 1 cup, 319 g

Blueberries—Canned—Heavy Syrup Solids And Liquids ☞ Vitamin K = 16.4 mcg; Serving size: 1 cup, 256 g

Blueberries—Canned—Light Syrup Drained ➤ Vitamin K = 48.6 mcg; Serving size: 1 cup, 244 g

Blueberries—Frozen—Sweetened ➤ Vitamin K = 40.7 mcg; Serving size: 1 cup, thawed, 230 g

Bosc Pear ➤ Vitamin K = 7.3 mcg; Serving size: 1 cup, sliced, 140 g

Boysenberries (Frozen) ➤ Vitamin K = 10.3 mcg; Serving size: 1 cup, unthawed, 132 g

Breadfruit ➤ Vitamin K = 1.1 mcg; Serving size: 1 cup, 220 g

Cabbage Red Pickled ➤ Vitamin K = 29.3 mcg; Serving size: 1 cup, 150 g

California Avocados ➤ Vitamin K = 48.3 mcg; Serving size: 1 cup, pureed, 230 g

Canned Orange Juice ➤ Vitamin K = 0.2 mcg; Serving size: 1 cup, 249 g

Cantaloupe Melons ➤ Vitamin K = 4.4 mcg; Serving size: 1 cup, balls, 177 g

Casaba Melon ➤ Vitamin K = 4.3 mcg; Serving size: 1 cup, cubes, 170 g

Cauliflower Pickled ➤ Vitamin K = 12.5 mcg; Serving size: 1 cup, 125 g

Celery Pickled ➤ Vitamin K = 38.6 mcg; Serving size: 1 cup, 150 g

Cherries (Sweet) ➤ Vitamin K = 2.9 mcg; Serving size: 1 cup, with pits, yields, 138 g

Cherries Sour Red—Canned—Heavy Syrup Pack—Solids And Liquids ➤ Vitamin K = 3.6 mcg; Serving size: 1 cup, 256 g

Cherries Sour Red—Canned—Water Pack—Solids And Liquids (Includes USDA Commodity Red Tart Cherries Canned) ➤ Vitamin K = 3.4 mcg; Serving size: 1 cup, 244 g

Cherries Sour—Canned—Water Pack—Drained ☛ Vitamin K = 13.6 mcg; Serving size: 1 cup, 168 g

Cherries Sweet—Canned—Juice—Pack—Solids And Liquids ☛ Vitamin K = 3.5 mcg; Serving size: 1 cup, pitted, 250 g

Cherries Sweet—Canned—Light Syrup Pack—Solids And Liquids ☛ Vitamin K = 3.5 mcg; Serving size: 1 cup, pitted, 252 g

Cherries Sweet—Canned—Pitted Heavy Syrup Drained ☛ Vitamin K = 1.6 mcg; Serving size: 1 cup, 179 g

Cherries Sweet—Canned—Pitted Heavy Syrup Pack—Solids And Liquids ☛ Vitamin K = 2.3 mcg; Serving size: 1 cup, 253 g

Cherries Sweet—Canned—Water Pack—Solids And Liquids ☛ Vitamin K = 3.5 mcg; Serving size: 1 cup, pitted, 248 g

Cherries Tart Dried Sweetened ☛ Vitamin K = 2 mcg; Serving size: 1/4 cup, 40 g

Chinese Preserved Sweet Vegetable ☛ Vitamin K = 0.2 mcg; Serving size: 1 slice, 12 g

Clementines ☛ Vitamin K = 0 mcg; Serving size: 1 fruit, 74 g

Corn Relish ☛ Vitamin K = 11.8 mcg; Serving size: 1 cup, 245 g

Cranberries ☛ Vitamin K = 5.5 mcg; Serving size: 1 cup, chopped, 110 g

Cranberry Juice—Blend 100% Juice—Bottled—With Added Vitamin C And Calcium ☛ Vitamin K = 0 mcg; Serving size: 6 (3/4) fl oz, 200 g

Cranberry Juice—Unsweetened ☛ Vitamin K = 12.9 mcg; Serving size: 1 cup, 253 g

Cranberry Salad Congealed ☛ Vitamin K = 10.1 mcg; Serving size: 1 cup, 253 g

Cranberry Sauce—Canned—Sweetened ☛ Vitamin K = 3.9 mcg; Serving size: 1 cup, 277 g

Cranberry-Orange Relish Uncooked ☞ Vitamin K = 7.4 mcg; Serving size: 1 cup, 275 g

Cranberry-Raspberry Sauce ☞ Vitamin K = 8.2 mcg; Serving size: 1 container (12 oz), 340 g

Dates (Deglet Noor) ☞ Vitamin K = 4 mcg; Serving size: 1 cup, chopped, 147 g

Dried Apples ☞ Vitamin K = 2.6 mcg; Serving size: 1 cup, 86 g

Dried Apricots ☞ Vitamin K = 4 mcg; Serving size: 1 cup, halves, 130 g

Dried Bananas ☞ Vitamin K = 2 mcg; Serving size: 1 cup, 100 g

Dried Blueberries (Sweetened) ☞ Vitamin K = 23.8 mcg; Serving size: 1/4 cup, 40 g

Dried Cranberries (Sweetened) ☞ Vitamin K = 3 mcg; Serving size: 1/4 cup, 40 g

Dried Figs ☞ Vitamin K = 23.2 mcg; Serving size: 1 cup, 149 g

Dried Litchis ☞ Vitamin K = 0 mcg; Serving size: 1 fruit, 2.5 g

Dried Peaches ☞ Vitamin K = 25.1 mcg; Serving size: 1 cup, halves, 160 g

Dried Pears ☞ Vitamin K = 36.7 mcg; Serving size: 1 cup, halves, 180 g

Feijoa ☞ Vitamin K = 8.5 mcg; Serving size: 1 cup, pureed, 243 g

Fig Dried Cooked With Sugar ☞ Vitamin K = 16.2 mcg; Serving size: 1 cup, 270 g

Figs ☞ Vitamin K = 3 mcg; Serving size: 1 large (2-1/2 inch dia), 64 g

Figs Dried Stewed ☞ Vitamin K = 17.4 mcg; Serving size: 1 cup, 259 g

Figs—Canned—Heavy Syrup Pack—Solids And Liquids ☞ Vitamin K = 13.7 mcg; Serving size: 1 cup, 259 g

Figs—Canned—Light Syrup Pack—Solids And Liquids ☞ Vitamin K

= 10.6 mcg; Serving size: 1 cup, 252 g

Figs—Canned—Water Pack—Solids And Liquids ☞ Vitamin K = 8.2 mcg; Serving size: 1 cup, 248 g

Florida Oranges ☞ Vitamin K = 0 mcg; Serving size: 1 cup sections, without membranes, 185 g

Fried Dwarf Banana Puerto Rican Style ☞ Vitamin K = 3.7 mcg; Serving size: 1 banana (4" x 1-1/2" x 1-1/2"), 36 g

Fried Dwarf Banana With Cheese Puerto Rican Style ☞ Vitamin K = 4.7 mcg; Serving size: 1 banana (4" x 1-1/2" x 1-1/2"), 40 g

Fried Yellow Plantains ☞ Vitamin K = 53.7 mcg; Serving size: 1 cup, 169 g

Frozen Strawberries ☞ Vitamin K = 4.9 mcg; Serving size: 1 cup, thawed, 221 g

Fruit Cocktail (Peach, Pineapple, Pear, Grape And Cherry)—Canned—Heavy Syrup Solids And Liquids ☞ Vitamin K = 6.4 mcg; Serving size: 1 cup, 248 g

Fruit Cocktail (Peach, Pineapple, Pear, Grape and Cherry)—Canned—Juice—Pack—Solids And Liquids ☞ Vitamin K = 6.2 mcg; Serving size: 1 cup, 237 g

Fruit Cocktail (Peach, Pineapple, Pear, Grape and Cherry)—Canned—Light Syrup Solids And Liquids ☞ Vitamin K = 6.3 mcg; Serving size: 1 cup, 242 g

Fruit Cocktail (Peach, Pineapple, Pear, Grape and Cherry)—Canned—Water Pack—Solids And Liquids ☞ Vitamin K = 6.2 mcg; Serving size: 1 cup, 237 g

Fruit Cocktail—Canned—Heavy Syrup Drained ☞ Vitamin K = 8.3 mcg; Serving size: 1 cup, 214 g

Fruit Cocktail—Or Mix Frozen ☞ Vitamin K = 8.6 mcg; Serving size: 1 cup, 215 g

Fruit Dessert With Cream And/or Pudding And Nuts ☞ Vitamin K = 3.4 mcg; Serving size: 1 cup, 178 g

Fruit Juice—Smoothie Bolthouse Farms Green Goodness ☞ Vitamin K = 18.6 mcg; Serving size: 1 cup, 230 g

Fruit Juice—Smoothie Bolthouse Farms Strawberry Banana ☞ Vitamin K = 2.1 mcg; Serving size: 1 cup, 233 g

Fruit Juice—Smoothie Naked Juice—Green Machine ☞ Vitamin K = 58.3 mcg; Serving size: 1 cup, 275 g

Fruit Juice—Smoothie Naked Juice—Strawberry Banana ☞ Vitamin K = 4.8 mcg; Serving size: 1 cup, 228 g

Fruit Juice—Smoothie Odwalla Original Superfood ☞ Vitamin K = 11.4 mcg; Serving size: 1 cup, 227 g

Fruit Juice—Smoothie Odwalla Strawberry Banana ☞ Vitamin K = 1.9 mcg; Serving size: 1 cup, 233 g

Fruit Salad—Excluding Citrus Fruits With Marshmallows ☞ Vitamin K = 56.4 mcg; Serving size: 1 cup, 171 g

Fruit Salad—Excluding Citrus Fruits With Nondairy Whipped Topping ☞ Vitamin K = 6.3 mcg; Serving size: 1 cup, 175 g

Fruit Salad—Excluding Citrus Fruits With Pudding ☞ Vitamin K = 4.9 mcg; Serving size: 1 cup, 182 g

Fruit Salad—Excluding Citrus Fruits With Salad Dressing Or Mayonnaise ☞ Vitamin K = 65.8 mcg; Serving size: 1 cup, 188 g

Fruit Salad—Excluding Citrus Fruits With Whipped Cream ☞ Vitamin K = 6 mcg; Serving size: 1 cup, 182 g

Fruit Salad—Fresh Or Raw Excluding Citrus Fruits No Dressing ☞ Vitamin K = 5.8 mcg; Serving size: 1 cup, 175 g

Fruit Salad—Fresh Or Raw Including Citrus Fruits No Dressing ☞ Vitamin K = 4.6 mcg; Serving size: 1 cup, 175 g

Fruit Salad—Including Citrus Fruit With Whipped Cream ☞ Vitamin K = 5.6 mcg; Serving size: 1 cup, 182 g

Fruit Salad—Including Citrus Fruits With Marshmallows ☞ Vitamin K = 55.1 mcg; Serving size: 1 cup, 171 g

Fruit Salad—Including Citrus Fruits With Nondairy Whipped Topping ☞ Vitamin K = 5.8 mcg; Serving size: 1 cup, 175 g

Fruit Salad—Including Citrus Fruits With Pudding ☞ Vitamin K = 4.6 mcg; Serving size: 1 cup, 182 g

Fruit Salad—Including Citrus Fruits With Salad Dressing Or Mayonnaise ☞ Vitamin K = 64.3 mcg; Serving size: 1 cup, 188 g

Fruit Salad—Puerto Rican Style ☞ Vitamin K = 2.2 mcg; Serving size: 1 cup, 247 g

Fuji Apples ☞ Vitamin K = 1.1 mcg; Serving size: 1 cup, sliced, 109 g

Fuyu Persimmon ☞ Vitamin K = 4.4 mcg; Serving size: 1 fruit (2-1/2 inch dia), 168 g

Gala Apples ☞ Vitamin K = 1.4 mcg; Serving size: 1 cup, sliced, 109 g

Golden Delicious Apples ☞ Vitamin K = 2 mcg; Serving size: 1 cup, sliced, 109 g

Golden Seedless Raisins ☞ Vitamin K = 5.8 mcg; Serving size: 1 cup, packed, 165 g

Granny Smith Apples ☞ Vitamin K = 3.5 mcg; Serving size: 1 cup, sliced, 109 g

Grape Juice ☞ Vitamin K = 1 mcg; Serving size: 1 cup, 253 g

Grape Juice—(With Added Vitamin C) ☞ Vitamin K = 1 mcg; Serving size: 1 cup, 253 g

Grape Juice—Canned—Or Bottled—Unsweetened—With Added Ascorbic Acid And Calcium ☞ Vitamin K = 1 mcg; Serving size: 1 cup, 253 g

Grapefruit ☛ Vitamin K = 0 mcg; Serving size: 1 cup sections, with juice, 230 g

Grapefruit And Orange Sections Cooked—Canned—Or—Frozen—In Light Syrup ☛ Vitamin K = 0 mcg; Serving size: 1 cup, 254 g

Grapefruit And Orange Sections Cooked—Canned—Or—Frozen—Unsweetened Water Pack ☛ Vitamin K = 0 mcg; Serving size: 1 cup, 244 g

Grapefruit And Orange Sections Raw ☛ Vitamin K = 0 mcg; Serving size: 1 section, 16 g

Grapefruit Juice ☛ Vitamin K = 0 mcg; Serving size: 8 fl oz, 240 g

Grapefruit Juice—100% With Calcium Added ☛ Vitamin K = 0 mcg; Serving size: 1 fl oz (no ice), 31 g

Grapefruit Juice—White—Canned—Or Bottled Unsweetened ☛ Vitamin K = 0 mcg; Serving size: 1 cup, 247 g

Grapefruit Juice—White—Canned—Sweetened ☛ Vitamin K = 0 mcg; Serving size: 1 cup, 250 g

Grapefruit Juice—White—Frozen—Concentrate—Unsweetened—Diluted With 3 Volume Water ☛ Vitamin K = 0 mcg; Serving size: 1 cup, 247 g

Grapefruit Juice—White—Frozen—Concentrate—Unsweetened—Undiluted ☛ Vitamin K = 0.2 mcg; Serving size: 1 can (6 fl oz), 207 g

Grapefruit Sections—Canned—Juice—Pack—Solids And Liquids ☛ Vitamin K = 0 mcg; Serving size: 1 cup, 249 g

Grapefruit Sections—Canned—Light Syrup Pack—Solids And Liquids ☛ Vitamin K = 0 mcg; Serving size: 1 cup, 254 g

Grapefruit Sections—Canned—Water Pack—Solids And Liquids ☛ Vitamin K = 0 mcg; Serving size: 1 cup, 244 g

Grapes ☛ Vitamin K = 13.4 mcg; Serving size: 1 cup, 92 g

Grapes—Canned—Thompson Seedless Heavy Syrup Pack—Solids And Liquids ☛ Vitamin K = 25.1 mcg; Serving size: 1 cup, 256 g

Grapes—Canned—Thompson Seedless Water Pack—Solids And Liquids ☛ Vitamin K = 24 mcg; Serving size: 1 cup, 245 g

Green Anjou Pear ☛ Vitamin K = 6 mcg; Serving size: 1 cup, sliced, 140 g

Green Olives ☛ Vitamin K = 0 mcg; Serving size: 1 olive, 2.7 g

Guanabana Nectar Canned ☛ Vitamin K = 0 mcg; Serving size: 1 cup, 251 g

Guava Nectar With Sucralose Canned ☛ Vitamin K = 3.4 mcg; Serving size: fl oz, 335 g

Guava Nectar—Canned—With Added Ascorbic Acid ☛ Vitamin K = 2.5 mcg; Serving size: 1 cup, 251 g

Guava Sauce Cooked ☛ Vitamin K = 4.5 mcg; Serving size: 1 cup, 238 g

Guava Shell—Canned—In Heavy Syrup ☛ Vitamin K = 5.6 mcg; Serving size: 1 cup, 310 g

Guavas ☛ Vitamin K = 4.3 mcg; Serving size: 1 cup, 165 g

Honeydew Melon ☛ Vitamin K = 4.9 mcg; Serving size: 1 cup, diced, 170 g

Juice—Apple And Grape Blend—With Added Ascorbic Acid ☛ Vitamin K = 0.5 mcg; Serving size: 8 fl oz, 250 g

Juice—Apple Grape And Pear Blend—With Added Ascorbic Acid And Calcium ☛ Vitamin K = 0 mcg; Serving size: 8 fl oz, 250 g

Jumbo Olives ☛ Vitamin K = 0.2 mcg; Serving size: 1 super colossal, 15 g

Kiwifruit ☛ Vitamin K = 72.5 mcg; Serving size: 1 cup, sliced, 180 g

Kiwifruit Zespri Sungold Raw ☛ Vitamin K = 4.9 mcg; Serving size: 1 fruit, 81 g

Kumquat Cooked Or—Canned—In Syrup ☛ Vitamin K = 0 mcg; Serving size: 1 kumquat, 14 g

Kumquats ☛ Vitamin K = 0 mcg; Serving size: 1 fruit without refuse, 19 g

Lemon Juice—From Concentrate Bottled Real Lemon ☛ Vitamin K = 0 mcg; Serving size: 1 tbsp, 15 g

Lemon Juice—From Concentrate—Canned—Or Bottled ☛ Vitamin K = 0 mcg; Serving size: 1 tbsp, 15 g

Lemon Juice—Raw ☛ Vitamin K = 0 mcg; Serving size: 1 cup, 244 g

Lemon Peel Raw ☛ Vitamin K = 0 mcg; Serving size: 1 tbsp, 6 g

Lemons ☛ Vitamin K = 0 mcg; Serving size: 1 cup, sections, 212 g

Lime Juice ☛ Vitamin K = 1.5 mcg; Serving size: 1 cup, 242 g

Lime Juice—Canned—Or Bottled Unsweetened ☛ Vitamin K = 1.2 mcg; Serving size: 1 cup, 246 g

Limes ☛ Vitamin K = 0.4 mcg; Serving size: 1 fruit (2 inch dia), 67 g

Litchis ☛ Vitamin K = 0.8 mcg; Serving size: 1 cup, 190 g

Loganberries (Frozen) ☛ Vitamin K = 11.5 mcg; Serving size: 1 cup, unthawed, 147 g

Lychee Cooked Or—Canned—In Sugar Or Syrup ☛ Vitamin K = 0.1 mcg; Serving size: 1 lychee with liquid, 21 g

Mango Cooked ☛ Vitamin K = 1.2 mcg; Serving size: 1 oz, 28 g

Mango Nectar Canned ☛ Vitamin K = 2 mcg; Serving size: 1 cup, 251 g

Mango Pickled ☛ Vitamin K = 0.8 mcg; Serving size: 1 slice, 28 g

Mangos ☛ Vitamin K = 6.9 mcg; Serving size: 1 cup pieces, 165 g

Maraschino Cherries (Canned) ☛ Vitamin K = 0.1 mcg; Serving size: 1 cherry (nlea serving), 5 g

Medjool Dates ☛ Vitamin K = 0.6 mcg; Serving size: 1 date, pitted, 24 g

Mulberries ☛ Vitamin K = 10.9 mcg; Serving size: 1 cup, 140 g

Mushrooms Pickled ☛ Vitamin K = 0 mcg; Serving size: 1 cup, 156 g

Nance—Frozen—Unsweetened ☛ Vitamin K = 13.3 mcg; Serving size: 1 cup without pits, thawed, 112 g

Naranjilla (Lulo) Pulp—Frozen—Unsweetened ☛ Vitamin K = 17.5 mcg; Serving size: 1 cup thawed, 120 g

Navel Oranges ☛ Vitamin K = 0 mcg; Serving size: 1 cup sections, without membranes, 165 g

Nectarine Cooked ☛ Vitamin K = 5.5 mcg; Serving size: 1 cup, 262 g

Nectarines ☛ Vitamin K = 3.1 mcg; Serving size: 1 cup slices, 143 g

Okra Pickled ☛ Vitamin K = 3 mcg; Serving size: 1 pod, 11 g

Olives ☛ Vitamin K = 0.1 mcg; Serving size: 1 tbsp, 8.4 g

Olives Black ☛ Vitamin K = 0 mcg; Serving size: 1 slice, 1 g

Olives Green Stuffed ☛ Vitamin K = 3.5 mcg; Serving size: 1 cup, 147 g

Orange Juice ☛ Vitamin K = 0.2 mcg; Serving size: 1 cup, 248 g

Orange Juice—100% ☛ Vitamin K = 0 mcg; Serving size: 1 fl oz (no ice), 31 g

Orange Juice—Chilled Includes From Concentrate—With Added Calcium And Vitamins A D E ☛ Vitamin K = 0 mcg; Serving size: 1 cup, 249 g

Orange Juice—From Concentrate ☛ Vitamin K = 0 mcg; Serving size: 1 cup, 249 g

Orange Juice—Frozen—Concentrate—Unsweetened—Diluted With 3 Volume Water ☛ Vitamin K = 0.2 mcg; Serving size: 1 cup, 249 g

Orange Juice—Frozen—Concentrate—Unsweetened—Diluted With 3 Volume Water—With Added Calcium ☛ Vitamin K = 0.2 mcg; Serving size: 1 cup, 249 g

Orange Juice—Frozen—Concentrate—Unsweetened—Undiluted ☛ Vitamin K = 1 mcg; Serving size: 1 cup, 262 g

Orange Juice—Frozen—Concentrate—Unsweetened—Undiluted— With Added Calcium ☛ Vitamin K = 1 mcg; Serving size: 1 cup, 262 g

Orange Juice—With Added Calcium ☛ Vitamin K = 0 mcg; Serving size: 1 cup, 249 g

Orange Juice—With Added Calcium And Vitamin D ☛ Vitamin K = 0 mcg; Serving size: 1 cup, 249 g

Orange Pineapple Juice—Blend ☛ Vitamin K = 0.2 mcg; Serving size: 8 fl oz, 246 g

Orange Sections—Canned—Juice—Pack ☛ Vitamin K = 0 mcg; Serving size: 1 cup, 204 g

Orange-Grapefruit Juice—Canned—Or Bottled Unsweetened ☛ Vitamin K = 0.2 mcg; Serving size: 1 cup, 247 g

Oranges ☛ Vitamin K = 0 mcg; Serving size: 1 cup, sections, 180 g

Papaya ☛ Vitamin K = 3.8 mcg; Serving size: 1 cup 1 inch pieces, 145 g

Papaya Cooked Or—Canned—In Sugar Or Syrup ☛ Vitamin K = 4.1 mcg; Serving size: 1 cup, 244 g

Papaya Dried ☛ Vitamin K = 2 mcg; Serving size: 1 strip, 23 g

Papaya Green Cooked ☛ Vitamin K = 6.3 mcg; Serving size: 1 cup, 244 g

Papaya Nectar Canned ☛ Vitamin K = 2 mcg; Serving size: 1 cup, 250 g

Papaya—Canned—Heavy Syrup Drained ☛ Vitamin K = 0.1 mcg; Serving size: 1 piece, 39 g

Passion Fruit (Granadilla) ☛ Vitamin K = 1.7 mcg; Serving size: 1 cup, 236 g

Peach Dried Cooked With Sugar ☛ Vitamin K = 12.2 mcg; Serving size: 1 cup, 270 g

Peach Nectar—Canned—Without Added Ascorbic Acid ☛ Vitamin K = 3 mcg; Serving size: 1 cup, 249 g

Peach Pickled ☛ Vitamin K = 1.6 mcg; Serving size: 1 fruit, 88 g

Peaches Dried Sulfured Stewed Without Added Sugar ☛ Vitamin K = 12.9 mcg; Serving size: 1 cup, 258 g

Peaches Spiced—Canned—Heavy Syrup Pack—Solids And Liquids ☛ Vitamin K = 4.1 mcg; Serving size: 1 cup, whole, 242 g

Peaches—Canned—Heavy Syrup Drained ☛ Vitamin K = 5.3 mcg; Serving size: 1 cup, 222 g

Peaches—Canned—Heavy Syrup Pack—Solids And Liquids ☛ Vitamin K = 4.5 mcg; Serving size: 1 cup, 262 g

Peaches—Canned—Juice—Pack—Solids And Liquids ☛ Vitamin K = 4.3 mcg; Serving size: 1 cup, 250 g

Peaches—Canned—Light Syrup Pack—Solids And Liquids ☛ Vitamin K = 4.3 mcg; Serving size: 1 cup, halves or slices, 251 g

Peaches—Canned—Water Pack—Solids And Liquids ☛ Vitamin K = 4.1 mcg; Serving size: 1 cup, halves or slices, 244 g

Peaches—Frozen—Sliced Sweetened ☛ Vitamin K = 5.5 mcg; Serving size: 1 cup, thawed, 250 g

Pear Dried Cooked With Sugar ☛ Vitamin K = 24.6 mcg; Serving size: 1 cup, 280 g

Pear Nectar—Canned—Without Added Ascorbic Acid ☞ Vitamin K = 4.5 mcg; Serving size: 1 cup, 250 g

Pears ☞ Vitamin K = 6.2 mcg; Serving size: 1 cup, slices, 140 g

Pears Dried Sulfured Stewed Without Added Sugar ☞ Vitamin K = 25.2 mcg; Serving size: 1 cup, halves, 255 g

Pears—Canned—Heavy Syrup Drained ☞ Vitamin K = 0.6 mcg; Serving size: 1 cup, 201 g

Pears—Canned—Heavy Syrup Pack—Solids And Liquids ☞ Vitamin K = 0.8 mcg; Serving size: 1 cup, 266 g

Pears—Canned—Juice—Pack—Solids And Liquids ☞ Vitamin K = 0.7 mcg; Serving size: 1 cup, halves, 248 g

Pears—Canned—Light Syrup Pack—Solids And Liquids ☞ Vitamin K = 0.8 mcg; Serving size: 1 cup, halves, 251 g

Pears—Canned—Water Pack—Solids And Liquids ☞ Vitamin K = 0.7 mcg; Serving size: 1 cup, halves, 244 g

Peppers Pickled ☞ Vitamin K = 6.2 mcg; Serving size: 1 cup, 135 g

Pickled Green Bananas Puerto Rican Style ☞ Vitamin K = 27 mcg; Serving size: 1 cup, 150 g

Pineapple ☞ Vitamin K = 1.2 mcg; Serving size: 1 cup, chunks, 165 g

Pineapple (Traditional) ☞ Vitamin K = 1.2 mcg; Serving size: 1 cup, chunks, 165 g

Pineapple Dried ☞ Vitamin K = 0.6 mcg; Serving size: 1 piece, 28 g

Pineapple Juice—Canned—Or Bottled—Unsweetened—With Added Ascorbic Acid ☞ Vitamin K = 0.8 mcg; Serving size: 1 cup, 250 g

Pineapple Juice—Canned—Or Bottled—Unsweetened—Without Added Ascorbic Acid ☞ Vitamin K = 0.8 mcg; Serving size: 1 cup, 250 g

Pineapple   Juice—Frozen—Concentrate—Unsweetened—Diluted
With 3 Volume Water ☞ Vitamin K = 0.8 mcg; Serving size: 1 cup,
250 g

Pineapple Juice—Frozen—Concentrate—Unsweetened—Undiluted
☞ Vitamin K = 2.2 mcg; Serving size: 1 can (6 fl oz), 216 g

Pineapple Raw Extra Sweet Variety ☞ Vitamin K = 1.2 mcg; Serving
size: 1 cup, chunks, 165 g

Pineapple Salad With Dressing ☞ Vitamin K = 24.8 mcg; Serving size:
1 serving (lettuce, 1 cup diced pineapple, dressing), 184 g

Pineapple—Canned—Heavy Syrup Pack—Solids And Liquids ☞
Vitamin K = 0.8 mcg; Serving size: 1 cup, crushed, sliced, or chunks,
254 g

Pineapple—Canned—Juice—Pack—Drained ☞ Vitamin K = 1.3 mcg;
Serving size: 1 cup, chunks, 181 g

Pineapple—Canned—Juice—Pack—Solids And Liquids ☞ Vitamin
K = 0.7 mcg; Serving size: 1 cup, crushed, sliced, or chunks, 249 g

Pineapple—Canned—Light Syrup Pack—Solids And Liquids ☞
Vitamin K = 0.8 mcg; Serving size: 1 cup, crushed, sliced, or chunks,
252 g

Pineapple—Canned—Water Pack—Solids And Liquids ☞ Vitamin K
= 0.7 mcg; Serving size: 1 cup, crushed, sliced, or chunks, 246 g

Pineapple—Frozen—Chunks Sweetened ☞ Vitamin K = 1.7 mcg;
Serving size: 1 cup, chunks, 245 g

Pink Grapefruit ☞ Vitamin K = 0 mcg; Serving size: 1 cup sections,
with juice, 230 g

Plantains ☞ Vitamin K = 42.6 mcg; Serving size: 1 cup, sliced, 148 g

Plantains Cooked ☞ Vitamin K = 25.8 mcg; Serving size: 1 cup,
mashed, 200 g

Plum Pickled ☛ Vitamin K = 1.2 mcg; Serving size: 1 plum, 28 g

Plums ☛ Vitamin K = 10.6 mcg; Serving size: 1 cup, sliced, 165 g

Plums Dried (Prunes) Stewed Without Added Sugar ☛ Vitamin K = 64.7 mcg; Serving size: 1 cup, pitted, 248 g

Plums—Canned—Heavy Syrup Drained ☛ Vitamin K = 11.7 mcg; Serving size: 1 cup, with pits, yields, 183 g

Plums—Canned—Purple Heavy Syrup Pack—Solids And Liquids ☛ Vitamin K = 11.1 mcg; Serving size: 1 cup, pitted, 258 g

Plums—Canned—Purple Juice—Pack—Solids And Liquids ☛ Vitamin K = 10.8 mcg; Serving size: 1 cup, pitted, 252 g

Plums—Canned—Purple Light Syrup Pack—Solids And Liquids ☛ Vitamin K = 10.8 mcg; Serving size: 1 cup, pitted, 252 g

Plums—Canned—Purple Water Pack—Solids And Liquids ☛ Vitamin K = 10.7 mcg; Serving size: 1 cup, pitted, 249 g

Pomegranate Juice—Bottled ☛ Vitamin K = 25.9 mcg; Serving size: 1 cup, 249 g

Pomegranates ☛ Vitamin K = 14.3 mcg; Serving size: 1/2 cup arils (seed/juice sacs), 87 g

Prune Dried Cooked With Sugar ☛ Vitamin K = 2.3 mcg; Serving size: 1 prune, 10 g

Prune Whip ☛ Vitamin K = 23.3 mcg; Serving size: 1 cup, 130 g

Prunes (Dried Plums) ☛ Vitamin K = 103.5 mcg; Serving size: 1 cup, pitted, 174 g

Purple Passion Fruit Juice ☛ Vitamin K = 1 mcg; Serving size: 1 cup, 247 g

Raisins ☛ Vitamin K = 5.8 mcg; Serving size: 1 cup, packed, 165 g

Raisins Cooked ☛ Vitamin K = 4.7 mcg; Serving size: 1 cup, 295 g

Raspberries ☞ Vitamin K = 9.6 mcg; Serving size: 1 cup, 123 g

Raspberries Cooked Or—Canned—Unsweetened Water Pack ☞ Vitamin K = 12.6 mcg; Serving size: 1 cup, 243 g

Raspberries—Canned—Red Heavy Syrup Pack—Solids And Liquids ☞ Vitamin K = 13.3 mcg; Serving size: 1 cup, 256 g

Raspberries—Frozen—Red Sweetened ☞ Vitamin K = 16.3 mcg; Serving size: 1 cup, thawed, 250 g

Raspberries—Frozen—Unsweetened ☞ Vitamin K = 19.5 mcg; Serving size: 1 cup, 250 g

Red And White Currants ☞ Vitamin K = 12.3 mcg; Serving size: 1 cup, 112 g

Red Anjou Pears ☞ Vitamin K = 6.2 mcg; Serving size: 1 small, 126 g

Red Delicious Apples ☞ Vitamin K = 2.8 mcg; Serving size: 1 cup, sliced, 109 g

Red Or Green Grapes (European) ☞ Vitamin K = 22 mcg; Serving size: 1 cup, 151 g

Rhubarb ☞ Vitamin K = 35.7 mcg; Serving size: 1 cup, diced, 122 g

Rhubarb Cooked Or—Canned—Drained Solids ☞ Vitamin K = 50.6 mcg; Serving size: 1 cup, 240 g

Rhubarb Cooked Or—Canned—In Light Syrup ☞ Vitamin K = 62.9 mcg; Serving size: 1 cup, 240 g

Rhubarb Cooked Or—Canned—Unsweetened ☞ Vitamin K = 70.3 mcg; Serving size: 1 cup, 240 g

Rhubarb—Frozen—Cooked With Sugar ☞ Vitamin K = 50.6 mcg; Serving size: 1 cup, 240 g

Rhubarb—Frozen—Uncooked ☞ Vitamin K = 40.1 mcg; Serving size: 1 cup, diced, 137 g

Sauerkraut Cooked Fat Added In Cooking ☞ Vitamin K = 20 mcg; Serving size: 1 cup, 147 g

Seaweed Pickled ☞ Vitamin K = 13.5 mcg; Serving size: 1 cup, 150 g

Shredded Coconut Meat (Sweetened) ☞ Vitamin K = 8.7 mcg; Serving size: 1 cup, 256 g

Sour Red Cherries ☞ Vitamin K = 3.3 mcg; Serving size: 1 cup, without pits, 155 g

Sour Red Cherries (Frozen) ☞ Vitamin K = 2.3 mcg; Serving size: 1 cup, unthawed, 155 g

Soursop ☞ Vitamin K = 0.9 mcg; Serving size: 1 cup, pulp, 225 g

Starfruit (Carambola) ☞ Vitamin K = 0 mcg; Serving size: 1 cup, cubes, 132 g

Starfruit Cooked With Sugar ☞ Vitamin K = 0 mcg; Serving size: 1 cup, 205 g

Strawberries ☞ Vitamin K = 3.3 mcg; Serving size: 1 cup, halves, 152 g

Strawberries Cooked Or—Canned—Unsweetened Water Pack ☞ Vitamin K = 3.6 mcg; Serving size: 1 cup, 242 g

Strawberries Raw With Sugar ☞ Vitamin K = 3.4 mcg; Serving size: 1 cup, 160 g

Strawberries—Canned—Heavy Syrup Pack—Solids And Liquids ☞ Vitamin K = 3.8 mcg; Serving size: 1 cup, 254 g

Strawberries—Frozen—Sweetened Sliced ☞ Vitamin K = 4.3 mcg; Serving size: 1 cup, thawed, 255 g

Tamarind Nectar Canned ☞ Vitamin K = 0.3 mcg; Serving size: 1 cup, 251 g

Tamarinds ☞ Vitamin K = 3.4 mcg; Serving size: 1 cup, pulp, 120 g

Tangerine Juice ☞ Vitamin K = 0 mcg; Serving size: 1 cup, 247 g

Tangerines ☞ Vitamin K = 0 mcg; Serving size: 1 cup, sections, 195 g

Tangerines (Mandarin Oranges)—Canned—Juice—Pack ☞ Vitamin K = 0 mcg; Serving size: 1 cup, 249 g

Tangerines (Mandarin Oranges)—Canned—Juice—Pack—Drained ☞ Vitamin K = 0 mcg; Serving size: 1 cup, 189 g

Tangerines (Mandarin Oranges)—Canned—Light Syrup Pack ☞ Vitamin K = 0 mcg; Serving size: 1 cup, 252 g

Tomato Green Pickled ☞ Vitamin K = 5.6 mcg; Serving size: 1 tomato (2-3/8" dia), 74 g

Tsukemono Japanese Pickles ☞ Vitamin K = 85.3 mcg; Serving size: 1 cup, 135 g

Turnip Pickled ☞ Vitamin K = 0.6 mcg; Serving size: 1 cup, 155 g

Vegetable Relish ☞ Vitamin K = 16.8 mcg; Serving size: 1 cup, 140 g

Vegetables Pickled ☞ Vitamin K = 17.8 mcg; Serving size: 1 cup, 163 g

Vegetables Pickled Hawaiian Style ☞ Vitamin K = 55.7 mcg; Serving size: 1 cup, 150 g

Watermelon ☞ Vitamin K = 0.2 mcg; Serving size: 1 cup, balls, 154 g

White Grapefruit ☞ Vitamin K = 0 mcg; Serving size: 1 cup sections, with juice, 230 g

White Grapefruit Juice ☞ Vitamin K = 0 mcg; Serving size: 1 cup, 247 g

Yellow Passion Fruit Juice ☞ Vitamin K = 1 mcg; Serving size: 1 cup, 247 g

Yellow Peaches ☞ Vitamin K = 4 mcg; Serving size: 1 cup slices, 154 g

Zante Currants ☞ Vitamin K = 4.8 mcg; Serving size: 1 cup, 144 g

Zucchini Pickled ☞ Vitamin K = 5.3 mcg; Serving size: 1 cup, 170 g

21

GRAINS AND PASTA

Pasta—Whole Wheat ☞ Vitamin K = 0.7 mcg; Serving size: 1 cup spaghetti not packed, 117 g

Amaranth Grain Uncooked ☞ Vitamin K = 0 mcg; Serving size: 1 cup, 193 g

Barley (Cooked with Fat) ☞ Vitamin K = 3.6 mcg; Serving size: 1 cup, cooked, 170 g

Barley (Cooked without Fat) ☞ Vitamin K = 1.4 mcg; Serving size: 1 cup, cooked, 170 g

Barley Flour Or Meal ☞ Vitamin K = 3.3 mcg; Serving size: 1 cup, 148 g

Barley Hulled ☞ Vitamin K = 4 mcg; Serving size: 1 cup, 184 g

Barley Malt Flour ☞ Vitamin K = 3.6 mcg; Serving size: 1 cup, 162 g

Barley Pearled Raw ☞ Vitamin K = 4.4 mcg; Serving size: 1 cup, 200 g

Brown Rice ☞ Vitamin K = 0.4 mcg; Serving size: 1 cup, 202 g

Buckwheat Flour Whole-Groat ☛ Vitamin K = 8.4 mcg; Serving size: 1 cup, 120 g

Buckwheat Groats (Cooked with Fat) ☛ Vitamin K = 10.9 mcg; Serving size: 1 cup, cooked, 170 g

Buckwheat Groats (Cooked without Fat) ☛ Vitamin K = 3.2 mcg; Serving size: 1 cup, cooked, 170 g

Bulgur (Cooked with Fat) ☛ Vitamin K = 9.9 mcg; Serving size: 1 cup, cooked, 140 g

Bulgur (Cooked without Fat) ☛ Vitamin K = 0.7 mcg; Serving size: 1 cup, cooked, 140 g

Bulgur (Cooked) ☛ Vitamin K = 0.9 mcg; Serving size: 1 cup, 182 g

Bulgur Dry ☛ Vitamin K = 2.7 mcg; Serving size: 1 cup, 140 g

Canned Hominy ☛ Vitamin K = 0.3 mcg; Serving size: 1 cup, 165 g

Congee ☛ Vitamin K = 0 mcg; Serving size: 1 cup, 249 g

Corn Bran Crude ☛ Vitamin K = 0.2 mcg; Serving size: 1 cup, 76 g

Corn Flour Masa—Enriched White ☛ Vitamin K = 0 mcg; Serving size: 1 cup, 114 g

Corn Flour Masa—Unenriched White ☛ Vitamin K = 0 mcg; Serving size: 1 cup, 114 g

Corn Flour Whole-Grain White ☛ Vitamin K = 0.4 mcg; Serving size: 1 cup, 117 g

Corn Flour Whole-Grain Yellow ☛ Vitamin K = 0.4 mcg; Serving size: 1 cup, 117 g

Corn Flour Yellow Degermed—Unenriched ☛ Vitamin K = 0.4 mcg; Serving size: 1 cup, 126 g

Corn Grain Yellow ☛ Vitamin K = 0.5 mcg; Serving size: 1 cup, 166 g

Cornmeal—Degermed—Enriched White ☞ Vitamin K = 0 mcg; Serving size: 1 cup, 157 g

Cornmeal—Degermed—Enriched Yellow ☞ Vitamin K = 0 mcg; Serving size: 1 cup, 157 g

Cornmeal—Degermed—Unenriched White ☞ Vitamin K = 0 mcg; Serving size: 1 cup, 157 g

Cornmeal—Degermed—Unenriched Yellow ☞ Vitamin K = 0 mcg; Serving size: 1 cup, 157 g

Cornstarch ☞ Vitamin K = 0 mcg; Serving size: 1 cup, 128 g

Couscous (Cooked) ☞ Vitamin K = 0.2 mcg; Serving size: 1 cup, cooked, 157 g

Couscous Plain Cooked ☞ Vitamin K = 0.2 mcg; Serving size: 1 cup, cooked, 160 g

Egg Noodles (Cooked) ☞ Vitamin K = 0 mcg; Serving size: 1 cup, 160 g

Macaroni Vegetable—Enriched Cooked ☞ Vitamin K = 0.4 mcg; Serving size: 1 cup spiral shaped, 134 g

Millet (Cooked with Fat) ☞ Vitamin K = 9.4 mcg; Serving size: 1 cup, cooked, 170 g

Millet (Cooked without Fat) ☞ Vitamin K = 0.5 mcg; Serving size: 1 cup, cooked, 170 g

Millet (Cooked) ☞ Vitamin K = 0.5 mcg; Serving size: 1 cup, 174 g

Millet Flour ☞ Vitamin K = 1 mcg; Serving size: 1 cup, 119 g

Millet Raw ☞ Vitamin K = 1.8 mcg; Serving size: 1 cup, 200 g

Noodles Chinese Chow Mein ☞ Vitamin K = 1.5 mcg; Serving size: 1/2 cup dry, 28 g

Noodles Cooked ☞ Vitamin K = 0 mcg; Serving size: 1 cup, cooked, 160 g

Noodles Egg Cooked—Enriched—With Added Salt ☞ Vitamin K = 0 mcg; Serving size: 1 cup, 160 g

Noodles Egg Cooked—Unenriched—With Added Salt ☞ Vitamin K = 0 mcg; Serving size: 1 cup, 160 g

Noodles Egg Dry—Enriched ☞ Vitamin K = 0.2 mcg; Serving size: 1 cup, 38 g

Noodles Egg Dry—Unenriched ☞ Vitamin K = 0.2 mcg; Serving size: 1 cup, 38 g

Noodles Egg—Unenriched Cooked—Without Added Salt ☞ Vitamin K = 0 mcg; Serving size: 1 cup, 160 g

Noodles Flat Crunchy Chinese Restaurant ☞ Vitamin K = 2.8 mcg; Serving size: 1 cup, 45 g

Noodles Vegetable Cooked ☞ Vitamin K = 160.8 mcg; Serving size: 1 cup, cooked, 160 g

Noodles Whole Grain Cooked ☞ Vitamin K = 1 mcg; Serving size: 1 cup, cooked, 160 g

Oat Bran ☞ Vitamin K = 3 mcg; Serving size: 1 cup, 94 g

Oat Flour Partially Debranned ☞ Vitamin K = 3.3 mcg; Serving size: 1 cup, 104 g

Oatmeal (Cooked) ☞ Vitamin K = 0.7 mcg; Serving size: 1 cup, 234 g

Pasta—Cooked ☞ Vitamin K = 0 mcg; Serving size: 1 cup, cooked, 140 g

Pasta—Cooked—Enriched—With Added Salt ☞ Vitamin K = 0 mcg; Serving size: 1 cup spaghetti not packed, 124 g

Pasta—Cooked—Enriched—Without Added Salt ☞ Vitamin K = 0 mcg; Serving size: 1 cup spaghetti not packed, 124 g

Pasta—Cooked—Unenriched—With Added Salt ☞ Vitamin K = 0 mcg; Serving size: 1 cup spaghetti not packed, 124 g

Pasta—Dry—Enriched ☛ Vitamin K = 0.1 mcg; Serving size: 1 cup spaghetti, 91 g

Pasta—Dry—Unenriched ☛ Vitamin K = 0.1 mcg; Serving size: 1 cup spaghetti, 91 g

Pasta—Gluten-Free Corn And Rice Flour Cooked ☛ Vitamin K = 0 mcg; Serving size: 1 cup spaghetti, 141 g

Pasta—Gluten-Free Corn Flour And Quinoa Flour Cooked ☛ Vitamin K = 0 mcg; Serving size: 1 cup spaghetti packed, 166 g

Pasta—Unenriched (Cooked) ☛ Vitamin K = 0 mcg; Serving size: 1 cup spaghetti not packed, 124 g

Pasta—Vegetable Cooked ☛ Vitamin K = 0.4 mcg; Serving size: 1 cup, cooked, 140 g

Pasta—Whole Grain 51% Whole Wheat Remaining—Enriched Semolina Cooked ☛ Vitamin K = 0.2 mcg; Serving size: 1 cup spaghetti not packed, 116 g

Pasta—Whole Grain 51% Whole Wheat Remaining—Enriched Semolina Dry ☛ Vitamin K = 0.8 mcg; Serving size: 1 cup spaghetti, 91 g

Pasta—Whole Grain 51% Whole Wheat Remaining—Unenriched Semolina Dry ☛ Vitamin K = 0.8 mcg; Serving size: 1 cup spaghetti, 91 g

Pasta—Whole Grain Cooked ☛ Vitamin K = 0.8 mcg; Serving size: 1 cup, cooked, 140 g

Pasta—Whole-Wheat Dry ☛ Vitamin K = 1.3 mcg; Serving size: 1 cup spaghetti, 91 g

Pearled Barley (Cooked) ☛ Vitamin K = 1.3 mcg; Serving size: 1 cup, 157 g

Quinoa (Cooked with Fat) ☛ Vitamin K = 8.5 mcg; Serving size: 1 cup, cooked, 170 g

Quinoa (Cooked without Fat) 🐄 Vitamin K = 0 mcg; Serving size: 1 cup, cooked, 170 g

Quinoa Cooked 🐄 Vitamin K = 0 mcg; Serving size: 1 cup, 185 g

Quinoa Uncooked 🐄 Vitamin K = 0 mcg; Serving size: 1 cup, 170 g

Rice—Bran 🐄 Vitamin K = 2.2 mcg; Serving size: 1 cup, 118 g

Rice—Brown And Wild Cooked (Cooked with Fat) 🐄 Vitamin K = 4.7 mcg; Serving size: 1 cup, cooked, 155 g

Rice—Brown And Wild Cooked (Cooked without Fat) 🐄 Vitamin K = 0.3 mcg; Serving size: 1 cup, cooked, 151 g

Rice—Brown Cooked (Cooked with Fat) Prepared With Butter 🐄 Vitamin K = 0.8 mcg; Serving size: 1 cup, cooked, 196 g

Rice—Brown Cooked (Cooked with Fat) Prepared With Margarine 🐄 Vitamin K = 5.1 mcg; Serving size: 1 cup, cooked, 196 g

Rice—Brown Cooked (Cooked with Fat) Prepared With Oil 🐄 Vitamin K = 5.7 mcg; Serving size: 1 cup, cooked, 196 g

Rice—Brown Long-Grain Raw 🐄 Vitamin K = 1.1 mcg; Serving size: 1 cup, 185 g

Rice—Brown Parboiled Cooked Uncle Bens 🐄 Vitamin K = 0.6 mcg; Serving size: 1 cup, 155 g

Rice—Brown Parboiled Dry Uncle Bens 🐄 Vitamin K = 0.4 mcg; Serving size: 1/4 cup, 48 g

Rice—Cooked—With Milk 🐄 Vitamin K = 0.4 mcg; Serving size: 1 cup, cooked, 200 g

Rice—Flour White—Unenriched 🐄 Vitamin K = 0 mcg; Serving size: 1 cup, 158 g

Rice—Noodles (Cooked) 🐄 Vitamin K = 0 mcg; Serving size: 1 cup, 176 g

Rice—Noodles Dry ☛ Vitamin K = 0 mcg; Serving size: 2 oz, 57 g

Rice—Sweet Cooked—With Honey ☛ Vitamin K = 0 mcg; Serving size: 1 cup, cooked, 175 g

Rice—White Cooked (Cooked with Fat) Prepared With Butter ☛ Vitamin K = 0.3 mcg; Serving size: 1 cup, cooked, 163 g

Rice—White Cooked (Cooked with Fat) Prepared With Margarine ☛ Vitamin K = 4.9 mcg; Serving size: 1 cup, cooked, 163 g

Rice—White Cooked (Cooked with Fat) Prepared With Oil ☛ Vitamin K = 5.4 mcg; Serving size: 1 cup, cooked, 163 g

Rice—White Cooked (Cooked without Fat) ☛ Vitamin K = 0 mcg; Serving size: 1 cup, cooked, 158 g

Rice—White Cooked Glutinous ☛ Vitamin K = 0 mcg; Serving size: 1 cup, cooked, 174 g

Rice—White Cooked—With Fat Puerto Rican Style ☛ Vitamin K = 10.9 mcg; Serving size: 1 cup, cooked, 155 g

Rice—White Glutinous—Unenriched Cooked ☛ Vitamin K = 0 mcg; Serving size: 1 cup, 174 g

Rice—White Long-Grain Parboiled—Enriched Cooked ☛ Vitamin K = 0 mcg; Serving size: 1 cup, 158 g

Rice—White Long-Grain Parboiled—Enriched Dry ☛ Vitamin K = 0.2 mcg; Serving size: 1 cup, 185 g

Rice—White Long-Grain Parboiled—Unenriched Cooked ☛ Vitamin K = 0 mcg; Serving size: 1 cup, 158 g

Rice—White Long-Grain Parboiled—Unenriched Dry ☛ Vitamin K = 0.2 mcg; Serving size: 1 cup, 185 g

Rice—White Long-Grain Precooked Or Instant—Enriched Dry ☛ Vitamin K = 0.1 mcg; Serving size: 1 cup, 95 g

Rice—White Long-Grain Precooked Or Instant—Enriched Prepared ☞ Vitamin K = 0 mcg; Serving size: 1 cup, 165 g

Rice—White Long-Grain Regular Cooked—Enriched—With Salt ☞ Vitamin K = 0 mcg; Serving size: 1 cup, 158 g

Rice—White Long-Grain Regular Cooked—Unenriched—With Salt ☞ Vitamin K = 0 mcg; Serving size: 1 cup, 158 g

Rice—White Long-Grain Regular Raw—Enriched ☞ Vitamin K = 0.2 mcg; Serving size: 1 cup, 185 g

Rice—White Long-Grain Regular Raw—Unenriched ☞ Vitamin K = 0.2 mcg; Serving size: 1 cup, 185 g

Rice—White Long-Grain Regular—Unenriched Cooked—Without Salt ☞ Vitamin K = 0 mcg; Serving size: 1 cup, 158 g

Rice—Wild 100% Cooked (Cooked with Fat) ☞ Vitamin K = 5.9 mcg; Serving size: 1 cup, cooked, 164 g

Rice—Wild 100% Cooked (Cooked without Fat) ☞ Vitamin K = 0.8 mcg; Serving size: 1 cup, cooked, 164 g

Roasted Buckwheat Groats ☞ Vitamin K = 3.2 mcg; Serving size: 1 cup, 168 g

Rye Flour Dark ☞ Vitamin K = 7.6 mcg; Serving size: 1 cup, 128 g

Rye Flour Light ☞ Vitamin K = 6 mcg; Serving size: 1 cup, 102 g

Rye Flour Medium ☞ Vitamin K = 6 mcg; Serving size: 1 cup, 102 g

Rye Grain ☞ Vitamin K = 10 mcg; Serving size: 1 cup, 169 g

Spaghetti Spinach Dry ☞ Vitamin K = 86.4 mcg; Serving size: 2 oz, 57 g

Spelt Uncooked ☞ Vitamin K = 6.3 mcg; Serving size: 1 cup, 174 g

Spinach Egg Noodles (Cooked) ☞ Vitamin K = 161.8 mcg; Serving size: 1 cup, 160 g

Tapioca Pearl Dry ☛ Vitamin K = 0 mcg; Serving size: 1 cup, 152 g

Teff Uncooked ☛ Vitamin K = 3.7 mcg; Serving size: 1 cup, 193 g

Uncooked Whole-Grain Cornmeal ☛ Vitamin K = 0.4 mcg; Serving size: 1 cup, 122 g

Uncooked Yellow Cornmeal ☛ Vitamin K = 0.4 mcg; Serving size: 1 cup, 122 g

Vermicelli Made From Soybeans ☛ Vitamin K = 2 mcg; Serving size: 1 cup, 140 g

Wheat Bran Crude ☛ Vitamin K = 1.1 mcg; Serving size: 1 cup, 58 g

Wheat Flour White All-Purpose—Enriched Unbleached ☛ Vitamin K = 0.4 mcg; Serving size: 1 cup, 125 g

Wheat Flour White All-Purpose—Unenriched ☛ Vitamin K = 0.4 mcg; Serving size: 1 cup, 125 g

Wheat Flour White Cake—Enriched ☛ Vitamin K = 0.4 mcg; Serving size: 1 cup unsifted, dipped, 137 g

Wheat Flour White Tortilla Mix—Enriched ☛ Vitamin K = 1.2 mcg; Serving size: 1 cup, 111 g

Wheat Flours Bread—Unenriched ☛ Vitamin K = 0.4 mcg; Serving size: 1 cup unsifted, dipped, 137 g

Wheat Hard White ☛ Vitamin K = 3.6 mcg; Serving size: 1 cup, 192 g

Wheat Kamut Khorasan Uncooked ☛ Vitamin K = 3.3 mcg; Serving size: 1 cup, 186 g

Wheat Soft White ☛ Vitamin K = 3.2 mcg; Serving size: 1 cup, 168 g

Wheat—Flour White All-Purpose Self-Rising—Enriched ☛ Vitamin K = 0.4 mcg; Serving size: 1 cup, 125 g

Wheat—Flour White All-Purpose—Enriched Bleached ☛ Vitamin K = 0.4 mcg; Serving size: 1 cup, 125 g

Wheat—Flour White Bread—Enriched ☞ Vitamin K = 0.4 mcg; Serving size: 1 cup, 137 g

Wheat—Flour Whole-Grain ☞ Vitamin K = 2.3 mcg; Serving size: 1 cup, 120 g

Wheat—Hard Red Spring ☞ Vitamin K = 3.6 mcg; Serving size: 1 cup, 192 g

Wheat—Hard Red Winter ☞ Vitamin K = 3.6 mcg; Serving size: 1 cup, 192 g

White Rice ☞ Vitamin K = 0 mcg; Serving size: 1 cup, 158 g

Whole Grain Sorghum Flour ☞ Vitamin K = 7.7 mcg; Serving size: 1 cup, 121 g

Wild Rice (Cooked) ☞ Vitamin K = 0.8 mcg; Serving size: 1 cup, 164 g

Wild Rice Raw ☞ Vitamin K = 3 mcg; Serving size: 1 cup, 160 g

Yellow Cornmeal—(Grits) ☞ Vitamin K = 0 mcg; Serving size: 1 cup, 233 g

Yellow Rice Cooked (Cooked with Fat) ☞ Vitamin K = 4.1 mcg; Serving size: 1 cup, cooked, 163 g

Yellow Rice Cooked (Cooked without Fat) ☞ Vitamin K = 0.3 mcg; Serving size: 1 cup, cooked, 158 g

22

MEATS

Armadillo—Cooked ☛ Vitamin K = 0.4 mcg; Serving size: 1 oz, boneless, cooked, 28 g

Bacon—And Beef Sticks ☛ Vitamin K = 0.4 mcg; Serving size: 1 oz, 28 g

Bacon—Turkey Low Sodium ☛ Vitamin K = 1.6 mcg; Serving size: 1 serving, 15 g

Bear—Cooked ☛ Vitamin K = 0.5 mcg; Serving size: 1 oz, boneless, cooked, 28 g

Beaver—Cooked ☛ Vitamin K = 0.4 mcg; Serving size: 1 oz, boneless, cooked, 28 g

Beef—Baloney (Bologna) ☛ Vitamin K = 0.7 mcg; Serving size: 1 slice, 30 g

Beef—Bottom Sirloin Tri-Tip Roast—Separable Lean Only—Trimmed To 0 Inch Fat All Grades—Raw ☛ Vitamin K = 1 mcg; Serving size: 3 oz, 85 g

Beef—Brisket Flat Half Boneless—Separable Lean And Fat—

Trimmed To 0 Inch Fat All Grades—Raw ☞ Vitamin K = 1.3 mcg; Serving size: 3 oz, 85 g

Beef—Brisket Flat Half—Separable Lean And Fat—Trimmed To 0 Inch Fat All Grades—Cooked Braised ☞ Vitamin K = 1.4 mcg; Serving size: 3 oz, 85 g

Beef—Brisket Whole—Separable Lean And Fat—Trimmed To 0 Inch Fat All Grades—Cooked Braised ☞ Vitamin K = 1.5 mcg; Serving size: 3 oz, 85 g

Beef—Brisket—Cooked—Lean And Fat Eaten ☞ Vitamin K = 0.4 mcg; Serving size: 1 thin slice, 21 g

Beef—Burgundy ☞ Vitamin K = 15.6 mcg; Serving size: 1 cup, 244 g

Beef—Chuck Arm Pot Roast—Separable Lean And Fat—Trimmed To 0 Inch Fat All Grades—Cooked Braised ☞ Vitamin K = 1.5 mcg; Serving size: 3 oz, 85 g

Beef—Chuck Blade Roast—Separable Lean And Fat—Trimmed To 0 Inch Fat All Grades—Cooked Braised ☞ Vitamin K = 4.7 mcg; Serving size: 1 piece, cooked, 235 g

Beef—Chuck Eye Country-Style Ribs Boneless—Separable Lean And Fat—Trimmed To 0 Inch Fat All Grades—Cooked Braised ☞ Vitamin K = 1.4 mcg; Serving size: 3 oz, 85 g

Beef—Chuck Eye Roast Boneless Americas Beef—Roast—Separable Lean And Fat—Trimmed To 0 Inch Fat All Grades—Cooked Roasted ☞ Vitamin K = 1.4 mcg; Serving size: 3 oz, 85 g

Beef—Chuck Eye Steak Boneless—Separable Lean And Fat—Trimmed To 0 Inch Fat All Grades—Cooked Grilled ☞ Vitamin K = 1.4 mcg; Serving size: 3 oz, 85 g

Beef—Chuck Mock Tender Steak Boneless—Separable Lean Only—Trimmed To 0 Inch Fat All Grades—Raw ☞ Vitamin K = 1.3 mcg; Serving size: 3 oz, 85 g

Beef—Chuck Short Ribs Boneless—Separable Lean Only—Trimmed To 0 Inch Fat All Grades—Raw ☛ Vitamin K = 1.3 mcg; Serving size: 3 oz, 85 g

Beef—Composite Of—Trimmed Retail Cuts—Separable Lean And Fat—Trimmed To 0 Inch Fat All Grades—Cooked ☛ Vitamin K = 1.3 mcg; Serving size: 3 oz, 85 g

Beef—Cow Head—Cooked ☛ Vitamin K = 0.4 mcg; Serving size: 1 oz, boneless, cooked, 28 g

Beef—Flank Steak—Separable Lean And Fat—Trimmed To 0 Inch Fat All Grades—Cooked Broiled ☛ Vitamin K = 1.2 mcg; Serving size: 3 oz, 85 g

Beef—Goulash ☛ Vitamin K = 4 mcg; Serving size: 1 cup, 249 g

Beef—Ground 70% Lean Meat / 30% Fat Loaf—Cooked Baked ☛ Vitamin K = 2.5 mcg; Serving size: 3 oz, 85 g

Beef—Ground 80% Lean Meat / 20% Fat Loaf—Cooked Baked ☛ Vitamin K = 1.3 mcg; Serving size: 3 oz, 85 g

Beef—Ground 90% Lean Meat / 10% Fat Loaf—Cooked Baked ☛ Vitamin K = 0.9 mcg; Serving size: 3 oz, 85 g

Beef—Ground 97% Lean Meat / 3% Fat Loaf—Cooked Baked ☛ Vitamin K = 1.3 mcg; Serving size: 3 oz, 85 g

Beef—Liver Braised ☛ Vitamin K = 0.6 mcg; Serving size: 1 oz, raw, 19 g

Beef—Loin Bottom Sirloin Butt Tri-Tip Roast—Separable Lean Only—Trimmed To 0 Inch Fat All Grades—Cooked Roasted ☛ Vitamin K = 1.1 mcg; Serving size: 1 serving, 85 g

Beef—Loin Tenderloin Roast Boneless—Separable Lean And Fat—Trimmed To 0 Inch Fat All Grades—Cooked Roasted ☛ Vitamin K = 1.4 mcg; Serving size: 3 oz, 85 g

Beef—Loin Tenderloin Steak Boneless—Separable Lean And Fat—

Trimmed To 0 Inch Fat All Grades—Cooked Grilled ☛ Vitamin K = 1.4 mcg; Serving size: 3 oz, 85 g

Beef—Neck Bones—Cooked ☛ Vitamin K = 0.2 mcg; Serving size: 1 oz, with bone, cooked, 11 g

Beef—Oxtails—Cooked ☛ Vitamin K = 0.3 mcg; Serving size: 1 oz, with bone, cooked, 16 g

Beef—Rib Back Ribs Bone-In—Separable Lean And Fat—Trimmed To 0 Inch Fat All Grades—Cooked Braised ☛ Vitamin K = 1.4 mcg; Serving size: 3 oz, 85 g

Beef—Roast Roasted—Lean Only Eaten ☛ Vitamin K = 0.4 mcg; Serving size: 1 thin slice, 21 g

Beef—Round Bottom Round Roast—Separable Lean And Fat— Trimmed To 0 Inch Fat All Grades—Cooked Roasted ☛ Vitamin K = 1.1 mcg; Serving size: 3 oz, 85 g

Beef—Round Tip Round Roast—Separable Lean And Fat— Trimmed To 0 Inch Fat All Grades—Cooked Roasted ☛ Vitamin K = 1.1 mcg; Serving size: 3 oz, 85 g

Beef—Sausage ☛ Vitamin K = 0.7 mcg; Serving size: 1 patty, 35 g

Beef—Shortribs—Cooked—Lean And Fat Eaten ☛ Vitamin K = 0.7 mcg; Serving size: 1 small rib, 28 g

Bockwurst Pork Veal—Raw ☛ Vitamin K = 63.9 mcg; Serving size: 1 sausage, 91 g

Chicken Breast—Baked Broiled Or Roasted With Marinade—Skin Eaten From—Raw ☛ Vitamin K = 3.9 mcg; Serving size: 1 cup, cooked, diced, 135 g

Chicken Breast—Tenders Breaded—Uncooked ☛ Vitamin K = 2.2 mcg; Serving size: 1 piece, 15 g

Chicken Wings—Boneless With Hot Sauce From Fast Food / Restaurant ☛ Vitamin K = 2.2 mcg; Serving size: 1 boneless wing, 35 g

Chicken—Back ☛ Vitamin K = 5.4 mcg; Serving size: 1 small back, 110 g

Chicken—Canned—Meat Only With Broth ☛ Vitamin K = 2.6 mcg; Serving size: 1 can (5 oz), 142 g

Chicken—Capons—Meat and Skin—Raw ☛ Vitamin K = 2 mcg; Serving size: 3 oz, 85 g

Chicken—Drumstick—Baked Broiled Or Roasted—Skin Eaten From —Raw ☛ Vitamin K = 4.3 mcg; Serving size: 1 cup, cooked, diced, 135 g

Chicken—Fillet—Grilled ☛ Vitamin K = 4.8 mcg; Serving size: 1 fillet, 100 g

Chicken—Leg Drumstick And Thigh—Baked Coated Skin / Coating Eaten ☛ Vitamin K = 7.2 mcg; Serving size: 1 cup, cooked, diced, 135 g

Chicken—Leg Drumstick And Thigh—Baked Coated Skin / Coating Not Eaten ☛ Vitamin K = 8.1 mcg; Serving size: 1 cup, cooked, diced, 135 g

Chicken—Leg Drumstick And Thigh—Baked Or Broiled—Skin Eaten ☛ Vitamin K = 4.3 mcg; Serving size: 1 cup, cooked, diced, 135 g

Chicken—Leg Drumstick And Thigh—Baked Or Broiled—Skin Not Eaten ☛ Vitamin K = 5 mcg; Serving size: 1 cup, cooked, diced, 135 g

Chicken—Leg Drumstick And Thigh—Fried Coated Skin / Coating Eaten ☛ Vitamin K = 14.6 mcg; Serving size: 1 cup, cooked, diced, 135 g

Chicken—Leg Drumstick And Thigh—Fried Coated Skin / Coating Not Eaten ☛ Vitamin K = 8.1 mcg; Serving size: 1 cup, cooked, diced, 135 g

Chicken—Leg Drumstick And Thigh—Grilled With Sauce—Skin Eaten ☛ Vitamin K = 8.6 mcg; Serving size: 1 cup, cooked, diced, 165 g

Chicken—Leg Drumstick And Thigh—Grilled With Sauce—Skin

Not Eaten ☛ Vitamin K = 9.2 mcg; Serving size: 1 cup, cooked, diced, 165 g

Chicken—Leg Drumstick And Thigh—Grilled Without Sauce—Skin Eaten ☛ Vitamin K = 7.4 mcg; Serving size: 1 cup, cooked, diced, 135 g

Chicken—Leg Drumstick And Thigh—Grilled Without Sauce—Skin Not Eaten ☛ Vitamin K = 8.1 mcg; Serving size: 1 cup, cooked, diced, 135 g

Chicken—Leg Drumstick And Thigh—Sauteed—Skin Eaten ☛ Vitamin K = 7.4 mcg; Serving size: 1 cup, cooked, diced, 135 g

Chicken—Leg Drumstick And Thigh—Sauteed—Skin Not Eaten ☛ Vitamin K = 8.1 mcg; Serving size: 1 cup, cooked, diced, 135 g

Chicken—Liver—Fried ☛ Vitamin K = 0.3 mcg; Serving size: 1 oz, raw, 19 g

Chicken—Neck Or Ribs ☛ Vitamin K = 1.4 mcg; Serving size: 1 neck, 35 g

Chicken—Nuggets From Frozen ☛ Vitamin K = 1.8 mcg; Serving size: 1 nugget, 16 g

Chicken—Nuggets From Other Sources ☛ Vitamin K = 1.3 mcg; Serving size: 1 nugget, 16 g

Chicken—Patty Frozen—Cooked ☛ Vitamin K = 2.5 mcg; Serving size: 1 patty, 60 g

Chicken—Patty Frozen—Uncooked ☛ Vitamin K = 6.7 mcg; Serving size: 1 patty, 60 g

Chicken—Patty Or Nuggets Boneless Breaded With Pasta And Tomato Sauce Fruit Dessert Frozen Meal ☛ Vitamin K = 10.2 mcg; Serving size: 1 meal (6.80 oz), 193 g

Chicken—Patty Parmigiana Breaded With Vegetable Diet Frozen Meal ☛ Vitamin K = 32.8 mcg; Serving size: 1 meal (8 oz), 226 g

Chicken—Roasting Dark Meat—Meat Only—Raw ☛ Vitamin K = 2.7 mcg; Serving size: 1 unit, 113 g

Chicken—Roasting Light Meat—Meat Only—Raw ☛ Vitamin K = 2.4 mcg; Serving size: 1 unit, 99 g

Chicken—Roasting—Meat Only—Raw ☛ Vitamin K = 2 mcg; Serving size: 3 oz, 85 g

Chicken—Skin ☛ Vitamin K = 0.5 mcg; Serving size: 1 oz, raw, 20 g

Chicken—Stewing Dark Meat—Meat Only—Raw ☛ Vitamin K = 2.5 mcg; Serving size: 1 unit, 105 g

Chicken—Stewing Light Meat—Meat Only—Raw ☛ Vitamin K = 2.1 mcg; Serving size: 1 unit, 89 g

Chicken—Stewing—Meat and Skin And Giblets And Neck—Cooked —Stewed ☛ Vitamin K = 1.6 mcg; Serving size: 3 oz, 85 g

Chicken—Stewing—Meat and Skin—Raw ☛ Vitamin K = 2 mcg; Serving size: 3 oz, 85 g

Chicken—Stewing—Meat Only—Cooked—Stewed ☛ Vitamin K = 4.3 mcg; Serving size: 1 cup, chopped or diced, 140 g

Chicken—Stewing—Meat Only—Raw ☛ Vitamin K = 1.7 mcg; Serving size: 3 oz, 85 g

Chicken—Tenders Or Strips Breaded From Other Sources ☛ Vitamin K = 5.5 mcg; Serving size: 1 tender, strip, or finger, 50 g

Chicken—Tenders Or Strips Breaded From Restaurant ☛ Vitamin K = 3.9 mcg; Serving size: 1 tender, strip, or finger, 50 g

Chicken—Thigh—Baked Broiled Or Roasted—Skin Eaten From— Raw ☛ Vitamin K = 4.5 mcg; Serving size: 1 cup, cooked, diced, 135 g

Chicken—Thigh—Baked Broiled Or Roasted—Skin Not Eaten From —Raw ☛ Vitamin K = 5.3 mcg; Serving size: 1 cup, cooked, diced, 135 g

Chicken—Thigh—Baked Coated Skin / Coating Eaten ☛ Vitamin K = 7.2 mcg; Serving size: 1 cup, cooked, diced, 135 g

Chicken—Thigh—Baked Coated Skin / Coating Not Eaten ☛ Vitamin K = 8.2 mcg; Serving size: 1 cup, cooked, diced, 135 g

Chicken—Thigh—Grilled With Sauce—Skin Eaten ☛ Vitamin K = 8.7 mcg; Serving size: 1 cup, cooked, diced, 165 g

Chicken—Wing—Baked Coated ☛ Vitamin K = 1.5 mcg; Serving size: 1 wing, any size, 55 g

Chicken—Wing—Baked Or Broiled From Fast Food / Restaurant ☛ Vitamin K = 0.9 mcg; Serving size: 1 wing, 35 g

Chicken—Wing—Fried Coated From Fast Food ☛ Vitamin K = 3.4 mcg; Serving size: 1 wing, any size, 55 g

Chicken—Wing—Fried Coated From Pre-Cooked ☛ Vitamin K = 5.3 mcg; Serving size: 1 wing, any size, 55 g

Chicken—Wing—Fried Coated From Restaurant ☛ Vitamin K = 3.4 mcg; Serving size: 1 wing, any size, 55 g

Chicken—Wing—Fried Coated From—Raw ☛ Vitamin K = 4.7 mcg; Serving size: 1 wing, any size, 55 g

Chuck Steak (Mock Tender) ☛ Vitamin K = 2.3 mcg; Serving size: 1 steak, 141 g

Cornish Game Hen Roasted—Skin Eaten ☛ Vitamin K = 7.3 mcg; Serving size: 1 hen (1-1/4 lb, raw), 305 g

Cornish Game Hen Roasted—Skin Not Eaten ☛ Vitamin K = 6 mcg; Serving size: 1 hen (1-1/4 lb, raw) (yield after cooking, bone and skin removed), 250 g

Cornish Game Hen—Cooked—Skin Eaten ☛ Vitamin K = 7.3 mcg; Serving size: 1 hen (1-1/4 lb, raw), 305 g

Cornish Game Hen—Cooked—Skin Not Eaten ☛ Vitamin K = 6

mcg; Serving size: 1 hen (1-1/4 lb, raw) (yield after cooking, bone and skin removed), 250 g

Deer Chop—Cooked ☛ Vitamin K = 1 mcg; Serving size: 1 oz, with bone, cooked, 23 g

Dove Fried ☛ Vitamin K = 5 mcg; Serving size: 1 dove, 110 g

Dove—Cooked (Includes Squab) ☛ Vitamin K = 5.6 mcg; Serving size: 1 cup, chopped or diced, 140 g

Duck—Coated Fried ☛ Vitamin K = 6 mcg; Serving size: 1 leg (drumstick and thigh), 115 g

Duck—Cooked—Skin Eaten ☛ Vitamin K = 19.4 mcg; Serving size: 1/2 Duck—(yield after cooking, bone removed), 380 g

Duck—Cooked—Skin Not Eaten ☛ Vitamin K = 8.4 mcg; Serving size: 1/2 Duck—(yield after cooking, bone and skin removed), 220 g

Duck—Domesticated—Meat and Skin—Cooked Roasted ☛ Vitamin K = 7.1 mcg; Serving size: 1 cup, chopped or diced, 140 g

Duck—Domesticated—Meat and Skin—Raw ☛ Vitamin K = 4.7 mcg; Serving size: 3 oz, 85 g

Duck—Pressed Chinese ☛ Vitamin K = 1.6 mcg; Serving size: 1 oz, cooked, 28 g

Duck—Roasted—Skin Eaten ☛ Vitamin K = 19.4 mcg; Serving size: 1/2 Duck—(yield after cooking, bone removed), 380 g

Duck—Roasted—Skin Not Eaten ☛ Vitamin K = 8.4 mcg; Serving size: 1/2 Duck—(yield after cooking, bone and skin removed), 220 g

Frankfurter—Beef Low Fat ☛ Vitamin K = 1 mcg; Serving size: 1 frankfurter, 57 g

Frankfurter—Beef Pork And Turkey Fat-free ☛ Vitamin K = 1 mcg; Serving size: 1 frank 1 nlea serving, 57 g

Frankfurter—Beef—Heated ☛ Vitamin K = 0.9 mcg; Serving size: 1

frankfurter, 48 g

Frankfurter—Beef—Unheated ☞ Vitamin K = 0.9 mcg; Serving size: 1 frankfurter, 50 g

Frankfurter—Meat And Poultry—Cooked Boiled ☞ Vitamin K = 0.9 mcg; Serving size: 1 frankfurter, 50 g

Frankfurter—Or Hot Dog Cheese-Filled ☞ Vitamin K = 1 mcg; Serving size: 1 frankfurter, 57 g

Frankfurter—Or Hot Dog Meat And Poultry Fat-free ☞ Vitamin K = 1.1 mcg; Serving size: 1 frankfurter, 57 g

Frankfurter—Or Hot Dog With Chili No Bun ☞ Vitamin K = 4.1 mcg; Serving size: 1 frankfurter with sauce, 125 g

Frankfurters Or Hot Dogs And Sauerkraut ☞ Vitamin K = 7.4 mcg; Serving size: 1 frankfurter with sauerkraut, 120 g

Frankfurters Or Hot Dogs With Tomato-Based Sauce ☞ Vitamin K = 5.4 mcg; Serving size: 1 cup, 244 g

Fried Chicken Chunks—Puerto Rican Style ☞ Vitamin K = 1.2 mcg; Serving size: 1 piece (1-1/2" x 1" each, boneless), 25 g

Game Meat Bear—Cooked Simmered ☞ Vitamin K = 1.5 mcg; Serving size: 3 oz, 85 g

Game Meat Beaver—Cooked Roasted ☞ Vitamin K = 1.4 mcg; Serving size: 3 oz, 85 g

Game Meat Caribou—Cooked Roasted ☞ Vitamin K = 1.2 mcg; Serving size: 3 oz, 85 g

Game Meat Deer Ground—Raw ☞ Vitamin K = 1 mcg; Serving size: 1 patty (cooked from 4 oz raw), 85 g

Game Meat Opossum—Cooked Roasted ☞ Vitamin K = 1.4 mcg; Serving size: 3 oz, 85 g

Game Meat Rabbit—Domesticated Composite Of Cuts—Cooked

Stewed ☛ Vitamin K = 1.4 mcg; Serving size: 3 oz, 85 g

Game Meat Rabbit—Wild—Cooked Stewed ☛ Vitamin K = 1.3 mcg; Serving size: 3 oz, 85 g

Game Meat Raccoon—Cooked Roasted ☛ Vitamin K = 1.4 mcg; Serving size: 3 oz, 85 g

Game Meat Squirrel—Cooked Roasted ☛ Vitamin K = 1.2 mcg; Serving size: 3 oz, 85 g

Goat Baked ☛ Vitamin K = 0.3 mcg; Serving size: 1 oz, boneless, cooked, 28 g

Goat Boiled ☛ Vitamin K = 0.3 mcg; Serving size: 1 oz, boneless, cooked, 28 g

Goat Ribs—Cooked ☛ Vitamin K = 0.6 mcg; Serving size: 1 rib, 46 g

Goose Domesticated—Meat and Skin—Cooked Roasted ☛ Vitamin K = 7.1 mcg; Serving size: 1 cup, chopped or diced, 140 g

Goose Wild Roasted ☛ Vitamin K = 7.1 mcg; Serving size: 1 cup, cooked, diced, 140 g

Ham—Breaded Or Floured Fried—Lean And Fat Eaten ☛ Vitamin K = 1.1 mcg; Serving size: 1 thin slice, 21 g

Ham—Croquette ☛ Vitamin K = 14.8 mcg; Serving size: 1 croquette (1-1/2" dia, 2" high), 62 g

Ham—Fried—Lean And Fat Eaten ☛ Vitamin K = 1.3 mcg; Serving size: 1 thin slice, 21 g

Ham—Fried—Lean Only Eaten ☛ Vitamin K = 1.3 mcg; Serving size: 1 thin slice, 21 g

Ham—Or Pork Salad ☛ Vitamin K = 80.6 mcg; Serving size: 1 cup, 182 g

Ham—Or Pork With Mushroom Sauce ☛ Vitamin K = 9.5 mcg; Serving size: 1 cup, 244 g

Ham—Or Pork With Stuffing ☛ Vitamin K = 14.6 mcg; Serving size: 1 cup, 200 g

Ham—Pot Pie ☛ Vitamin K = 61.3 mcg; Serving size: 1 pie, 632 g

Ham—Stroganoff ☛ Vitamin K = 20 mcg; Serving size: 1 cup, 244 g

Italian Sausage ☛ Vitamin K = 1.2 mcg; Serving size: 1 patty, 35 g

Lamb—Ground Or Patty—Cooked ☛ Vitamin K = 4.1 mcg; Serving size: 1 patty (4 oz, raw), 77 g

Lamb—Ground—Raw ☛ Vitamin K = 1 mcg; Serving size: 1 oz, 28.4 g

Lamb—Hocks—Cooked ☛ Vitamin K = 0.8 mcg; Serving size: 1 oz, with bone, cooked, 19 g

Lamb—Loin Chop—CookedLean And Fat Eaten ☛ Vitamin K = 3.4 mcg; Serving size: 1 small (4 oz, with bone, raw), 71 g

Lamb—Or Mutton Goulash ☛ Vitamin K = 8 mcg; Serving size: 1 cup, 249 g

Lamb—Or Mutton Loaf ☛ Vitamin K = 9.8 mcg; Serving size: 1 small or thin slice, 86 g

Lamb—Ribs—CookedLean And Fat Eaten ☛ Vitamin K = 2.4 mcg; Serving size: 1 rib, 46 g

Lamb—Roast—CookedLean And Fat Eaten ☛ Vitamin K = 0.6 mcg; Serving size: 1 thin slice, 14 g

Lamb—Shoulder Chop—CookedLean And Fat Eaten ☛ Vitamin K = 4.6 mcg; Serving size: 1 small (5.5 oz, with bone, raw), 100 g

Meat Loaf—Prepared With Beef ☛ Vitamin K = 0.9 mcg; Serving size: 1 small or thin slice, 86 g

Meat Loaf—Prepared With Ham ☛ Vitamin K = 5 mcg; Serving size: 1 small or thin slice, 86 g

Meat Loaf—Prepared With Venison/deer ☛ Vitamin K = 0.9 mcg;

Serving size: 1 small or thin slice, 86 g

Meat Loaf—Puerto Rican Style ☛ Vitamin K = 8.6 mcg; Serving size: 1 serving (3" x 1" x 2"), 95 g

Meatballs—Frozen Italian Style ☛ Vitamin K = 7 mcg; Serving size: 3 oz, 85 g

Meatballs—Puerto Rican Style ☛ Vitamin K = 4.4 mcg; Serving size: 1 meatball with sauce, 50 g

Moose—Cooked ☛ Vitamin K = 0.3 mcg; Serving size: 1 oz, boneless, cooked, 28 g

Mortadella Beef Pork ☛ Vitamin K = 0.5 mcg; Serving size: 1 oz, 28.4 g

Ostrich Top Loin—Cooked ☛ Vitamin K = 2.9 mcg; Serving size: 1 serving (3 oz), 85 g

Ostrich—Cooked ☛ Vitamin K = 1 mcg; Serving size: 1 oz, cooked, 28 g

Pepperoni ☛ Vitamin K = 4.9 mcg; Serving size: 3 oz, 85 g

Pheasant—Cooked ☛ Vitamin K = 6.4 mcg; Serving size: 1/2 pheasant breast, 130 g

Pheasant—Cooked Total Edible ☛ Vitamin K = 6.9 mcg; Serving size: 1 cup, chopped or diced, 140 g

Pork—Bratwurst ☛ Vitamin K = 2.9 mcg; Serving size: 1 link cooked, 85 g

Pork—Ground Or Patty Breaded—Cooked ☛ Vitamin K = 2.4 mcg; Serving size: 1 oz, raw, 25 g

Pork—Hash ☛ Vitamin K = 27.2 mcg; Serving size: 1 cup, 190 g

Pork—Roll Cured Fried ☛ Vitamin K = 0.4 mcg; Serving size: 1 slice (1 oz), 28 g

Pork—Sausage—Link/patty Fully—Cooked Microwaved ☛ Vitamin

K = 0.9 mcg; Serving size: 1 patty, 30 g

Pork—Steak Or Cutlet Battered Fried—Lean And Fat Eaten ☞ Vitamin K = 0.4 mcg; Serving size: 1 oz, with bone, raw, 18 g

Pork—Tenderloin Battered Fried ☞ Vitamin K = 0.6 mcg; Serving size: 1 oz, boneless, raw, 25 g

Quail—Cooked ☞ Vitamin K = 3.2 mcg; Serving size: 1 quail, 75 g

Quail—Cooked Total Edible ☞ Vitamin K = 1.2 mcg; Serving size: 1 oz, 28.4 g

Rabbit—Wild—Cooked ☞ Vitamin K = 0.3 mcg; Serving size: 1 oz, with bone, cooked, 23 g

Raccoon—Cooked ☞ Vitamin K = 0.5 mcg; Serving size: 1 oz, boneless, cooked, 28 g

Ribeye Steak (Filet) ☞ Vitamin K = 2.1 mcg; Serving size: 1 fillet, 129 g

Ripe Plantain Meat Pie—Puerto Rican Style ☞ Vitamin K = 47.1 mcg; Serving size: 1 piece (4" x 2" x 2"), 190 g

Salami—Cooked Beef ☞ Vitamin K = 0.3 mcg; Serving size: 1 slice, 26 g

Salami—Cooked Beef And Pork ☞ Vitamin K = 0.4 mcg; Serving size: 1 slice round, 12.3 g

Salisbury Steak—Baked With Tomato Sauce Vegetable Diet Frozen Meal ☞ Vitamin K = 8.1 mcg; Serving size: 1 meal (9.5 oz), 269 g

Salisbury Steak—With Gravy Macaroni And Cheese Frozen Meal ☞ Vitamin K = 10.5 mcg; Serving size: 1 meal (10 oz), 284 g

Salisbury Steak—With Gravy Macaroni And Cheese Vegetable Frozen Meal ☞ Vitamin K = 60.3 mcg; Serving size: 1 meal (11.5 oz), 326 g

Salisbury Steak—With Gravy Potatoes Vegetable Dessert Frozen Meal ☞ Vitamin K = 30 mcg; Serving size: 1 meal (16.5 oz), 468 g

Salisbury Steak—With Gravy Potatoes Vegetable Frozen Meal ☞ Vitamin K = 13.1 mcg; Serving size: 1 armour meal (11 oz), 312 g

Salisbury Steak—With Gravy Potatoes Vegetable Soup Or Macaroni And Cheese Dessert Frozen Meal ☞ Vitamin K = 11.9 mcg; Serving size: 1 meal (15.5 oz), 439 g

Salisbury Steak—With Gravy Whipped Potatoes Vegetable Dessert Frozen Meal ☞ Vitamin K = 6.9 mcg; Serving size: 1 swanson salisbury steak dinner (11 oz), 312 g

Sausage—Italian Pork—Cooked ☞ Vitamin K = 2.8 mcg; Serving size: 1 link, 4/lb, 83 g

Squirrel—Cooked ☞ Vitamin K = 0.3 mcg; Serving size: 1 oz, with bone, cooked, 23 g

Turkey—All Classes Back—Meat and Skin—Cooked Roasted ☞ Vitamin K = 6.3 mcg; Serving size: 1 cup, chopped or diced, 140 g

Turkey—Light Meat—Breaded Baked Or Fried—Skin Eaten ☞ Vitamin K = 1.4 mcg; Serving size: 1 small or thin slice, 30 g

Turkey—Light Meat—Breaded Baked Or Fried—Skin Not Eaten ☞ Vitamin K = 1.4 mcg; Serving size: 1 small or thin slice, 30 g

Turkey—Nuggets ☞ Vitamin K = 2.7 mcg; Serving size: 1 nugget, 20 g

Turkey—Sausage—Fresh—Cooked ☞ Vitamin K = 0.9 mcg; Serving size: 1 serving, 57 g

Turkey—Tetrazzini Frozen Meal ☞ Vitamin K = 21.6 mcg; Serving size: 1 meal (10 oz), 284 g

Veal—Chop Broiled—Lean And Fat Eaten ☞ Vitamin K = 4.3 mcg; Serving size: 1 small chop (4.75 oz, with bone, raw), 78 g

Veal—Composite Of Trimmed Retail Cuts—Separable Lean And Fat —Cooked ☞ Vitamin K = 5.6 mcg; Serving size: 3 oz, 85 g

Veal—Composite Of Trimmed Retail Cuts—Separable Lean Only—

Cooked ☛ Vitamin K = 5.6 mcg; Serving size: 3 oz, 85 g

Veal—Cordon Bleu ☛ Vitamin K = 64.3 mcg; Serving size: 1 roll (with ham and sauce), 229 g

Veal—Cutlet Or Steak Broiled—Lean And Fat Eaten ☛ Vitamin K = 1.5 mcg; Serving size: 1 oz, boneless, cooked, 28 g

Veal—Cutlet Or Steak Broiled—Lean Only Eaten ☛ Vitamin K = 1.4 mcg; Serving size: 1 oz, boneless, cooked, lean only, 28 g

Veal—Cutlet Or Steak Fried—Lean Only Eaten ☛ Vitamin K = 1.4 mcg; Serving size: 1 oz, boneless, cooked, lean only, 28 g

Veal—Foreshank Osso Buco—Separable Lean And Fat—Cooked Braised ☛ Vitamin K = 1.3 mcg; Serving size: 3 oz, 85 g

Veal—Foreshank Osso Buco—Separable Lean Only—Cooked Braised ☛ Vitamin K = 1.2 mcg; Serving size: 3 oz, 85 g

Veal—Fricassee—Puerto Rican Style ☛ Vitamin K = 11.3 mcg; Serving size: 1 cup, 230 g

Veal—Ground Or Patty—Cooked ☛ Vitamin K = 0.6 mcg; Serving size: 1 small patty (3.2 oz, raw, 5 patties per lb), 54 g

Veal—Ground—Cooked Broiled ☛ Vitamin K = 1 mcg; Serving size: 3 oz, 85 g

Veal—Ground—Cooked Pan-Fried ☛ Vitamin K = 1.3 mcg; Serving size: 3 oz, 85 g

Veal—Ground—Raw ☛ Vitamin K = 1.2 mcg; Serving size: 3 oz, 85 g

Veal—Leg (Top Round)—Separable Lean And Fat—Cooked Braised ☛ Vitamin K = 6 mcg; Serving size: 3 oz, 85 g

Veal—Leg Top Round Cap Off Cutlet Boneless—Cooked Grilled ☛ Vitamin K = 1.1 mcg; Serving size: 3 oz, 85 g

Veal—Leg Top Round Cap Off Cutlet Boneless—Raw ☛ Vitamin K = 0.9 mcg; Serving size: 3 oz, 85 g

Veal—Loin—Separable Lean Only—Cooked Roasted ☛ Vitamin K = 4.7 mcg; Serving size: 3 oz, 85 g

Veal—Loin—Separable Lean Only—Raw ☛ Vitamin K = 0.9 mcg; Serving size: 3 oz, 85 g

Veal—Marsala ☛ Vitamin K = 18.7 mcg; Serving size: 1 slice with sauce, 96 g

Veal—Parmigiana ☛ Vitamin K = 10.4 mcg; Serving size: 1 patty with sauce and cheese, 182 g

Veal—Parmigiana With Vegetable Fettuccine Alfredo Dessert Frozen Meal ☛ Vitamin K = 36.5 mcg; Serving size: 1 meal (12.75 oz), 361 g

Veal—Patty Breaded—Cooked ☛ Vitamin K = 3.4 mcg; Serving size: 1 small patty (3.2 oz, raw, 5 patties per lb), 64 g

Veal—Rib—Separable Lean And Fat—Cooked Braised ☛ Vitamin K = 6 mcg; Serving size: 3 oz, 85 g

Veal—Roasted—Lean And Fat Eaten ☛ Vitamin K = 1.4 mcg; Serving size: 1 thin slice, 21 g

Veal—Roasted—Lean Only Eaten ☛ Vitamin K = 1.2 mcg; Serving size: 1 thin slice, 21 g

Veal—Scallopini ☛ Vitamin K = 15 mcg; Serving size: 1 slice with sauce, 96 g

Veal—Shoulder Arm—Separable Lean And Fat—Raw ☛ Vitamin K = 1.3 mcg; Serving size: 1 oz, 28.4 g

Veal—Shoulder Blade Chop—Separable Lean And Fat—Cooked Grilled ☛ Vitamin K = 1.2 mcg; Serving size: 3 oz, 85 g

Veal—Shoulder Blade—Separable Lean Only—Cooked Braised ☛ Vitamin K = 5.8 mcg; Serving size: 3 oz, 85 g

Veal—Shoulder Whole (Arm And Blade)—Separable Lean And Fat—Cooked Braised ☛ Vitamin K = 5 mcg; Serving size: 3 oz, 85 g

Veal—Shoulder Whole (Arm And Blade)—Separable Lean And Fat
—Raw ☞ Vitamin K = 1.3 mcg; Serving size: 1 oz, 28.4 g

Veal—Sirloin—Separable Lean And Fat—Cooked Roasted ☞
Vitamin K = 5.6 mcg; Serving size: 3 oz, 85 g

Veal—Sirloin—Separable Lean And Fat—Raw ☞ Vitamin K = 1.3
mcg; Serving size: 1 oz, 28.4 g

Veal—Variety Meats And By-Products—Liver—Cooked Braised ☞
Vitamin K = 1.1 mcg; Serving size: 1 slice, 80 g

Venison Or Deer And Noodles With Cream Or White Sauce ☞
Vitamin K = 4 mcg; Serving size: 1 cup, 249 g

Venison Or Deer With Gravy ☞ Vitamin K = 2.9 mcg; Serving size: 1
cup, 244 g

Venison Or Deer With Tomato-Based Sauce ☞ Vitamin K = 4.7 mcg;
Serving size: 1 cup, 249 g

Venison/deer—Cured ☞ Vitamin K = 0.4 mcg; Serving size: 1 oz,
boneless, cooked, 28 g

Venison/deer—Jerky ☞ Vitamin K = 0.3 mcg; Serving size: 1 strip or
stick (4" long), 14 g

Venison/deer—Ribs—Cooked ☞ Vitamin K = 0.3 mcg; Serving size: 1
oz, with bone, raw, 17 g

Venison/deer—Roasted ☞ Vitamin K = 0.4 mcg; Serving size: 1 oz,
boneless, cooked, 28 g

Venison/deer—Stewed ☞ Vitamin K = 0.4 mcg; Serving size: 1 oz,
boneless, cooked, 28 g

Vienna Sausages Stewed—With Potatoes—Puerto Rican Style ☞
Vitamin K = 23.5 mcg; Serving size: 1 cup, 175 g

Wild Pig Smoked ☞ Vitamin K = 0.4 mcg; Serving size: 1 oz, boneless,
cooked, 28 g

23

NUTS AND SEEDS

Almond Butter ☞ Vitamin K = 0 mcg; Serving size: 1 tbsp, 16 g

Almond Butter Plain—With Salt Added ☞ Vitamin K = 0 mcg; Serving size: 1 tbsp, 16 g

Almond Paste ☞ Vitamin K = 0 mcg; Serving size: 1 oz, 28.4 g

Almonds ☞ Vitamin K = 0 mcg; Serving size: 1 cup, whole, 143 g

Almonds Blanched ☞ Vitamin K = 0 mcg; Serving size: 1 cup whole kernels, 145 g

Almonds Dry—Roasted—With Salt Added ☞ Vitamin K = 0 mcg; Serving size: 1 cup whole kernels, 138 g

Almonds Flavored ☞ Vitamin K = 0 mcg; Serving size: 1 nut, 1 g

Almonds Honey—Roasted ☞ Vitamin K = 0.1 mcg; Serving size: 1 nut, 1 g

Almonds Oil—Roasted Lightly—Salted ☞ Vitamin K = 0 mcg; Serving size: 1 cup whole kernels, 157 g

Almonds Oil—Roasted—With Salt Added ☞ Vitamin K = 0 mcg; Serving size: 1 cup whole kernels, 157 g

Almonds Oil—Roasted—Without Salt Added ☞ Vitamin K = 0 mcg; Serving size: 1 cup whole kernels, 157 g

Almonds—Salted ☞ Vitamin K = 0 mcg; Serving size: 1 nut, 1 g

Almonds—Unsalted ☞ Vitamin K = 0 mcg; Serving size: 1 nut, 1 g

Black Wal Dried ☞ Vitamin K = 3.4 mcg; Serving size: 1 cup, chopped, 125 g

Brazilnuts ☞ Vitamin K = 0 mcg; Serving size: 1 cup, whole, 133 g

Cashew Butter Plain—With Salt Added ☞ Vitamin K = 4.8 mcg; Serving size: 1 tbsp, 16 g

Cashew Dry—Roasted—With Salt Added ☞ Vitamin K = 47.5 mcg; Serving size: 1 cup, halves and whole, 137 g

Cashew Oil—Roasted—With Salt Added ☞ Vitamin K = 44.8 mcg; Serving size: 1 cup, whole, 129 g

Cashews Lightly—Salted ☞ Vitamin K = 0.7 mcg; Serving size: 1 nut, 2 g

Cashews—Unsalted ☞ Vitamin K = 0.7 mcg; Serving size: 1 nut, 2 g

Cashews, Raw ☞ Vitamin K = 9.7 mcg; Serving size: 1 oz, 28.4 g

Coconut Cream Canned Sweetened ☞ Vitamin K = 0 mcg; Serving size: 1 tbsp, 19 g

Coconut Dried ☞ Vitamin K = 0.1 mcg; Serving size: 1 oz, 28.4 g

Coconut Meat Dried—Sweetened Flaked Packaged ☞ Vitamin K = 0 mcg; Serving size: 1 cup, 85 g

Coconut Meat Raw ☞ Vitamin K = 0.2 mcg; Serving size: 1 cup, shredded, 80 g

Coconut Milk, Raw ☛ Vitamin K = 0.2 mcg; Serving size: 1 cup, 240 g

Coconut Water ☛ Vitamin K = 0 mcg; Serving size: 1 cup, 240 g

Dry-Roasted Cashews ☛ Vitamin K = 47.5 mcg; Serving size: 1 cup, halves and whole, 137 g

Dry-Roasted Mixed—Salted ☛ Vitamin K = 15.7 mcg; Serving size: 1 cup, 131 g

Dry—Roasted Almonds ☛ Vitamin K = 0 mcg; Serving size: 1 cup whole kernels, 138 g

Dry—Roasted Macadamia Nuts ☛ Vitamin K = 0 mcg; Serving size: 1 cup, whole or halves, 132 g

Dry—Roasted Peanuts ☛ Vitamin K = 0 mcg; Serving size: 1 cup, 146 g

Dry—Roasted Pistachio Nuts ☛ Vitamin K = 16.2 mcg; Serving size: 1 cup, 123 g

Dry—Roasted Sunflower Seeds ☛ Vitamin K = 3.5 mcg; Serving size: 1 cup, 128 g

Dry—Roasted Sunflower—With Salt ☛ Vitamin K = 3.5 mcg; Serving size: 1 cup, 128 g

Flax Seeds ☛ Vitamin K = 0.4 mcg; Serving size: 1 tbsp, whole, 10.3 g

Hazelnuts ☛ Vitamin K = 16.3 mcg; Serving size: 1 cup, chopped, 115 g

Macadamia Dry—Roasted—With Salt Added ☛ Vitamin K = 0 mcg; Serving size: 1 cup, whole or halves, 132 g

Mixed Dry—Roasted—With PeaSalt Added Chosen Roaster ☛ Vitamin K = 5.7 mcg; Serving size: 1 cup, 132 g

Mixed Dry—Roasted—With PeaSalt Added Planters Pistachio Blend ☛ Vitamin K = 13.1 mcg; Serving size: 1 cup, 147 g

Mixed Dry—Roasted—With PeaWith Salt Added ☞ Vitamin K = 17.7 mcg; Serving size: 1 cup, 137 g

Mixed Honey—Roasted ☞ Vitamin K = 20.4 mcg; Serving size: 1 cup, 142 g

Mixed Oil—Roasted—With PeaLightly—Salted ☞ Vitamin K = 1.6 mcg; Serving size: 1 oz, 28.4 g

Mixed Oil—Roasted—With PeaWith Salt Added ☞ Vitamin K = 7.6 mcg; Serving size: 1 cup, 134 g

Mixed Oil—Roasted—With PeaWithout Salt Added ☞ Vitamin K = 7.6 mcg; Serving size: 1 cup, 134 g

Mixed Oil—Roasted—Without PeaWith Salt Added ☞ Vitamin K = 25.8 mcg; Serving size: 1 cup, 144 g

Mixed Seeds ☞ Vitamin K = 4.6 mcg; Serving size: 1 cup, 145 g

Mixed Unroasted ☞ Vitamin K = 19 mcg; Serving size: 1 cup, 142 g

Mixed—With PeaUnsalted ☞ Vitamin K = 16.6 mcg; Serving size: 1 cup, 142 g

Mixed—Without PeaSalted ☞ Vitamin K = 23.4 mcg; Serving size: 1 cup, 142 g

Mixed—Without PeaUnsalted ☞ Vitamin K = 23.6 mcg; Serving size: 1 cup, 142 g

Oil—Roasted Cashews ☞ Vitamin K = 44.8 mcg; Serving size: 1 cup, whole, 129 g

PeaDry—Roasted Lightly—Salted ☞ Vitamin K = 0 mcg; Serving size: 1 peanut, without shell, 1 g

Peanut Butter—And Chocolate Spread ☞ Vitamin K = 0 mcg; Serving size: 1 tablespoon, 16 g

Peanut Butter—And Jelly ☞ Vitamin K = 0 mcg; Serving size: 1 tablespoon, 16 g

Peanut Butter—Reduced Sodium And Reduced Sugar ☞ Vitamin K = 0.1 mcg; Serving size: 1 tablespoon, 16 g

Pecans ☞ Vitamin K = 3.8 mcg; Serving size: 1 cup, chopped, 109 g

Pecans Honey—Roasted ☞ Vitamin K = 0.3 mcg; Serving size: 1 nut, 2 g

Pecans—Salted ☞ Vitamin K = 0.1 mcg; Serving size: 1 nut, 2 g

Pecans—Unsalted ☞ Vitamin K = 0.1 mcg; Serving size: 1 nut, 2 g

Pine Dried ☞ Vitamin K = 72.8 mcg; Serving size: 1 cup, 135 g

Pistachio Dry—Roasted—With Salt Added ☞ Vitamin K = 16.2 mcg; Serving size: 1 cup, 123 g

Pistachio Lightly—Salted ☞ Vitamin K = 0.2 mcg; Serving size: 1 nut, 1 g

Pistachio—Salted ☞ Vitamin K = 0.2 mcg; Serving size: 1 nut, 1 g

Pistachio—Unsalted ☞ Vitamin K = 0.2 mcg; Serving size: 1 nut, 1 g

Pumpkin And Squash Seeds Dried ☞ Vitamin K = 9.4 mcg; Serving size: 1 cup, 129 g

Pumpkin—Salted ☞ Vitamin K = 6.3 mcg; Serving size: 1 cup, without shell, 144 g

Roasted Chestnuts ☞ Vitamin K = 11.2 mcg; Serving size: 1 cup, 143 g

Roasted Squash And Pumpkin—Salted ☞ Vitamin K = 5.3 mcg; Serving size: 1 cup, 118 g

Roasted Squash And Pumpkin—Unsalted ☞ Vitamin K = 5.3 mcg; Serving size: 1 cup, 118 g

Sesame Butter Tahini ☞ Vitamin K = 0 mcg; Serving size: 1 tbsp, 15 g

Sesame Seed Kernels Dried ☞ Vitamin K = 0 mcg; Serving size: 1 cup, 150 g

Sesame Seed Kernels Toasted—With Salt Added ☛ Vitamin K = 0 mcg; Serving size: 1 cup, 128 g

Sesame Seed Kernels Toasted—Without Salt Added ☛ Vitamin K = 0 mcg; Serving size: 1 cup, 128 g

Sesame Whole Dried ☛ Vitamin K = 0 mcg; Serving size: 1 cup, 144 g

Shredded Coconut Meat ☛ Vitamin K = 0.3 mcg; Serving size: 1 cup, shredded, 93 g

Sunflower Flavored ☛ Vitamin K = 3.7 mcg; Serving size: 1 cup, without shell, 144 g

Sunflower Plain—Salted ☛ Vitamin K = 3.9 mcg; Serving size: 1 cup, without shell, 144 g

Sunflower Seed Kernels Dry—Roasted—With Salt Added ☛ Vitamin K = 3.5 mcg; Serving size: 1 cup, 128 g

Sunflower Seed Kernels Oil—Roasted—With Salt Added ☛ Vitamin K = 4.2 mcg; Serving size: 1 cup, 135 g

Sunflower Seed Kernels Oil—Roasted—Without Salt ☛ Vitamin K = 4.2 mcg; Serving size: 1 cup, 135 g

Sunflower Seeds Dried ☛ Vitamin K = 0 mcg; Serving size: 1 cup, with hulls, edible yield, 46 g

Trail Mix—With And Fruit ☛ Vitamin K = 10.8 mcg; Serving size: 1 cup, 140 g

Trail Mix—With Chocolate ☛ Vitamin K = 10.4 mcg; Serving size: 1 cup, 140 g

Trail Mix—With Nuts ☛ Vitamin K = 13.9 mcg; Serving size: 1 cup, 140 g

Trail Mix—With Pretzels Cereal Or Granola ☛ Vitamin K = 9.9 mcg; Serving size: 1 cup, 140 g

WalDry—Roasted—With Salt Added ☞ Vitamin K = 0.9 mcg; Serving size: 1 oz, 28 g

WalHoney—Roasted ☞ Vitamin K = 0.3 mcg; Serving size: 1 nut, 2 g

Walnuts ☞ Vitamin K = 3.2 mcg; Serving size: 1 cup, chopped, 117 g

24

PREPARED MEALS

Rice And Vermicelli Mix—Beef Flavor—Unprepared ☞ Vitamin K = 1.5 mcg; Serving size: 1/ 3 cup, 61 g

Almond Chicken ☞ Vitamin K = 30.7 mcg; Serving size: 1 cup, 242 g

Beans String Green Cooked Szechuan-Style ☞ Vitamin K = 105.3 mcg; Serving size: 1 cup, 185 g

Beef And Broccoli ☞ Vitamin K = 135.8 mcg; Serving size: 1 cup, 217 g

Beef And Noodles—With Soy-Based Sauce ☞ Vitamin K = 41.3 mcg; Serving size: 1 cup, 249 g

Beef And Rice—With Soy-Based Sauce ☞ Vitamin K = 41.5 mcg; Serving size: 1 cup, 244 g

Beef And Vegetables—With Carrots Broccoli And/or Dark-Green Leafy; No Potatoes Soy-Based Sauce ☞ Vitamin K = 83.8 mcg; Serving size: 1 cup, 217 g

Beef And Vegetables—Without Carrots Broccoli And Dark-Green Leafy; No Potatoes Soy-Based Sauce ☞ Vitamin K = 44.7 mcg; Serving size: 1 cup, 217 g

Beef Chow Mein Or Chop Suey—No Noodles ☞ Vitamin K = 29.3 mcg; Serving size: 1 cup, 220 g

Beef Chow Mein Or Chop Suey—With Noodles ☞ Vitamin K = 26 mcg; Serving size: 1 cup, 220 g

Beef Corned Beef Hash—With Potato Canned ☞ Vitamin K = 4.2 mcg; Serving size: 1 cup, 236 g

Beef Egg Foo Yung ☞ Vitamin K = 16.3 mcg; Serving size: 1 patty, 86 g

Beef Enchilada Chili Gravy Rice Refried Beans—Frozen Meal ☞ Vitamin K = 10.6 mcg; Serving size: 1 meal (15 oz), 425 g

Beef Enchilada Dinner—Frozen Meal ☞ Vitamin K = 10.6 mcg; Serving size: 1 meal (15 oz), 425 g

Beef Macaroni—With Tomato Sauce—Frozen Entree Reduced Fat ☞ Vitamin K = 7 mcg; Serving size: 1 serving, 269 g

Beef Noodles And Vegetables—With Carrots Broccoli And/or Dark-Green Leafy; Soy-Based Sauce ☞ Vitamin K = 71.8 mcg; Serving size: 1 cup, 217 g

Beef Noodles And Vegetables—Without Carrots Broccoli And Dark-Green Leafy; Soy-Based Sauce ☞ Vitamin K = 38.2 mcg; Serving size: 1 cup, 217 g

Beef Pot Pie—Frozen Entree Prepared ☞ Vitamin K = 7.2 mcg; Serving size: 1 pie, cooked (average weight), 268 g

Beef Potatoes And Vegetables—With Carrots, Broccoli, Dark-Green Leafy, Soy-Based Sauce ☞ Vitamin K = 77.6 mcg; Serving size: 1 cup, 252 g

Beef Potatoes And Vegetables—Without Carrots Broccoli And Dark-Green Leafy; Soy-Based Sauce ☞ Vitamin K = 47.1 mcg; Serving size: 1 cup, 252 g

Beef Rice And Vegetables—With Carrots Broccoli And/or Dark-

Green Leafy; Soy-Based Sauce ☛ Vitamin K = 72.9 mcg; Serving size: 1 cup, 217 g

Beef Rice And Vegetables—Without Carrots Broccoli And Dark-Green Leafy; Soy-Based Sauce ☛ Vitamin K = 38.6 mcg; Serving size: 1 cup, 217 g

Beef Stew Canned Entree ☛ Vitamin K = 12.2 mcg; Serving size: 1 cup (1 serving), 196 g

Beef Tofu And Vegetables—With Carrots Broccoli And/or Dark-Green Leafy; No Potatoes Soy-Based Sauce ☛ Vitamin K = 81.4 mcg; Serving size: 1 cup, 217 g

Beef Tofu And Vegetables—Without Carrots Broccoli And Dark-Green Leafy; No Potatoes Soy-Based Sauce ☛ Vitamin K = 43.6 mcg; Serving size: 1 cup, 217 g

Beef—With Soy-Based Sauce ☛ Vitamin K = 50.3 mcg; Serving size: 1 cup, 244 g

Beef—With Sweet And Sour Sauce ☛ Vitamin K = 21.2 mcg; Serving size: 1 cup, 252 g

Bibimbap Korean ☛ Vitamin K = 133.8 mcg; Serving size: 1 cup, 162 g

Biryani—With Chicken ☛ Vitamin K = 10.6 mcg; Serving size: 1 cup, 196 g

Biryani—With Meat ☛ Vitamin K = 12.2 mcg; Serving size: 1 cup, 196 g

Biryani—With Vegetables ☛ Vitamin K = 4.8 mcg; Serving size: 1 cup, 172 g

Bread Stuffing Made—With Egg ☛ Vitamin K = 21.1 mcg; Serving size: 1 cup, 170 g

Burrito Bean And Cheese—Frozen ☛ Vitamin K = 9.8 mcg; Serving size: 1 burrito, 129 g

Burrito Beef And Bean Microwaved ☛ Vitamin K = 8.7 mcg; Serving size: 1 burrito cooked, 116 g

Burrito Beef And Bean—Frozen ☛ Vitamin K = 9.5 mcg; Serving size: 1 burrito frozen, 139 g

Burrito—With Beans And Rice Meatless ☛ Vitamin K = 10.4 mcg; Serving size: 1 small burrito, 182 g

Burrito—With Beans Meatless ☛ Vitamin K = 10.4 mcg; Serving size: 1 small burrito, 170 g

Burrito—With Beans Rice And Sour Cream Meatless ☛ Vitamin K = 10.8 mcg; Serving size: 1 small burrito, 208 g

Burrito—With Chicken ☛ Vitamin K = 5 mcg; Serving size: 1 small burrito, 142 g

Burrito—With Chicken And Beans ☛ Vitamin K = 7.7 mcg; Serving size: 1 small burrito, 153 g

Burrito—With Chicken And Sour Cream ☛ Vitamin K = 5.2 mcg; Serving size: 1 small burrito, 162 g

Burrito—With Chicken Beans And Rice ☛ Vitamin K = 7.6 mcg; Serving size: 1 small burrito, 165 g

Burrito—With Chicken Beans And Sour Cream ☛ Vitamin K = 8.1 mcg; Serving size: 1 small burrito, 179 g

Burrito—With Chicken Beans Rice And Sour Cream ☛ Vitamin K = 8 mcg; Serving size: 1 small burrito, 191 g

Burrito—With Meat ☛ Vitamin K = 6.1 mcg; Serving size: 1 small burrito, 161 g

Burrito—With Meat And Beans ☛ Vitamin K = 8.3 mcg; Serving size: 1 small burrito, 166 g

Burrito—With Meat And Sour Cream ☛ Vitamin K = 6.5 mcg; Serving size: 1 small burrito, 187 g

Burrito—With Meat Beans And Rice ☞ Vitamin K = 8.3 mcg; Serving size: 1 small burrito, 177 g

Burrito—With Meat Beans And Sour Cream ☞ Vitamin K = 8.6 mcg; Serving size: 1 small burrito, 192 g

Burrito—With Meat Beans And Sour Cream—From Fast Food ☞ Vitamin K = 5.8 mcg; Serving size: 1 small burrito, 192 g

Burrito—With Meat Beans Rice And Sour Cream ☞ Vitamin K = 8.7 mcg; Serving size: 1 small burrito, 203 g

Cake Made—With Glutinous Rice ☞ Vitamin K = 0 mcg; Serving size: 1 oz, 28 g

Cake Made—With Glutinous Rice And Dried Beans ☞ Vitamin K = 0 mcg; Serving size: 1 piece, 16 g

Cake Or Pancake Made—With Rice Flour And/or Dried Beans ☞ Vitamin K = 1.2 mcg; Serving size: 1 idli (2-1/4" dia), 38 g

Cannelloni Cheese- And Spinach-Filled No Sauce ☞ Vitamin K = 75.3 mcg; Serving size: 1 cannelloni, 74 g

Cannelloni Cheese-Filled—With Tomato Sauce Diet—Frozen Meal ☞ Vitamin K = 2.3 mcg; Serving size: 1 meal (9.125 oz), 259 g

Cheese Enchilada—Frozen Meal ☞ Vitamin K = 11.9 mcg; Serving size: 1 meal (10 oz), 284 g

Cheese Quiche Meatless ☞ Vitamin K = 6.3 mcg; Serving size: 1 piece (1/8 of 9" dia), 192 g

Cheese Turnover—Puerto Rican Style ☞ Vitamin K = 1.1 mcg; Serving size: 1 turnover, 21 g

Chicken Burritos Diet—Frozen Meal ☞ Vitamin K = 14.5 mcg; Serving size: 1 meal (10 oz), 284 g

Chicken Chow Mein—With Rice Diet—Frozen Meal ☞ Vitamin K = 18.8 mcg; Serving size: 1 lean cuisine meal (11.25 oz), 319 g

Chicken Egg Foo Yung ☛ Vitamin K = 15.9 mcg; Serving size: 1 patty, 86 g

Chicken Enchilada Diet—Frozen Meal ☛ Vitamin K = 7.2 mcg; Serving size: 1 meal (8.5 oz), 241 g

Chicken Fajitas Diet—Frozen Meal ☛ Vitamin K = 5.9 mcg; Serving size: 1 meal (6.75 oz), 191 g

Chicken In Orange Sauce—With Almond Rice Diet—Frozen Meal ☛ Vitamin K = 6.1 mcg; Serving size: 1 meal (8 oz), 227 g

Chicken In Soy-Based Sauce Rice And Vegetables—Frozen Meal ☛ Vitamin K = 21.9 mcg; Serving size: 1 meal (9 oz), 255 g

Chicken Nuggets Dark And White Meat Precooked—Frozen Not Reheated ☛ Vitamin K = 8.7 mcg; Serving size: 1 serving, 87 g

Chicken Nuggets White Meat Precooked—Frozen Not Reheated ☛ Vitamin K = 8.2 mcg; Serving size: 1 serving, 82 g

Chicken Or Turkey—And Noodles—With Soy-Based Sauce ☛ Vitamin K = 36.1 mcg; Serving size: 1 cup, 224 g

Chicken Or Turkey—And Rice—With Soy-Based Sauce ☛ Vitamin K = 40 mcg; Serving size: 1 cup, 244 g

Chicken Or Turkey—And Vegetables—Without Carrots Broccoli And Dark-Green Leafy; No Potatoes Soy-Based Sauce ☛ Vitamin K = 43.6 mcg; Serving size: 1 cup, 217 g

Chicken Or Turkey—Chow Mein Or Chop Suey—No Noodles ☛ Vitamin K = 27.7 mcg; Serving size: 1 cup, 220 g

Chicken Or Turkey—Chow Mein Or Chop Suey—With Noodles ☛ Vitamin K = 24.9 mcg; Serving size: 1 cup, 220 g

Chicken Or Turkey—Rice And Vegetables—With Carrots Broccoli And/or Dark-Green Leafy; Soy-Based Sauce ☛ Vitamin K = 71.8 mcg; Serving size: 1 cup, 217 g

Chicken Or Turkey—Rice And Vegetables—Without Carrots Broccoli And Dark-Green Leafy; Soy-Based Sauce ☛ Vitamin K = 37.8 mcg; Serving size: 1 cup, 217 g

Chicken Or Turkey—With Teriyaki ☛ Vitamin K = 0 mcg; Serving size: 1 cup, 244 g

Chicken Pot Pie—Frozen Entree Prepared ☛ Vitamin K = 32.3 mcg; Serving size: 1 pie, 302 g

Chicken Tenders Breaded—Frozen Prepared ☛ Vitamin K = 3.7 mcg; Serving size: 1 piece, 21 g

Chilaquiles Tortilla Casserole—With Salsa And Cheese No Egg ☛ Vitamin K = 21.1 mcg; Serving size: 1 cup, 232 g

Chilaquiles Tortilla Casserole—With Salsa Cheese And Egg ☛ Vitamin K = 21.6 mcg; Serving size: 1 cup, 232 g

Chiles Rellenos Cheese-Filled ☛ Vitamin K = 16.4 mcg; Serving size: 1 chili, 143 g

Chiles Rellenos Filled—With Meat And Cheese ☛ Vitamin K = 16.7 mcg; Serving size: 1 chili, 143 g

Chili Con Carne—With Beans Canned Entree ☛ Vitamin K = 11.1 mcg; Serving size: 1 cup, 242 g

Chili No Beans Canned Entree ☛ Vitamin K = 5.3 mcg; Serving size: 1 cup, 240 g

Chili—With Beans Microwavable Bowls ☛ Vitamin K = 9.5 mcg; Serving size: 1 cup, 244 g

Chimichanga Meatless ☛ Vitamin K = 13.1 mcg; Serving size: 1 small chimichanga, 128 g

Chimichanga Meatless—With Sour Cream ☛ Vitamin K = 12.8 mcg; Serving size: 1 small chimichanga, 136 g

Chimichanga—With Chicken ☛ Vitamin K = 11.7 mcg; Serving size: 1

small chimichanga, 97 g

Chimichanga—With Chicken And Sour Cream ☛ Vitamin K = 11.9 mcg; Serving size: 1 small chimichanga, 108 g

Chimichanga—With Meat ☛ Vitamin K = 12.1 mcg; Serving size: 1 small chimichanga, 105 g

Chimichanga—With Meat And Sour Cream ☛ Vitamin K = 10.2 mcg; Serving size: 1 small chimichanga, 92 g

Chow Fun Noodles—With Meat And Vegetables ☛ Vitamin K = 12 mcg; Serving size: 1 cup, 152 g

Chow Fun Noodles—With Vegetables Meatless ☛ Vitamin K = 15 mcg; Serving size: 1 cup, 152 g

Chow Mein Or Chop Suey—Meatless—With Noodles ☛ Vitamin K = 35 mcg; Serving size: 1 cup, 220 g

Chow Mein Or Chop Suey—Various Types Of Meat—With Noodles ☛ Vitamin K = 25.3 mcg; Serving size: 1 cup, 220 g

Congee—With Meat Poultry And/or Seafood ☛ Vitamin K = 0.2 mcg; Serving size: 1 cup, 249 g

Congee—With Meat Poultry And/or Seafood And Vegetables ☛ Vitamin K = 4.2 mcg; Serving size: 1 cup, 249 g

Congee—With Vegetables ☛ Vitamin K = 4.5 mcg; Serving size: 1 cup, 249 g

Corn Dogs—Frozen Prepared ☛ Vitamin K = 4.5 mcg; Serving size: 1 corndog, 78 g

Crepe Filled—With Meat Poultry Or Seafood No Sauce ☛ Vitamin K = 13.4 mcg; Serving size: 1 crepe with filling, any size, 125 g

Crepe Filled—With Meat Poultry Or Seafood—With Sauce ☛ Vitamin K = 4.2 mcg; Serving size: 1 crepe with filling, any size, 155 g

Dirty Rice ☛ Vitamin K = 5.9 mcg; Serving size: 1 cup, 198 g

Dosa Indian—With Filling ☛ Vitamin K = 6.4 mcg; Serving size: 1 small, 113 g

Dukboki Or Tteokbokki Korean ☛ Vitamin K = 14.8 mcg; Serving size: 1 cup, 250 g

Dumpling Fried—Puerto Rican Style ☛ Vitamin K = 2 mcg; Serving size: 1 small dumpling, 16 g

Dumpling Meat-Filled ☛ Vitamin K = 9.1 mcg; Serving size: 1 dumpling, any size, 97 g

Dumpling Potato- Or Cheese-Filled—Frozen ☛ Vitamin K = 9 mcg; Serving size: 3 pieces pierogies, 114 g

Dumpling Vegetable ☛ Vitamin K = 30.6 mcg; Serving size: 1 dumpling, any size, 97 g

Egg Foo Yung ☛ Vitamin K = 15.7 mcg; Serving size: 1 patty, 86 g

Egg Roll Meatless ☛ Vitamin K = 6 mcg; Serving size: 1 miniature egg roll, 13 g

Egg Roll—With Beef And/or Pork ☛ Vitamin K = 3.9 mcg; Serving size: 1 miniature roll, 13 g

Egg Roll—With Chicken Or Turkey ☛ Vitamin K = 4.1 mcg; Serving size: 1 miniature egg roll, 13 g

Egg Roll—With Shrimp ☛ Vitamin K = 6 mcg; Serving size: 1 miniature egg roll, 13 g

Egg Rolls Chicken Refrigerated Heated ☛ Vitamin K = 19 mcg; Serving size: 1 roll, 80 g

Egg Rolls Pork Refrigerated Heated ☛ Vitamin K = 19.2 mcg; Serving size: 1 roll, 85 g

Egg Rolls Vegetable—Frozen Prepared ☛ Vitamin K = 26.8 mcg; Serving size: 1 egg roll, 68 g

Empanada Mexican Turnover Filled—With Cheese And Vegetables ☞ Vitamin K = 6.4 mcg; Serving size: 1 small/appetizer, 81 g

Empanada Mexican Turnover Filled—With Chicken And Vegetables ☞ Vitamin K = 6 mcg; Serving size: 1 small/appetizer, 81 g

Enchilada Just Cheese Meatless No Beans Green-Chile Or Enchilada Sauce ☞ Vitamin K = 11 mcg; Serving size: 1 enchilada, any size, 111 g

Enchilada Just Cheese Meatless No Beans Red-Chile Or Enchilada Sauce ☞ Vitamin K = 5.5 mcg; Serving size: 1 enchilada, any size, 119 g

Enchilada—With Beans Green-Chile Or Enchilada Sauce ☞ Vitamin K = 13.9 mcg; Serving size: 1 enchilada, any size, 132 g

Enchilada—With Beans Meatless Red-Chile Or Enchilada Sauce ☞ Vitamin K = 8.3 mcg; Serving size: 1 enchilada, any size, 141 g

Enchilada—With Chicken And Beans Green-Chile Or Enchilada Sauce ☞ Vitamin K = 13.1 mcg; Serving size: 1 enchilada, any size, 132 g

Enchilada—With Chicken And Beans Red-Chile Or Enchilada Sauce ☞ Vitamin K = 6.7 mcg; Serving size: 1 enchilada, any size, 132 g

Enchilada—With Chicken Green-Chile Or Enchilada Sauce ☞ Vitamin K = 10.5 mcg; Serving size: 1 enchilada, any size, 114 g

Enchilada—With Chicken Red-Chile Or Enchilada Sauce ☞ Vitamin K = 4.9 mcg; Serving size: 1 enchilada, any size, 123 g

Enchilada—With Meat And Beans Green-Chile Or Enchilada Sauce ☞ Vitamin K = 12.3 mcg; Serving size: 1 enchilada, any size, 123 g

Enchilada—With Meat And Beans Red-Chile Or Enchilada Sauce ☞ Vitamin K = 6.9 mcg; Serving size: 1 enchilada, any size, 132 g

Enchilada—With Meat Green-Chile Or Enchilada Sauce ☞ Vitamin K = 10.8 mcg; Serving size: 1 enchilada, any size, 114 g

Enchilada—With Meat Red-Chile Or Enchilada Sauce ☞ Vitamin K = 5.4 mcg; Serving size: 1 enchilada, any size, 122 g

Fajita—With Vegetables ☞ Vitamin K = 8.6 mcg; Serving size: 1 fajita, 141 g

Fish And Vegetables—With Carrots Broccoli And/or Dark-Green Leafy; No Potatoes Soy-Based Sauce ☞ Vitamin K = 82.5 mcg; Serving size: 1 cup, 217 g

Fish And Vegetables—Without Carrots Broccoli And Dark-Green Leafy; No Potatoes Soy-Based Sauce ☞ Vitamin K = 43.4 mcg; Serving size: 1 cup, 217 g

Flavored Rice And Pasta Mixture ☞ Vitamin K = 7.2 mcg; Serving size: 1 cup, beef flavor, 184 g

Flavored Rice And Pasta Mixture Reduced Sodium ☞ Vitamin K = 18.8 mcg; Serving size: 1 cup, 196 g

Flavored Rice Brown And Wild ☞ Vitamin K = 5.2 mcg; Serving size: 1 cup, 217 g

Flavored Rice Mixture ☞ Vitamin K = 9.4 mcg; Serving size: 1 cup, 218 g

Flavored Rice Mixture—With Cheese ☞ Vitamin K = 16.1 mcg; Serving size: 1 cup, 230 g

Fried Rice—Puerto Rican Style ☞ Vitamin K = 2.2 mcg; Serving size: 1 cup, 173 g

Fried Stuffed Potatoes—Puerto Rican Style ☞ Vitamin K = 11.3 mcg; Serving size: 1 fritter (4" x 2-1/4" x 3/4"), 95 g

Gnocchi Cheese ☞ Vitamin K = 4.9 mcg; Serving size: 1 cup, 70 g

Gnocchi Potato ☞ Vitamin K = 2.6 mcg; Serving size: 1 cup, 188 g

Gordita Sope Or Chalupa—With Beans ☞ Vitamin K = 14.7 mcg; Serving size: 1 small, 150 g

Gordita Sope Or Chalupa—With Beans And Sour Cream ☛ Vitamin K = 15 mcg; Serving size: 1 small, 165 g

Gordita Sope Or Chalupa—With Chicken ☛ Vitamin K = 12.8 mcg; Serving size: 1 small, 115 g

Gordita Sope Or Chalupa—With Chicken And Sour Cream ☛ Vitamin K = 12.4 mcg; Serving size: 1 small, 124 g

Gordita Sope Or Chalupa—With Meat ☛ Vitamin K = 12.7 mcg; Serving size: 1 small, 115 g

Gordita Sope Or Chalupa—With Meat And Sour Cream ☛ Vitamin K = 13.3 mcg; Serving size: 1 small, 132 g

Grape Leaves Stuffed—With Rice ☛ Vitamin K = 34.9 mcg; Serving size: 1 roll, 56 g

Ground Beef—With Tomato Sauce And Taco Seasonings On A Cornbread Crust ☛ Vitamin K = 5.5 mcg; Serving size: 1 cup, 179 g

Hopping John ☛ Vitamin K = 45.7 mcg; Serving size: 1 cup, 224 g

Hot Pockets Croissant Pockets Chicken Broccoli And Cheddar Stuffed Sandwich—Frozen ☛ Vitamin K = 1 mcg; Serving size: 1 serving (1 hot pocket), 127 g

Hot Pockets Ham N Cheese Stuffed Sandwich—Frozen ☛ Vitamin K = 1 mcg; Serving size: 1 serving (1 hot pocket), 127 g

Hot Pockets Meatballs & Mozzarella Stuffed Sandwich—Frozen ☛ Vitamin K = 13.7 mcg; Serving size: 1 hot pocket, 127 g

Jalapeno Pepper Stuffed—With Cheese—Breaded Or Battered Fried ☛ Vitamin K = 4.8 mcg; Serving size: 1 jalapeno pepper, 25 g

Jambalaya—With Meat And Rice ☛ Vitamin K = 8.8 mcg; Serving size: 1 cup, 244 g

Kishke Stuffed Derma ☛ Vitamin K = 0.1 mcg; Serving size: 1 cubic inch, cooked, 18 g

Knish Cheese ☛ Vitamin K = 11.1 mcg; Serving size: 1 knish, 60 g

Knish Meat ☛ Vitamin K = 8.7 mcg; Serving size: 1 knish, 50 g

Knish Potato ☛ Vitamin K = 12.4 mcg; Serving size: 1 knish, 61 g

Kung Pao Beef ☛ Vitamin K = 21.7 mcg; Serving size: 1 cup, 162 g

Kung Pao Pork ☛ Vitamin K = 20.4 mcg; Serving size: 1 cup, 162 g

Kung Pao Shrimp ☛ Vitamin K = 20.7 mcg; Serving size: 1 cup, 162 g

Lasagna—Cheese—Frozen Prepared ☛ Vitamin K = 20.5 mcg; Serving size: 1 cup 1 serving, 225 g

Lasagna—Cheese—Frozen—Unprepared ☛ Vitamin K = 7.3 mcg; Serving size: 1 cup 1 serving, 237 g

Lasagna—Meatless Spinach Noodles ☛ Vitamin K = 109 mcg; Serving size: 1 piece, 227 g

Lasagna—Meatless Whole Wheat Noodles ☛ Vitamin K = 41.8 mcg; Serving size: 1 piece, 227 g

Lasagna—Meatless—With Vegetables ☛ Vitamin K = 41.8 mcg; Serving size: 1 piece, 227 g

Lasagna—Vegetable—Frozen Baked ☛ Vitamin K = 40.4 mcg; Serving size: 1 serving, 227 g

Lasagna—With Cheese And Meat Sauce Diet—Frozen Meal ☛ Vitamin K = 5.6 mcg; Serving size: 1 weight watchers meal (11 oz), 312 g

Lasagna—With Cheese And Sauce Diet—Frozen Meal ☛ Vitamin K = 9 mcg; Serving size: 1 meal (11 oz), 312 g

Lasagna—With Chicken Or Turkey ☛ Vitamin K = 9.5 mcg; Serving size: 1 piece, 206 g

Lasagna—With Chicken Or Turkey—And Spinach ☛ Vitamin K = 36.3 mcg; Serving size: 1 piece, 206 g

Lasagna—With Meat ☛ Vitamin K = 13.6 mcg; Serving size: 1 piece, 206 g

Lasagna—With Meat & Sauce—Frozen Entree ☛ Vitamin K = 7.9 mcg; Serving size: 1 piece side, 134 g

Lasagna—With Meat And Spinach ☛ Vitamin K = 36.7 mcg; Serving size: 1 piece, 206 g

Lasagna—With Meat Home Recipe ☛ Vitamin K = 4.1 mcg; Serving size: 1 piece, 206 g

Lasagna—With Meat Sauce—Frozen Prepared ☛ Vitamin K = 8.6 mcg; Serving size: 1 piece side, 123 g

Lasagna—With Meat Spinach Noodles ☛ Vitamin K = 70.7 mcg; Serving size: 1 piece, 206 g

Lasagna—With Meat-Whole Wheat Noodles ☛ Vitamin K = 10.1 mcg; Serving size: 1 piece, 206 g

Lean Pockets Ham N Cheddar ☛ Vitamin K = 2.2 mcg; Serving size: 1 hot pocket, 127 g

Lean Pockets Meatballs & Mozzarella ☛ Vitamin K = 4.5 mcg; Serving size: 1 each, 128 g

Lefse Norwegian ☛ Vitamin K = 3.6 mcg; Serving size: 1 lefse, any size, 80 g

Linguini—With Vegetables And Seafood In White Wine Sauce Diet —Frozen Meal ☛ Vitamin K = 47.6 mcg; Serving size: 1 meal (9.5 oz), 269 g

Lo Mein—With Beef ☛ Vitamin K = 21.2 mcg; Serving size: 1 cup, 200 g

Lo Mein—With Chicken ☛ Vitamin K = 20.4 mcg; Serving size: 1 cup, 200 g

Lo Mein—With Pork ☛ Vitamin K = 20.4 mcg; Serving size: 1 cup, 200 g

Lo Mein—With Shrimp ☛ Vitamin K = 20.2 mcg; Serving size: 1 cup, 200 g

Macaroni And Cheese Box—Mix—With Cheese Sauce—Unprepared ☛ Vitamin K = 1.5 mcg; Serving size: 1 serving (3.5 oz), 25 g

Macaroni And Cheese Canned Entree ☛ Vitamin K = 0.5 mcg; Serving size: 1 serving, 244 g

Macaroni And Cheese Diet—Frozen Meal ☛ Vitamin K = 0.8 mcg; Serving size: 1 meal (9 oz), 255 g

Macaroni And Cheese Dinner—With Dry Sauce Mix Boxed Uncooked ☛ Vitamin K = 0.1 mcg; Serving size: 1 serving (makes roughly 1 cup prepared), 70 g

Macaroni And Cheese Dry Mix Prepared—With 2% Milk And 80% Stick Margarine—From Dry Mix ☛ Vitamin K = 12.7 mcg; Serving size: 1 cup, 198 g

Macaroni And Cheese—Frozen Entree ☛ Vitamin K = 7 mcg; Serving size: 1 cup, 137 g

Macaroni Or Noodles—Creamed—With Cheese ☛ Vitamin K = 0.9 mcg; Serving size: 1 cup, 230 g

Macaroni Or Noodles—Creamed—With Cheese And Tuna ☛ Vitamin K = 0.9 mcg; Serving size: 1 cup, 230 g

Macaroni Or Noodles—With Cheese ☛ Vitamin K = 7.1 mcg; Serving size: 1 cup, 230 g

Macaroni Or Noodles—With Cheese And Chicken Or Turkey ☛ Vitamin K = 6 mcg; Serving size: 1 cup, 230 g

Macaroni Or Noodles—With Cheese And Egg ☛ Vitamin K = 11 mcg; Serving size: 1 cup, 230 g

Macaroni Or Noodles—With Cheese And Frankfurters Or Hot Dogs ☛ Vitamin K = 8.3 mcg; Serving size: 1 cup, 230 g

Macaroni Or Noodles—With Cheese And Meat ☛ Vitamin K = 7.4 mcg; Serving size: 1 cup, 230 g

Macaroni Or Noodles—With Cheese And Meat Prepared—From Hamburger Helper Mix ☛ Vitamin K = 1.8 mcg; Serving size: 1 cup, 230 g

Macaroni Or Noodles—With Cheese And Tomato ☛ Vitamin K = 11 mcg; Serving size: 1 cup, 230 g

Macaroni Or Noodles—With Cheese And Tuna ☛ Vitamin K = 7.4 mcg; Serving size: 1 cup, 230 g

Macaroni Or Noodles—With Cheese Easy Mac Type ☛ Vitamin K = 0.2 mcg; Serving size: 1 cup, 230 g

Macaroni Or Noodles—With Cheese Made—From Packaged Mix ☛ Vitamin K = 9 mcg; Serving size: 1 cup, 230 g

Macaroni Or Noodles—With Cheese Made—From Reduced Fat Packaged Mix ☛ Vitamin K = 6.2 mcg; Serving size: 1 cup, 230 g

Macaroni Or Noodles—With Cheese Made—From Reduced Fat Packaged Mix—Unprepared ☛ Vitamin K = 2.2 mcg; Serving size: 1 serving (3.5 oz), 99 g

Macaroni Or Noodles—With Cheese Microwaveable—Unprepared ☛ Vitamin K = 0.1 mcg; Serving size: 1 serving 1 pouch, 61 g

Macaroni Or Pasta Salad Made—With Any Type Of Fat-free Dressing ☛ Vitamin K = 16.5 mcg; Serving size: 1 cup, 204 g

Macaroni Or Pasta Salad Made—With Creamy Dressing ☛ Vitamin K = 45.3 mcg; Serving size: 1 cup, 204 g

Macaroni Or Pasta Salad Made—With Italian Dressing ☛ Vitamin K = 25.5 mcg; Serving size: 1 cup, 204 g

Macaroni Or Pasta Salad Made—With Light Creamy Dressing ☛ Vitamin K = 12.6 mcg; Serving size: 1 cup, 204 g

Macaroni Or Pasta Salad Made—With Light Italian Dressing ☛ Vitamin K = 14.9 mcg; Serving size: 1 cup, 204 g

Macaroni Or Pasta Salad Made—With Light Mayonnaise ☛ Vitamin K = 25.3 mcg; Serving size: 1 cup, 204 g

Macaroni Or Pasta Salad Made—With Light Mayonnaise-Type Salad Dressing ☛ Vitamin K = 25.3 mcg; Serving size: 1 cup, 204 g

Macaroni Or Pasta Salad Made—With Mayonnaise ☛ Vitamin K = 56.5 mcg; Serving size: 1 cup, 204 g

Macaroni Or Pasta Salad Made—With Mayonnaise-Type Salad Dressing ☛ Vitamin K = 21.4 mcg; Serving size: 1 cup, 204 g

Macaroni Or Pasta Salad—With Cheese ☛ Vitamin K = 49.8 mcg; Serving size: 1 cup, 204 g

Macaroni Or Pasta Salad—With Chicken ☛ Vitamin K = 47.9 mcg; Serving size: 1 cup, 204 g

Macaroni Or Pasta Salad—With Crab Meat ☛ Vitamin K = 48.1 mcg; Serving size: 1 cup, 204 g

Macaroni Or Pasta Salad—With Egg ☛ Vitamin K = 51.4 mcg; Serving size: 1 cup, 204 g

Macaroni Or Pasta Salad—With Meat ☛ Vitamin K = 47.7 mcg; Serving size: 1 cup, 204 g

Macaroni Or Pasta Salad—With Shrimp ☛ Vitamin K = 48.3 mcg; Serving size: 1 cup, 204 g

Macaroni Or Pasta Salad—With Tuna ☛ Vitamin K = 47.9 mcg; Serving size: 1 cup, 204 g

Macaroni Or Pasta Salad—With Tuna And Egg ☛ Vitamin K = 44.3 mcg; Serving size: 1 cup, 204 g

Macaroni—With Tuna—Puerto Rican Style ☞ Vitamin K = 9.2 mcg; Serving size: 1 cup, 225 g

Manicotti Cheese-Filled No Sauce ☞ Vitamin K = 1 mcg; Serving size: 1 manicotti, 127 g

Manicotti Cheese-Filled—With Meat Sauce ☞ Vitamin K = 2.9 mcg; Serving size: 1 manicotti, 143 g

Manicotti Cheese-Filled—With Tomato Sauce Diet—Frozen Meal ☞ Vitamin K = 3.4 mcg; Serving size: 1 meal (9.25 oz), 262 g

Manicotti Cheese-Filled—With Tomato Sauce Meatless ☞ Vitamin K = 2.9 mcg; Serving size: 1 manicotti, 143 g

Manicotti Vegetable- And Cheese-Filled—With Tomato Sauce Meatless ☞ Vitamin K = 46.6 mcg; Serving size: 1 manicotti, 143 g

Meat Turnover—Puerto Rican Style ☞ Vitamin K = 2.7 mcg; Serving size: 1 turnover, 28 g

Mexican Casserole Made—With Ground Beef Beans Tomato Sauce Cheese Taco Seasonings And Corn Chips ☞ Vitamin K = 8.2 mcg; Serving size: 1 cup, 144 g

Mexican Casserole Made—With Ground Beef Tomato Sauce Cheese Taco Seasonings And Corn Chips ☞ Vitamin K = 6.3 mcg; Serving size: 1 cup, 144 g

Moo Goo Gai Pan ☞ Vitamin K = 33.5 mcg; Serving size: 1 cup, 216 g

Moo Shu Pork—Without Chinese Pancake ☞ Vitamin K = 52.7 mcg; Serving size: 1 cup, 151 g

Nachos—With Cheese And Sour Cream ☞ Vitamin K = 0.4 mcg; Serving size: 1 nacho, 7 g

Nachos—With Chicken And Cheese ☞ Vitamin K = 0.4 mcg; Serving size: 1 nacho, 7 g

Nachos—With Chicken Cheese And Sour Cream ☞ Vitamin K = 0.3 mcg; Serving size: 1 nacho, 7 g

Nachos—With Chili ☞ Vitamin K = 0.4 mcg; Serving size: 1 nacho, 7 g

Nachos—With Meat And Cheese ☞ Vitamin K = 0.4 mcg; Serving size: 1 nacho, 7 g

Nachos—With Meat Cheese And Sour Cream ☞ Vitamin K = 0.4 mcg; Serving size: 1 nacho, 7 g

Noodle Pudding ☞ Vitamin K = 7.5 mcg; Serving size: 1 cup, 144 g

Noodles—With Vegetables In Tomato-Based Sauce Diet—Frozen Meal ☞ Vitamin K = 6 mcg; Serving size: 1 meal (10 oz), 284 g

Pad Thai Meatless ☞ Vitamin K = 41 mcg; Serving size: 1 cup, 200 g

Pad Thai ☞ Vitamin K = 36.8 mcg; Serving size: 1 cup, 200 g

Pad Thai—With Chicken ☞ Vitamin K = 36.8 mcg; Serving size: 1 cup, 200 g

Pad Thai—With Meat ☞ Vitamin K = 38.2 mcg; Serving size: 1 cup, 200 g

Pad Thai—With Seafood ☞ Vitamin K = 38 mcg; Serving size: 1 cup, 200 g

Paella ☞ Vitamin K = 8.2 mcg; Serving size: 1 cup, 240 g

Paella—With Meat Valenciana Style ☞ Vitamin K = 7 mcg; Serving size: 1 cup, with bone (yield after bone removed), 137 g

Paella—With Seafood ☞ Vitamin K = 9.1 mcg; Serving size: 1 cup, 240 g

Pasta Meat-Filled—With Gravy Canned ☞ Vitamin K = 6.3 mcg; Serving size: 1 cup, 250 g

Pasta Mix—Classic Beef—Unprepared ☞ Vitamin K = 0.4 mcg; Serving size: 1 package, 122 g

Pasta Mix—Classic Cheeseburger Macaroni—Unprepared ☞ Vitamin K = 1.4 mcg; Serving size: 1 package, 123 g

Pasta Mix—Italian Lasagna—Unprepared ☞ Vitamin K = 18.2 mcg; Serving size: 1 package, 141 g

Pasta Whole Grain—With Cream Sauce And Added Vegetables Home Recipe ☞ Vitamin K = 3.3 mcg; Serving size: 1 cup, 250 g

Pasta Whole Grain—With Cream Sauce And Added Vegetables Ready-To-Heat ☞ Vitamin K = 8.5 mcg; Serving size: 1 cup, 250 g

Pasta Whole Grain—With Cream Sauce And Added Vegetables Restaurant ☞ Vitamin K = 23 mcg; Serving size: 1 cup, 250 g

Pasta Whole Grain—With Cream Sauce And Meat Home Recipe ☞ Vitamin K = 2.5 mcg; Serving size: 1 cup, 250 g

Pasta Whole Grain—With Cream Sauce And Meat Ready-To-Heat ☞ Vitamin K = 7.8 mcg; Serving size: 1 cup, 250 g

Pasta Whole Grain—With Cream Sauce And Meat Restaurant ☞ Vitamin K = 22.5 mcg; Serving size: 1 cup, 250 g

Pasta Whole Grain—With Cream Sauce And Poultry Home Recipe ☞ Vitamin K = 2 mcg; Serving size: 1 cup, 250 g

Pasta Whole Grain—With Cream Sauce And Poultry Ready-To-Heat ☞ Vitamin K = 7.3 mcg; Serving size: 1 cup, 250 g

Pasta Whole Grain—With Cream Sauce And Poultry Restaurant ☞ Vitamin K = 22 mcg; Serving size: 1 cup, 250 g

Pasta Whole Grain—With Cream Sauce And Seafood Home Recipe ☞ Vitamin K = 2 mcg; Serving size: 1 cup, 250 g

Pasta Whole Grain—With Cream Sauce And Seafood Ready-To-Heat ☞ Vitamin K = 7.3 mcg; Serving size: 1 cup, 250 g

Pasta Whole Grain—With Cream Sauce And Seafood Restaurant ☞ Vitamin K = 22 mcg; Serving size: 1 cup, 250 g

Pasta Whole Grain—With Cream Sauce Home Recipe ☛ Vitamin K = 2.3 mcg; Serving size: 1 cup, 250 g

Pasta Whole Grain—With Cream Sauce Meat And Added Vegetables Home Recipe ☛ Vitamin K = 3 mcg; Serving size: 1 cup, 250 g

Pasta Whole Grain—With Cream Sauce Meat And Added Vegetables Ready-To-Heat ☛ Vitamin K = 8.3 mcg; Serving size: 1 cup, 250 g

Pasta Whole Grain—With Cream Sauce Meat And Added Vegetables Restaurant ☛ Vitamin K = 23 mcg; Serving size: 1 cup, 250 g

Pasta Whole Grain—With Cream Sauce Poultry And Added Vegetables Home Recipe ☛ Vitamin K = 2.8 mcg; Serving size: 1 cup, 250 g

Pasta Whole Grain—With Cream Sauce Poultry And Added Vegetables Ready-To-Heat ☛ Vitamin K = 8 mcg; Serving size: 1 cup, 250 g

Pasta Whole Grain—With Cream Sauce Poultry And Added Vegetables Restaurant ☛ Vitamin K = 22.8 mcg; Serving size: 1 cup, 250 g

Pasta Whole Grain—With Cream Sauce Ready-To-Heat ☛ Vitamin K = 7.5 mcg; Serving size: 1 cup, 250 g

Pasta Whole Grain—With Cream Sauce Restaurant ☛ Vitamin K = 22.3 mcg; Serving size: 1 cup, 250 g

Pasta Whole Grain—With Cream Sauce Seafood And Added Vegetables Home Recipe ☛ Vitamin K = 2.8 mcg; Serving size: 1 cup, 250 g

Pasta Whole Grain—With Cream Sauce Seafood And Added Vegetables Ready-To-Heat ☛ Vitamin K = 8 mcg; Serving size: 1 cup, 250 g

Pasta Whole Grain—With Cream Sauce Seafood And Added Vegetables Restaurant ☛ Vitamin K = 22.8 mcg; Serving size: 1 cup, 250 g

Pasta Whole Grain—With Tomato-Based Sauce And Added Vegetables Home Recipe ☛ Vitamin K = 14.8 mcg; Serving size: 1 cup, 250 g

Pasta Whole Grain—With Tomato-Based Sauce And Added Vegetables Ready-To-Heat ☛ Vitamin K = 19.8 mcg; Serving size: 1 cup, 250 g

Pasta Whole Grain—With Tomato-Based Sauce And Added Vegetables Restaurant ☞ Vitamin K = 33.8 mcg; Serving size: 1 cup, 250 g

Pasta Whole Grain—With Tomato-Based Sauce And Meat Home Recipe ☞ Vitamin K = 14.8 mcg; Serving size: 1 cup, 250 g

Pasta Whole Grain—With Tomato-Based Sauce And Meat Ready-To-Heat ☞ Vitamin K = 19.8 mcg; Serving size: 1 cup, 250 g

Pasta Whole Grain—With Tomato-Based Sauce And Meat Restaurant ☞ Vitamin K = 34 mcg; Serving size: 1 cup, 250 g

Pasta Whole Grain—With Tomato-Based Sauce And Poultry Home Recipe ☞ Vitamin K = 14.3 mcg; Serving size: 1 cup, 250 g

Pasta Whole Grain—With Tomato-Based Sauce And Poultry Ready-To-Heat ☞ Vitamin K = 19.5 mcg; Serving size: 1 cup, 250 g

Pasta Whole Grain—With Tomato-Based Sauce And Poultry Restaurant ☞ Vitamin K = 33.5 mcg; Serving size: 1 cup, 250 g

Pasta Whole Grain—With Tomato-Based Sauce And Seafood Home Recipe ☞ Vitamin K = 14.5 mcg; Serving size: 1 cup, 250 g

Pasta Whole Grain—With Tomato-Based Sauce And Seafood Ready-To-Heat ☞ Vitamin K = 19.5 mcg; Serving size: 1 cup, 250 g

Pasta Whole Grain—With Tomato-Based Sauce And Seafood Restaurant ☞ Vitamin K = 33.5 mcg; Serving size: 1 cup, 250 g

Pasta Whole Grain—With Tomato-Based Sauce Home Recipe ☞ Vitamin K = 17.5 mcg; Serving size: 1 cup, 250 g

Pasta Whole Grain—With Tomato-Based Sauce Meat And Added Vegetables Home Recipe ☞ Vitamin K = 12.5 mcg; Serving size: 1 cup, 250 g

Pasta Whole Grain—With Tomato-Based Sauce Meat And Added Vegetables Ready-To-Heat ☞ Vitamin K = 17.5 mcg; Serving size: 1 cup, 250 g

Pasta Whole Grain—With Tomato-Based Sauce Meat And Added Vegetables Restaurant ☞ Vitamin K = 31.8 mcg; Serving size: 1 cup, 250 g

Pasta Whole Grain—With Tomato-Based Sauce Poultry And Added Vegetables Home Recipe ☞ Vitamin K = 12 mcg; Serving size: 1 cup, 250 g

Pasta Whole Grain—With Tomato-Based Sauce Poultry And Added Vegetables Ready-To-Heat ☞ Vitamin K = 17.3 mcg; Serving size: 1 cup, 250 g

Pasta Whole Grain—With Tomato-Based Sauce Poultry And Added Vegetables Restaurant ☞ Vitamin K = 31.5 mcg; Serving size: 1 cup, 250 g

Pasta Whole Grain—With Tomato-Based Sauce Ready-To-Heat ☞ Vitamin K = 22.5 mcg; Serving size: 1 cup, 250 g

Pasta Whole Grain—With Tomato-Based Sauce Restaurant ☞ Vitamin K = 36.5 mcg; Serving size: 1 cup, 250 g

Pasta Whole Grain—With Tomato-Based Sauce Seafood And Added Vegetables Home Recipe ☞ Vitamin K = 12.3 mcg; Serving size: 1 cup, 250 g

Pasta Whole Grain—With Tomato-Based Sauce Seafood And Added Vegetables Ready-To-Heat ☞ Vitamin K = 17.3 mcg; Serving size: 1 cup, 250 g

Pasta Whole Grain—With Tomato-Based Sauce Seafood And Added Vegetables Restaurant ☞ Vitamin K = 31.5 mcg; Serving size: 1 cup, 250 g

Pasta—With Cream Sauce And Added Vegetables Ready-To-Heat ☞ Vitamin K = 7.8 mcg; Serving size: 1 cup, 250 g

Pasta—With Cream Sauce And Added Vegetables Restaurant ☞ Vitamin K = 22.3 mcg; Serving size: 1 cup, 250 g

Pasta—With Cream Sauce And Added Vegetables—From Home Recipe ☛ Vitamin K = 2.3 mcg; Serving size: 1 cup, 250 g

Pasta—With Cream Sauce And Meat Home Recipe ☛ Vitamin K = 1.8 mcg; Serving size: 1 cup, 250 g

Pasta—With Cream Sauce And Meat Ready-To-Heat ☛ Vitamin K = 7 mcg; Serving size: 1 cup, 250 g

Pasta—With Cream Sauce And Meat Restaurant ☛ Vitamin K = 21.8 mcg; Serving size: 1 cup, 250 g

Pasta—With Cream Sauce And Poultry Home Recipe ☛ Vitamin K = 1.3 mcg; Serving size: 1 cup, 250 g

Pasta—With Cream Sauce And Poultry Ready-To-Heat ☛ Vitamin K = 6.5 mcg; Serving size: 1 cup, 250 g

Pasta—With Cream Sauce And Poultry Restaurant ☛ Vitamin K = 21.3 mcg; Serving size: 1 cup, 250 g

Pasta—With Cream Sauce And Seafood Home Recipe ☛ Vitamin K = 1.3 mcg; Serving size: 1 cup, 250 g

Pasta—With Cream Sauce And Seafood Ready-To-Heat ☛ Vitamin K = 6.5 mcg; Serving size: 1 cup, 250 g

Pasta—With Cream Sauce And Seafood Restaurant ☛ Vitamin K = 21.3 mcg; Serving size: 1 cup, 250 g

Pasta—With Cream Sauce Home Recipe ☛ Vitamin K = 1.5 mcg; Serving size: 1 cup, 250 g

Pasta—With Cream Sauce Meat And Added Vegetables Home Recipe ☛ Vitamin K = 2.3 mcg; Serving size: 1 cup, 250 g

Pasta—With Cream Sauce Meat And Added Vegetables Ready-To-Heat ☛ Vitamin K = 7.5 mcg; Serving size: 1 cup, 250 g

Pasta—With Cream Sauce Meat And Added Vegetables Restaurant ☛ Vitamin K = 22.3 mcg; Serving size: 1 cup, 250 g

Pasta—With Cream Sauce Poultry And Added Vegetables Home Recipe ☞ Vitamin K = 2 mcg; Serving size: 1 cup, 250 g

Pasta—With Cream Sauce Poultry And Added Vegetables Ready-To-Heat ☞ Vitamin K = 7.3 mcg; Serving size: 1 cup, 250 g

Pasta—With Cream Sauce Poultry And Added Vegetables Restaurant ☞ Vitamin K = 22 mcg; Serving size: 1 cup, 250 g

Pasta—With Cream Sauce Ready-To-Heat ☞ Vitamin K = 6.8 mcg; Serving size: 1 cup, 250 g

Pasta—With Cream Sauce Restaurant ☞ Vitamin K = 21.5 mcg; Serving size: 1 cup, 250 g

Pasta—With Cream Sauce Seafood And Added Vegetables Home Recipe ☞ Vitamin K = 2 mcg; Serving size: 1 cup, 250 g

Pasta—With Cream Sauce Seafood And Added Vegetables Ready-To-Heat ☞ Vitamin K = 7.3 mcg; Serving size: 1 cup, 250 g

Pasta—With Cream Sauce Seafood And Added Vegetables Restaurant ☞ Vitamin K = 22 mcg; Serving size: 1 cup, 250 g

Pasta—With Sauce And Meat—From School Lunch ☞ Vitamin K = 16.3 mcg; Serving size: 1 cup, 250 g

Pasta—With Sauce Meatless School Lunch ☞ Vitamin K = 17.5 mcg; Serving size: 1 cup, 250 g

Pasta—With Sauce ☞ Vitamin K = 14 mcg; Serving size: 1 cup, 250 g

Pasta—With Sliced Franks In Tomato Sauce Canned Entree ☞ Vitamin K = 4 mcg; Serving size: 1 serving (1 cup), 252 g

Pasta—With Tomato Sauce No Meat Canned ☞ Vitamin K = 3 mcg; Serving size: 1 serving, 252 g

Pasta—With Tomato-Based Sauce And Added Vegetables Home Recipe ☞ Vitamin K = 14 mcg; Serving size: 1 cup, 250 g

Pasta—With Tomato-Based Sauce And Added Vegetables Ready-To-Heat ➖ Vitamin K = 19 mcg; Serving size: 1 cup, 250 g

Pasta—With Tomato-Based Sauce And Added Vegetables Restaurant ➖ Vitamin K = 33.3 mcg; Serving size: 1 cup, 250 g

Pasta—With Tomato-Based Sauce And Beans Or Lentils ➖ Vitamin K = 16.6 mcg; Serving size: 1 cup, 227 g

Pasta—With Tomato-Based Sauce And Cheese ➖ Vitamin K = 27.5 mcg; Serving size: 1 cup, 250 g

Pasta—With Tomato-Based Sauce And Meat Home Recipe ➖ Vitamin K = 14 mcg; Serving size: 1 cup, 250 g

Pasta—With Tomato-Based Sauce And Meat Ready-To-Heat ➖ Vitamin K = 19 mcg; Serving size: 1 cup, 250 g

Pasta—With Tomato-Based Sauce And Meat Restaurant ➖ Vitamin K = 33.3 mcg; Serving size: 1 cup, 250 g

Pasta—With Tomato-Based Sauce And Poultry Home Recipe ➖ Vitamin K = 13.5 mcg; Serving size: 1 cup, 250 g

Pasta—With Tomato-Based Sauce And Poultry Ready-To-Heat ➖ Vitamin K = 18.8 mcg; Serving size: 1 cup, 250 g

Pasta—With Tomato-Based Sauce And Poultry Restaurant ➖ Vitamin K = 32.8 mcg; Serving size: 1 cup, 250 g

Pasta—With Tomato-Based Sauce And Seafood Home Recipe ➖ Vitamin K = 13.8 mcg; Serving size: 1 cup, 250 g

Pasta—With Tomato-Based Sauce And Seafood Ready-To-Heat ➖ Vitamin K = 18.8 mcg; Serving size: 1 cup, 250 g

Pasta—With Tomato-Based Sauce And Seafood Restaurant ➖ Vitamin K = 32.8 mcg; Serving size: 1 cup, 250 g

Pasta—With Tomato-Based Sauce Cheese And Meat ➖ Vitamin K = 3 mcg; Serving size: 1 cannelloni, 86 g

Pasta—With Tomato-Based Sauce Home Recipe ☛ Vitamin K = 16.8 mcg; Serving size: 1 cup, 250 g

Pasta—With Tomato-Based Sauce Meat And Added Vegetables Home Recipe ☛ Vitamin K = 11.8 mcg; Serving size: 1 cup, 250 g

Pasta—With Tomato-Based Sauce Meat And Added Vegetables Ready-To-Heat ☛ Vitamin K = 16.8 mcg; Serving size: 1 cup, 250 g

Pasta—With Tomato-Based Sauce Meat And Added Vegetables Restaurant ☛ Vitamin K = 31 mcg; Serving size: 1 cup, 250 g

Pasta—With Tomato-Based Sauce Poultry And Added Vegetables Home Recipe ☛ Vitamin K = 11.3 mcg; Serving size: 1 cup, 250 g

Pasta—With Tomato-Based Sauce Poultry And Added Vegetables Ready-To-Heat ☛ Vitamin K = 16.5 mcg; Serving size: 1 cup, 250 g

Pasta—With Tomato-Based Sauce Poultry And Added Vegetables Restaurant ☛ Vitamin K = 30.8 mcg; Serving size: 1 cup, 250 g

Pasta—With Tomato-Based Sauce Ready-To-Heat ☛ Vitamin K = 21.8 mcg; Serving size: 1 cup, 250 g

Pasta—With Tomato-Based Sauce Restaurant ☛ Vitamin K = 35.8 mcg; Serving size: 1 cup, 250 g

Pasta—With Tomato-Based Sauce Seafood And Added Vegetables Home Recipe ☛ Vitamin K = 11.5 mcg; Serving size: 1 cup, 250 g

Pasta—With Tomato-Based Sauce Seafood And Added Vegetables Ready-To-Heat ☛ Vitamin K = 16.5 mcg; Serving size: 1 cup, 250 g

Pasta—With Tomato-Based Sauce Seafood And Added Vegetables Restaurant ☛ Vitamin K = 30.8 mcg; Serving size: 1 cup, 250 g

Pasta—With Vegetables No Sauce Or Dressing ☛ Vitamin K = 30.9 mcg; Serving size: 1 cup, 150 g

Pastry Egg And Cheese Filled ☛ Vitamin K = 6 mcg; Serving size: 1 kolache, 142 g

Pastry Filled—With Potatoes And Peas Fried ☞ Vitamin K = 1.9 mcg; Serving size: 1 miniature samosa, 9 g

Pastry Meat / Poultry-Filled ☞ Vitamin K = 2.5 mcg; Serving size: 1 kolache, 85 g

Pizza Rolls—Frozen—Unprepared ☞ Vitamin K = 3.7 mcg; Serving size: 1 serving 6 rolls, 80 g

Pork And Onions—With Soy-Based Sauce ☞ Vitamin K = 36.9 mcg; Serving size: 1 cup, 256 g

Pork And Vegetables Hawaiian Style ☞ Vitamin K = 40.8 mcg; Serving size: 1 cup, 252 g

Pork And Vegetables—With Carrots Broccoli And/or Dark-Green Leafy; No Potatoes Soy-Based Sauce ☞ Vitamin K = 82.7 mcg; Serving size: 1 cup, 217 g

Pork And Vegetables—Without Carrots Broccoli And Dark- Green Leafy; No Potatoes Soy-Based Sauce ☞ Vitamin K = 43.6 mcg; Serving size: 1 cup, 217 g

Pork And Watercress—With Soy-Based Sauce ☞ Vitamin K = 198 mcg; Serving size: 1 cup, 162 g

Pork Chow Mein Or Chop Suey—No Noodles ☞ Vitamin K = 27.9 mcg; Serving size: 1 cup, 220 g

Pork Chow Mein Or Chop Suey—With Noodles ☞ Vitamin K = 24.9 mcg; Serving size: 1 cup, 220 g

Pork Egg Foo Yung ☞ Vitamin K = 15.6 mcg; Serving size: 1 patty, 86 g

Pork Or Ham—With Soy-Based Sauce ☞ Vitamin K = 48.6 mcg; Serving size: 1 cup, 244 g

Pork Rice And Vegetables—With Carrots Broccoli And/or Dark-Green Leafy; Soy-Based Sauce ☞ Vitamin K = 71.8 mcg; Serving size: 1 cup, 217 g

Pork Rice And Vegetables—Without Carrots Broccoli And Dark-Green Leafy; Soy-Based Sauce ☞ Vitamin K = 37.8 mcg; Serving size: 1 cup, 217 g

Pork Tofu And Vegetables—With Carrots Broccoli And/or Dark-Green Leafy; No Potatoes Soy-Base Sauce ☞ Vitamin K = 80.7 mcg; Serving size: 1 cup, 217 g

Pork Tofu And Vegetables—Without Carrots Broccoli And Dark-Green Leafy; No Potatoes Soy-Based Sauce ☞ Vitamin K = 43 mcg; Serving size: 1 cup, 217 g

Potato And Ham Fritters—Puerto Rican Style ☞ Vitamin K = 10.4 mcg; Serving size: 1 fritter (2-3/4" x 2-1/2" x 1"), 70 g

Potato Mashed ☞ Vitamin K = 3.8 mcg; Serving size: 1 cup, 250 g

Potato Mashed Ready-To-Heat—With Cheese ☞ Vitamin K = 6 mcg; Serving size: 1 cup, 250 g

Potato Mashed Ready-To-Heat—With Gravy ☞ Vitamin K = 5 mcg; Serving size: 1 cup, 250 g

Potato Mashed—From Dry Mix Made—With Milk ☞ Vitamin K = 9.3 mcg; Serving size: 1 cup, 250 g

Potato Mashed—From Dry Mix Made—With Milk—With Cheese ☞ Vitamin K = 8.8 mcg; Serving size: 1 cup, 250 g

Potato Mashed—From Dry Mix Made—With Milk—With Gravy ☞ Vitamin K = 7.8 mcg; Serving size: 1 cup, 250 g

Potato Mashed—From Dry Mix ☞ Vitamin K = 9.3 mcg; Serving size: 1 cup, 250 g

Potato Mashed—From Fast Food—With Gravy ☞ Vitamin K = 12 mcg; Serving size: 1 cup, 250 g

Potato Mashed—From Fresh Made—With Milk ☞ Vitamin K = 3.8 mcg; Serving size: 1 cup, 250 g

Potato Mashed—From Fresh Made—With Milk—With Cheese ☞ Vitamin K = 4 mcg; Serving size: 1 cup, 250 g

Potato Mashed—From Fresh Made—With Milk—With Gravy ☞ Vitamin K = 3.3 mcg; Serving size: 1 cup, 250 g

Potato Mashed—From Fresh ☞ Vitamin K = 3.8 mcg; Serving size: 1 cup, 250 g

Potato Mashed—From Restaurant ☞ Vitamin K = 8.5 mcg; Serving size: 1 cup, 250 g

Potato Mashed—From Restaurant—With Gravy ☞ Vitamin K = 7.3 mcg; Serving size: 1 cup, 250 g

Potato Mashed—From School Lunch ☞ Vitamin K = 9.3 mcg; Serving size: 1 cup, 250 g

Potato Pancake ☞ Vitamin K = 1.2 mcg; Serving size: 1 miniature/bite size pancake, 10 g

Potato Pudding ☞ Vitamin K = 10.5 mcg; Serving size: 1 cup, 228 g

Potato Salad German Style ☞ Vitamin K = 5.3 mcg; Serving size: 1 cup, 175 g

Potato Salad Made—With Any Type Of Fat-free Dressing ☞ Vitamin K = 21.7 mcg; Serving size: 1 cup, 275 g

Potato Salad Made—With Creamy Dressing ☞ Vitamin K = 69.6 mcg; Serving size: 1 cup, 275 g

Potato Salad Made—With Italian Dressing ☞ Vitamin K = 33 mcg; Serving size: 1 cup, 275 g

Potato Salad Made—With Light Creamy Dressing ☞ Vitamin K = 9.4 mcg; Serving size: 1 cup, 275 g

Potato Salad Made—With Light Italian Dressing ☞ Vitamin K = 13.5 mcg; Serving size: 1 cup, 275 g

Potato Salad Made—With Light Mayonnaise ☛ Vitamin K = 33.8 mcg; Serving size: 1 cup, 275 g

Potato Salad Made—With Light Mayonnaise-Type Salad Dressing ☛ Vitamin K = 33.8 mcg; Serving size: 1 cup, 275 g

Potato Salad Made—With Mayonnaise ☛ Vitamin K = 76.5 mcg; Serving size: 1 cup, 275 g

Potato Salad Made—With Mayonnaise-Type Salad Dressing ☛ Vitamin K = 28.6 mcg; Serving size: 1 cup, 275 g

Potato Salad—From Restaurant ☛ Vitamin K = 76.5 mcg; Serving size: 1 cup, 275 g

Potato Salad—With Egg ☛ Vitamin K = 17.9 mcg; Serving size: 1/2 cup, 125 g

Potato Salad—With Egg Made—With Any Type Of Fat-free Dressing ☛ Vitamin K = 19.3 mcg; Serving size: 1 cup, 275 g

Potato Salad—With Egg Made—With Creamy Dressing ☛ Vitamin K = 61.1 mcg; Serving size: 1 cup, 275 g

Potato Salad—With Egg Made—With Italian Dressing ☛ Vitamin K = 29.2 mcg; Serving size: 1 cup, 275 g

Potato Salad—With Egg Made—With Light Creamy Dressing ☛ Vitamin K = 8.3 mcg; Serving size: 1 cup, 275 g

Potato Salad—With Egg Made—With Light Italian Dressing ☛ Vitamin K = 11.8 mcg; Serving size: 1 cup, 275 g

Potato Salad—With Egg Made—With Light Mayonnaise ☛ Vitamin K = 30 mcg; Serving size: 1 cup, 275 g

Potato Salad—With Egg Made—With Light Mayonnaise-Type Salad Dressing ☛ Vitamin K = 30 mcg; Serving size: 1 cup, 275 g

Potato Salad—With Egg Made—With Mayonnaise-Type Salad Dressing ☛ Vitamin K = 25.3 mcg; Serving size: 1 cup, 275 g

Potato Salad—With Egg—From Restaurant ☞ Vitamin K = 67.1 mcg; Serving size: 1 cup, 275 g

Potato Scalloped Ready-To-Heat ☞ Vitamin K = 6.8 mcg; Serving size: 1 cup, 250 g

Potato Scalloped Ready-To-Heat—With Meat ☞ Vitamin K = 8 mcg; Serving size: 1 cup, 250 g

Potato Scalloped—From Dry Mix ☞ Vitamin K = 4.8 mcg; Serving size: 1 cup, 250 g

Potato Scalloped—From Dry Mix—With Meat ☞ Vitamin K = 4.8 mcg; Serving size: 1 cup, 250 g

Potato Scalloped—From Fast Food Or Restaurant ☞ Vitamin K = 9 mcg; Serving size: 1 cup, 250 g

Potato Scalloped—From Fresh ☞ Vitamin K = 4 mcg; Serving size: 1 cup, 250 g

Potato Scalloped—From Fresh—With Meat ☞ Vitamin K = 5.5 mcg; Serving size: 1 cup, 250 g

Potsticker Or Wonton Pork And Vegetable—Frozen—Unprepared ☞ Vitamin K = 79.8 mcg; Serving size: 5 pieces 1 serving, 145 g

Pulled Pork In Barbecue Sauce ☞ Vitamin K = 3.5 mcg; Serving size: 1 cup, 249 g

Pupusa Bean-Filled ☞ Vitamin K = 3 mcg; Serving size: 1 pupusa (about 5" dia), 126 g

Quesadilla Just Cheese Meatless ☞ Vitamin K = 1.4 mcg; Serving size: 1 slice or wedge, 18 g

Quesadilla Just Cheese—From Fast Food ☞ Vitamin K = 1.4 mcg; Serving size: 1 slice or wedge, 18 g

Quesadilla—With Meat ☞ Vitamin K = 1.5 mcg; Serving size: 1 slice or wedge, 20 g

Quesadilla—With Vegetables ☞ Vitamin K = 2.1 mcg; Serving size: 1 slice or wedge, 20 g

Quesadilla—With Vegetables And Chicken ☞ Vitamin K = 1.8 mcg; Serving size: 1 slice or wedge, 20 g

Quesadilla—With Vegetables And Meat ☞ Vitamin K = 1.8 mcg; Serving size: 1 slice or wedge, 20 g

Quiche—With Meat Poultry Or Fish ☞ Vitamin K = 5.6 mcg; Serving size: 1 piece (1/8 of 9" dia), 192 g

Ravioli—Cheese And Spinach Filled—With Tomato Sauce ☞ Vitamin K = 24.3 mcg; Serving size: 1 piece, 38 g

Ravioli—Cheese And Spinach-Filled No Sauce ☞ Vitamin K = 13.1 mcg; Serving size: 1 piece, 15 g

Ravioli—Cheese And Spinach-Filled—With Cream Sauce ☞ Vitamin K = 23.7 mcg; Serving size: 1 piece, 38 g

Ravioli—Cheese-Filled Canned ☞ Vitamin K = 5.6 mcg; Serving size: 1 cup, 242 g

Ravioli—Cheese-Filled No Sauce ☞ Vitamin K = 0.1 mcg; Serving size: 1 piece, 15 g

Ravioli—Cheese-Filled—With Cream Sauce ☞ Vitamin K = 1.5 mcg; Serving size: 1 piece, 38 g

Ravioli—Cheese-Filled—With Meat Sauce ☞ Vitamin K = 1.2 mcg; Serving size: 1 piece, 35 g

Ravioli—Cheese-Filled—With Tomato Sauce ☞ Vitamin K = 5.4 mcg; Serving size: 1 piece, 38 g

Ravioli—Cheese-Filled—With Tomato Sauce Diet—Frozen Meal ☞ Vitamin K = 3.8 mcg; Serving size: 1 meal (9 oz), 255 g

Ravioli—Cheese—With Tomato Sauce—Frozen Not Prepared

Includes Regular And Light Entrees ☞ Vitamin K = 25.6 mcg; Serving size: 1 cup, 159 g

Ravioli—Meat-Filled No Sauce ☞ Vitamin K = 0.1 mcg; Serving size: 1 piece, 15 g

Ravioli—Meat-Filled—With Cream Sauce ☞ Vitamin K = 1.3 mcg; Serving size: 1 piece, 35 g

Ravioli—Meat-Filled—With Tomato Sauce Or Meat Sauce ☞ Vitamin K = 1.2 mcg; Serving size: 1 piece, 35 g

Ravioli—Meat-Filled—With Tomato Sauce Or Meat Sauce Canned ☞ Vitamin K = 2.1 mcg; Serving size: 1 cup, 262 g

Red Beans And Rice ☞ Vitamin K = 17.5 mcg; Serving size: 1 cup, 224 g

Rice And Vermicelli Mix—Chicken Flavor—Unprepared ☞ Vitamin K = 0.3 mcg; Serving size: 1/3 cup, 56 g

Rice And Vermicelli Mix—Rice Pilaf Flavor—Unprepared ☞ Vitamin K = 0.3 mcg; Serving size: 1/3 cup, 68 g

Rice Bowl—With Chicken—Frozen Entree Prepared ☞ Vitamin K = 12.9 mcg; Serving size: 1 bowl, 340 g

Rice Brown—With Beans ☞ Vitamin K = 18.2 mcg; Serving size: 1 cup, 239 g

Rice Brown—With Beans And Tomatoes ☞ Vitamin K = 15.5 mcg; Serving size: 1 cup, 239 g

Rice Brown—With Carrots Fat Added In Cooking ☞ Vitamin K = 9.6 mcg; Serving size: 1 cup, 189 g

Rice Brown—With Corn Fat Not Added In Cooking ☞ Vitamin K = 0.4 mcg; Serving size: 1 cup, 188 g

Rice Brown—With Gravy Fat Added In Cooking ☞ Vitamin K = 5.2 mcg; Serving size: 1 cup, 237 g

Rice Brown—With Gravy Fat Not Added In Cooking ☞ Vitamin K = 0.7 mcg; Serving size: 1 cup, 237 g

Rice Brown—With Other Vegetables Fat Added In Cooking ☞ Vitamin K = 10.5 mcg; Serving size: 1 cup, 190 g

Rice Brown—With Other Vegetables Fat Not Added In Cooking ☞ Vitamin K = 6.5 mcg; Serving size: 1 cup, 186 g

Rice Brown—With Peas And Carrots Fat Added In Cooking ☞ Vitamin K = 11.8 mcg; Serving size: 1 cup, 190 g

Rice Brown—With Peas And Carrots Fat Not Added In Cooking ☞ Vitamin K = 7.9 mcg; Serving size: 1 cup, 187 g

Rice Brown—With Peas Fat Added In Cooking ☞ Vitamin K = 14.6 mcg; Serving size: 1 cup, 190 g

Rice Brown—With Peas Fat Not Added In Cooking ☞ Vitamin K = 10.7 mcg; Serving size: 1 cup, 187 g

Rice Brown—With Soy-Based Sauce Fat Added In Cooking ☞ Vitamin K = 5 mcg; Serving size: 1 cup, 237 g

Rice Brown—With Soy-Based Sauce Fat Not Added In Cooking ☞ Vitamin K = 0.5 mcg; Serving size: 1 cup, 237 g

Rice Brown—With Tomatoes And/or Tomato Based Sauce Fat Added In Cooking ☞ Vitamin K = 6.8 mcg; Serving size: 1 cup, 243 g

Rice Brown—With Tomatoes And/or Tomato Based Sauce Fat Not Added In Cooking ☞ Vitamin K = 2.2 mcg; Serving size: 1 cup, 243 g

Rice Brown—With Vegetables And Gravy Fat Added In Cooking ☞ Vitamin K = 17.5 mcg; Serving size: 1 cup, 292 g

Rice Brown—With Vegetables And Gravy Fat Not Added In Cooking ☞ Vitamin K = 13 mcg; Serving size: 1 cup, 288 g

Rice Brown—With Vegetables Cheese And/or Cream Based Sauce

Fat Added In Cooking ☛ Vitamin K = 17.9 mcg; Serving size: 1 cup, 293 g

Rice Brown—With Vegetables Cheese And/or Cream Based Sauce Fat Not Added In Cooking ☛ Vitamin K = 13.3 mcg; Serving size: 1 cup, 289 g

Rice Brown—With Vegetables Soy-Based Sauce Fat Added In Cooking ☛ Vitamin K = 17.1 mcg; Serving size: 1 cup, 290 g

Rice Brown—With Vegetables Soy-Based Sauce Fat Not Added In Cooking ☛ Vitamin K = 12.6 mcg; Serving size: 1 cup, 286 g

Rice Cooked—With Coconut Milk ☛ Vitamin K = 0.2 mcg; Serving size: 1 cup, 200 g

Rice Croquette ☛ Vitamin K = 19 mcg; Serving size: 1 croquette (1-1/2" dia, 2" high), 62 g

Rice Dessert Or Salad—With Fruit ☛ Vitamin K = 1.6 mcg; Serving size: 1 cup, 155 g

Rice Dressing ☛ Vitamin K = 12.5 mcg; Serving size: 1 cup, 167 g

Rice Fried—With Beef ☛ Vitamin K = 5.1 mcg; Serving size: 1 cup, 198 g

Rice Fried—With Chicken ☛ Vitamin K = 4.8 mcg; Serving size: 1 cup, 198 g

Rice Fried—With Pork ☛ Vitamin K = 4.8 mcg; Serving size: 1 cup, 198 g

Rice Fried—With Shrimp ☛ Vitamin K = 4.8 mcg; Serving size: 1 cup, 198 g

Rice Meal Fritter—Puerto Rican Style ☛ Vitamin K = 1.3 mcg; Serving size: 1 cruller (3" x 2" x 1/2"), 30 g

Rice Mix Cheese Flavor Dry Mix—Unprepared ☛ Vitamin K = 11.7 mcg; Serving size: 1/4 cup dry rice mix, 57 g

Rice Mix White And Wild Flavored—Unprepared ☛ Vitamin K = 0.3 mcg; Serving size: 2 oz (1/4 c dry rice mix and 4 tsp seasoning mix), 57 g

Rice White—With Corn Fat Added In Cooking ☛ Vitamin K = 4.2 mcg; Serving size: 1 cup, 161 g

Rice White—With Corn Fat Not Added In Cooking ☛ Vitamin K = 0.2 mcg; Serving size: 1 cup, 161 g

Rice White—With Dark Green Vegetables And Tomatoes And/or Tomato-Based Sauce Fat Added In Cooking ☛ Vitamin K = 32.2 mcg; Serving size: 1 cup, 172 g

Rice White—With Dark Green Vegetables And Tomatoes And/or Tomato-Based Sauce Fat Not Added In Cooking ☛ Vitamin K = 28.7 mcg; Serving size: 1 cup, 172 g

Rice White—With Dark Green Vegetables Fat Added In Cooking ☛ Vitamin K = 62.8 mcg; Serving size: 1 cup, 172 g

Rice White—With Dark Green Vegetables Fat Not Added In Cooking ☛ Vitamin K = 59.9 mcg; Serving size: 1 cup, 172 g

Rice White—With Gravy Fat Added In Cooking ☛ Vitamin K = 5.7 mcg; Serving size: 1 cup, 237 g

Rice White—With Gravy Fat Not Added In Cooking ☛ Vitamin K = 0.5 mcg; Serving size: 1 cup, 237 g

Rice White—With Lentils Fat Added In Cooking ☛ Vitamin K = 15.1 mcg; Serving size: 1 cup, 207 g

Rice White—With Lentils Fat Not Added In Cooking ☛ Vitamin K = 4.4 mcg; Serving size: 1 cup, 198 g

Rice White—With Other Vegetables Fat Added In Cooking ☛ Vitamin K = 10.8 mcg; Serving size: 1 cup, 172 g

Rice White—With Other Vegetables Fat Not Added In Cooking ☛ Vitamin K = 6.7 mcg; Serving size: 1 cup, 172 g

Rice White—With Peas And Carrots Fat Added In Cooking ☞ Vitamin K = 11.4 mcg; Serving size: 1 cup, 160 g

Rice White—With Peas And Carrots Fat Not Added In Cooking ☞ Vitamin K = 7.5 mcg; Serving size: 1 cup, 160 g

Rice White—With Peas Fat Added In Cooking ☞ Vitamin K = 14.1 mcg; Serving size: 1 cup, 160 g

Rice White—With Peas Fat Not Added In Cooking ☞ Vitamin K = 10.4 mcg; Serving size: 1 cup, 160 g

Rice White—With Soy-Based Sauce Fat Added In Cooking ☞ Vitamin K = 5.2 mcg; Serving size: 1 cup, 237 g

Rice White—With Soy-Based Sauce Fat Not Added In Cooking ☞ Vitamin K = 0 mcg; Serving size: 1 cup, 237 g

Rice White—With Tomatoes And/or Tomato-Based Sauce Fat Added In Cooking ☞ Vitamin K = 6.5 mcg; Serving size: 1 cup, 209 g

Rice White—With Tomatoes And/or Tomato-Based Sauce Fat Not Added In Cooking ☞ Vitamin K = 1.9 mcg; Serving size: 1 cup, 206 g

Rice White—With Vegetables And Gravy Fat Added In Cooking ☞ Vitamin K = 17.2 mcg; Serving size: 1 cup, 260 g

Rice White—With Vegetables And Gravy Fat Not Added In Cooking ☞ Vitamin K = 12.5 mcg; Serving size: 1 cup, 256 g

Rice White—With Vegetables Cheese And/or Cream Based Sauce Fat Added In Cooking ☞ Vitamin K = 17.6 mcg; Serving size: 1 cup, 262 g

Rice White—With Vegetables Cheese And/or Cream Based Sauce Fat Not Added In Cooking ☞ Vitamin K = 12.9 mcg; Serving size: 1 cup, 258 g

Rice White—With Vegetables Soy-Based Sauce Fat Added In Cooking ☞ Vitamin K = 16.8 mcg; Serving size: 1 cup, 258 g

Rice White—With Vegetables Soy-Based Sauce Fat Not Added In Cooking ☞ Vitamin K = 12.2 mcg; Serving size: 1 cup, 255 g

Rice—With Beans ☞ Vitamin K = 19.6 mcg; Serving size: 1 cup, 239 g

Rice—With Beans And Beef ☞ Vitamin K = 17.2 mcg; Serving size: 1 cup, 239 g

Rice—With Beans And Chicken ☞ Vitamin K = 16.5 mcg; Serving size: 1 cup, 239 g

Rice—With Beans And Pork ☞ Vitamin K = 16.5 mcg; Serving size: 1 cup, 239 g

Rice—With Beans And Tomatoes ☞ Vitamin K = 16.5 mcg; Serving size: 1 cup, 239 g

Rice—With Broccoli Cheese Sauce—Frozen Side Dish ☞ Vitamin K = 68.1 mcg; Serving size: 1 side dish (4.5 oz), 128 g

Rice—With Chicken—Puerto Rican Style ☞ Vitamin K = 10.4 mcg; Serving size: 1 cup, with bone (yield after bone removed), 157 g

Rice—With Green Beans Water Chestnuts In Sherry Mushroom Sauce—Frozen Side Dish ☞ Vitamin K = 28.7 mcg; Serving size: 1 side dish (10 oz), 284 g

Rice—With Onions—Puerto Rican Style ☞ Vitamin K = 17.2 mcg; Serving size: 1 cup, 165 g

Rice—With Raisins ☞ Vitamin K = 5.6 mcg; Serving size: 1 cup, 185 g

Rice—With Spanish Sausage—Puerto Rican Style ☞ Vitamin K = 11.7 mcg; Serving size: 1 cup, 180 g

Rice—With Squid—Puerto Rican Style ☞ Vitamin K = 15.5 mcg; Serving size: 1 cup, 160 g

Rice—With Stewed Beans—Puerto Rican Style ☞ Vitamin K = 7.9 mcg; Serving size: 1 cup, 188 g

Rice—With Vienna Sausage—Puerto Rican Style ☛ Vitamin K = 9.2 mcg; Serving size: 1 cup, 180 g

Rigatoni—With Meat Sauce And Cheese Diet—Frozen Meal ☛ Vitamin K = 4.7 mcg; Serving size: 1 meal (9.75 oz), 276 g

Roll—With Meat And/or Shrimp Vegetables And Rice Paper Not Fried ☛ Vitamin K = 20.4 mcg; Serving size: 1 roll (4-1/4" x 1-1/2" dia), 71 g

Salisbury Steak—With Gravy—Frozen ☛ Vitamin K = 1.1 mcg; Serving size: 1 patty, 63 g

Sausage Egg And Cheese Breakfast Biscuit ☛ Vitamin K = 2.3 mcg; Serving size: 1 biscuit, 126 g

Seafood Paella—Puerto Rican Style ☛ Vitamin K = 13.8 mcg; Serving size: 1 cup, 230 g

Seaweed Prepared—With Soy Sauce ☛ Vitamin K = 20.7 mcg; Serving size: 1 cup, 96 g

Shellfish Mixture And Vegetables—With Carrots Broccoli And/or Dark-Green Leafy; No Potatoes Soy-Based Sauce ☛ Vitamin K = 82.9 mcg; Serving size: 1 cup, 217 g

Shellfish Mixture And Vegetables—Without Carrots Broccoli And Dark-Green Leafy; No Potatoes Soy-Based Sauce ☛ Vitamin K = 43.8 mcg; Serving size: 1 cup, 217 g

Shrimp And Noodles—With Soy-Based Sauce ☛ Vitamin K = 36.3 mcg; Serving size: 1 cup, 224 g

Shrimp And Vegetables—With Carrots Broccoli And/or Dark-Green Leafy; No Potatoes Soy-Based Sauce ☛ Vitamin K = 82.9 mcg; Serving size: 1 cup, 217 g

Shrimp And Vegetables—Without Carrots Broccoli And Dark-Green Leafy; No Potatoes Soy-Based Sauce ☛ Vitamin K = 43.8 mcg; Serving size: 1 cup, 217 g

Shrimp Chow Mein Or Chop Suey—No Noodles ☞ Vitamin K = 27.5 mcg; Serving size: 1 cup, 220 g

Shrimp Chow Mein Or Chop Suey—With Noodles ☞ Vitamin K = 24.4 mcg; Serving size: 1 cup, 220 g

Shrimp Egg Foo Yung ☞ Vitamin K = 32 mcg; Serving size: 1 cup, 175 g

Shrimp Teriyaki ☞ Vitamin K = 0.8 mcg; Serving size: 1 cup, 201 g

Soft Taco—With Chicken And Beans ☞ Vitamin K = 8.5 mcg; Serving size: 1 small taco or tostada, 112 g

Soft Taco—With Chicken Beans And Sour Cream ☞ Vitamin K = 8.8 mcg; Serving size: 1 small taco or tostada, 127 g

Soft Taco—With Fish ☞ Vitamin K = 7.5 mcg; Serving size: 1 small taco or tostada, 94 g

Soft Taco—With Meat ☞ Vitamin K = 8.1 mcg; Serving size: 1 small taco or tostada, 103 g

Soft Taco—With Meat And Beans ☞ Vitamin K = 8.9 mcg; Serving size: 1 small taco or tostada, 117 g

Soft Taco—With Meat And Sour Cream—From Fast Food ☞ Vitamin K = 8 mcg; Serving size: 1 small taco or tostada, 117 g

Soft Taco—With Meat Beans And Sour Cream ☞ Vitamin K = 9.2 mcg; Serving size: 1 small taco or tostada, 132 g

Somen Salad—With Noodles Lettuce Egg Fish And Pork ☞ Vitamin K = 30.9 mcg; Serving size: 1 cup, 160 g

Spaghetti And Meatballs Dinner—Frozen Meal ☞ Vitamin K = 14.5 mcg; Serving size: 1 meal (12.5 oz), 354 g

Spaghetti And Meatballs—With Tomato Sauce Sliced Apples Bread —Frozen Meal ☞ Vitamin K = 3.6 mcg; Serving size: 1 meal (11.5 oz), 326 g

Spaghetti—With Corned Beef—Puerto Rican Style ☞ Vitamin K = 11.8 mcg; Serving size: 1 cup, 215 g

Spaghetti—With Meat And Mushroom Sauce Diet—Frozen Meal ☞ Vitamin K = 4.9 mcg; Serving size: 1 meal (11.5 oz), 326 g

Spaghetti—With Meat Sauce Diet—Frozen Meal ☞ Vitamin K = 12.2 mcg; Serving size: 1 meal (10.5 oz), 298 g

Spaghetti—With Meat Sauce—Frozen Entree ☞ Vitamin K = 2 mcg; Serving size: 1 serving, 283 g

Spaghetti—With Meatballs In Tomato Sauce Canned ☞ Vitamin K = 4.4 mcg; Serving size: 1 cup, 246 g

Spanakopitta ☞ Vitamin K = 25.5 mcg; Serving size: 1 cubic inch, 12 g

Spanish Rice Fat Added In Cooking ☞ Vitamin K = 8.3 mcg; Serving size: 1 cup, 243 g

Spanish Rice Fat Not Added In Cooking ☞ Vitamin K = 3.6 mcg; Serving size: 1 cup, 243 g

Spanish Rice Mix Dry Mix Prepared ☞ Vitamin K = 5.7 mcg; Serving size: 1 cup, 198 g

Spanish Rice Mix Dry Mix—Unprepared ☞ Vitamin K = 1.9 mcg; Serving size: 1/2 cup, 70 g

Spanish Rice—With Ground Beef ☞ Vitamin K = 6.9 mcg; Serving size: 1 cup, 230 g

Spinach Quiche Meatless ☞ Vitamin K = 163.3 mcg; Serving size: 1 piece (1/8 of 9" dia), 143 g

Steak Teriyaki ☞ Vitamin K = 3.4 mcg; Serving size: 1 cup, 244 g

Stewed Potatoes ☞ Vitamin K = 10 mcg; Serving size: 1 cup, 250 g

Stewed Potatoes—With Tomatoes ☞ Vitamin K = 11.3 mcg; Serving size: 1 cup, 250 g

Stewed Rice—Puerto Rican Style ☞ Vitamin K = 11.4 mcg; Serving size: 1 cup, 170 g

Stuffed Shells—Cheese- And Spinach- Filled No Sauce ☞ Vitamin K = 54 mcg; Serving size: 1 shell (jumbo), 60 g

Stuffed Shells—Cheese-Filled No Sauce ☞ Vitamin K = 0.4 mcg; Serving size: 1 shell (jumbo), 60 g

Stuffed Shells—Cheese-Filled—With Meat Sauce ☞ Vitamin K = 1.9 mcg; Serving size: 1 shell (jumbo), 85 g

Stuffed Shells—Cheese-Filled—With Tomato Sauce Meatless ☞ Vitamin K = 1.8 mcg; Serving size: 1 shell (jumbo), 85 g

Stuffed Shells—With Chicken—With Tomato Sauce ☞ Vitamin K = 1.6 mcg; Serving size: 1 shell (jumbo), 83 g

Stuffed Shells—With Fish And/or Shellfish—With Tomato Sauce ☞ Vitamin K = 1.6 mcg; Serving size: 1 shell (jumbo), 83 g

Sushi—Nfs ☞ Vitamin K = 0.4 mcg; Serving size: 1 piece, 30 g

Sushi—Roll Avocado ☞ Vitamin K = 1 mcg; Serving size: 1 piece, 30 g

Sushi—Roll California ☞ Vitamin K = 0.4 mcg; Serving size: 1 piece, 30 g

Sushi—Roll Eel ☞ Vitamin K = 0 mcg; Serving size: 1 piece, 30 g

Sushi—Roll Salmon ☞ Vitamin K = 0 mcg; Serving size: 1 piece, 30 g

Sushi—Roll Shrimp ☞ Vitamin K = 0 mcg; Serving size: 1 piece, 30 g

Sushi—Roll Tuna ☞ Vitamin K = 0 mcg; Serving size: 1 piece, 30 g

Sushi—Roll Vegetable ☞ Vitamin K = 0.7 mcg; Serving size: 1 piece, 22 g

Sushi—Topped—With Crab ☞ Vitamin K = 0 mcg; Serving size: 1 piece, 35 g

Sushi—Topped—With Eel ☞ Vitamin K = 0 mcg; Serving size: 1 piece, 35 g

Sushi—Topped—With Egg ☞ Vitamin K = 0.1 mcg; Serving size: 1 piece, 50 g

Sushi—Topped—With Salmon ☞ Vitamin K = 0 mcg; Serving size: 1 piece, 35 g

Sushi—Topped—With Shrimp ☞ Vitamin K = 0 mcg; Serving size: 1 piece, 35 g

Sushi—Topped—With Tuna ☞ Vitamin K = 0 mcg; Serving size: 1 piece, 35 g

Sweet And Sour Pork ☞ Vitamin K = 19.2 mcg; Serving size: 1 cup, 226 g

Sweet And Sour Pork—With Rice ☞ Vitamin K = 17.3 mcg; Serving size: 1 cup, 244 g

Sweet And Sour Shrimp ☞ Vitamin K = 18 mcg; Serving size: 1 cup, 176 g

Sweet Bread Dough Filled—With Meat Steamed ☞ Vitamin K = 1.5 mcg; Serving size: 1 manapua, 93 g

Tabbouleh ☞ Vitamin K = 161.4 mcg; Serving size: 1 cup, 160 g

Taco Or Tostada Salad Meatless ☞ Vitamin K = 30.4 mcg; Serving size: 1 small taco salad, 234 g

Taco Or Tostada Salad Meatless—With Sour Cream ☞ Vitamin K = 30.9 mcg; Serving size: 1 small taco salad, 266 g

Taco Or Tostada Salad—With Chicken ☞ Vitamin K = 30.5 mcg; Serving size: 1 small taco salad, 240 g

Taco Or Tostada Salad—With Chicken And Sour Cream ☞ Vitamin K = 31.1 mcg; Serving size: 1 small taco salad, 273 g

Taco Or Tostada Salad—With Meat ☞ Vitamin K = 30.8 mcg; Serving size: 1 small taco salad, 237 g

Taco Or Tostada Salad—With Meat And Sour Cream ☞ Vitamin K = 30.9 mcg; Serving size: 1 small taco salad, 264 g

Taco Or Tostada—With Beans ☞ Vitamin K = 9.6 mcg; Serving size: 1 small taco or tostada, 125 g

Taco Or Tostada—With Beans And Sour Cream ☞ Vitamin K = 9.8 mcg; Serving size: 1 small taco or tostada, 140 g

Taco Or Tostada—With Chicken ☞ Vitamin K = 6.8 mcg; Serving size: 1 small taco or tostada, 80 g

Taco Or Tostada—With Chicken And Beans ☞ Vitamin K = 8.2 mcg; Serving size: 1 small taco or tostada, 103 g

Taco Or Tostada—With Chicken And Sour Cream ☞ Vitamin K = 7.1 mcg; Serving size: 1 small taco or tostada, 96 g

Taco Or Tostada—With Chicken Beans And Sour Cream ☞ Vitamin K = 8.4 mcg; Serving size: 1 small taco or tostada, 118 g

Taco Or Tostada—With Fish ☞ Vitamin K = 1.7 mcg; Serving size: 1 miniature taco, 20 g

Taco Or Tostada—With Meat ☞ Vitamin K = 1.8 mcg; Serving size: 1 miniature taco, 22 g

Taco Or Tostada—With Meat And Beans ☞ Vitamin K = 8.7 mcg; Serving size: 1 small taco or tostada, 109 g

Taco Or Tostada—With Meat And Beans—From Fast Food ☞ Vitamin K = 15.9 mcg; Serving size: 1 small taco or tostada, 109 g

Taco Or Tostada—With Meat And Sour Cream ☞ Vitamin K = 8.1 mcg; Serving size: 1 small taco or tostada, 109 g

Taco Or Tostada—With Meat Beans And Sour Cream ☞ Vitamin K = 8.9 mcg; Serving size: 1 small taco or tostada, 124 g

Taco—With Crab Meat—Puerto Rican Style ☛ Vitamin K = 8 mcg; Serving size: 1 taco (4-1/2" dia), 121 g

Tamal In A Leaf—Puerto Rican Style ☛ Vitamin K = 3 mcg; Serving size: 1 tamal (6" x 2" x 1/2"), 41 g

Tamale Casserole—Puerto Rican Style ☛ Vitamin K = 9.7 mcg; Serving size: 1 cup, 237 g

Tamale Casserole—With Meat ☛ Vitamin K = 4.6 mcg; Serving size: 1 cup, 244 g

Tamale Meatless—With Sauce—Puerto Rican Or Caribbean Style ☛ Vitamin K = 0.1 mcg; Serving size: 1 tamale, 72 g

Tamale Plain Meatless No Sauce—Puerto Rican Style Or Carribean Style ☛ Vitamin K = 0 mcg; Serving size: 1 tamale, 36 g

Tamale—With Chicken ☛ Vitamin K = 0.3 mcg; Serving size: 1 small tamale, 84 g

Taquito Or Flauta—With Cheese ☛ Vitamin K = 0.3 mcg; Serving size: 1 small taquito, 36 g

Taquitos—Frozen—Beef And Cheese Oven-Heated ☛ Vitamin K = 9.2 mcg; Serving size: 1 piece, 42 g

Taquitos—Frozen—Chicken And Cheese Oven-Heated ☛ Vitamin K = 7.1 mcg; Serving size: 1 piece, 42 g

Tofu And Vegetables—With Carrots Broccoli And/or Dark-Green Leafy; No Potatoes—With Soy-Based Sauce ☛ Vitamin K = 76.4 mcg; Serving size: 1 cup, 217 g

Tofu And Vegetables—Without Carrots Broccoli And Dark-Green Leafy; No Potatoes—With Soy-Based Sauce ☛ Vitamin K = 41 mcg; Serving size: 1 cup, 217 g

Tortellini—Cheese-Filled Meatless—With Tomato Sauce ☛ Vitamin K = 17.5 mcg; Serving size: 1 cup, 250 g

Tortellini—Cheese-Filled Meatless—With Tomato Sauce Canned ☛ Vitamin K = 1 mcg; Serving size: 1 cup, 247 g

Tortellini—Cheese-Filled Meatless—With Vegetables And Vinaigrette Dressing ☛ Vitamin K = 54.6 mcg; Serving size: 1 cup, 169 g

Tortellini—Cheese-Filled Meatless—With Vinaigrette Dressing ☛ Vitamin K = 18.1 mcg; Serving size: 1 cup, 169 g

Tortellini—Cheese-Filled No Sauce ☛ Vitamin K = 1.5 mcg; Serving size: 1 cup, 150 g

Tortellini—Cheese-Filled—With Cream Sauce ☛ Vitamin K = 1.5 mcg; Serving size: 1 cup, 250 g

Tortellini—Meat-Filled No Sauce ☛ Vitamin K = 4.2 mcg; Serving size: 1 cup, 190 g

Tortellini—Meat-Filled—With Tomato Sauce ☛ Vitamin K = 6.7 mcg; Serving size: 1 cup, 210 g

Tortellini—Meat-Filled—With Tomato Sauce Canned ☛ Vitamin K = 3.3 mcg; Serving size: 1 cup, 233 g

Tortellini—Pasta—With Cheese Filling Fresh-Refrigerated As Purchased ☛ Vitamin K = 1.1 mcg; Serving size: 3/4 cup, 81 g

Tortellini—Spinach-Filled No Sauce ☛ Vitamin K = 53.3 mcg; Serving size: 1 cup, 122 g

Tortellini—Spinach-Filled—With Tomato Sauce ☛ Vitamin K = 94.4 mcg; Serving size: 1 cup, 200 g

Turkey Stuffing Mashed Potatoes W/gravy Assorted Vegetables—Frozen Microwaved ☛ Vitamin K = 44.3 mcg; Serving size: 1 serving, 385 g

Turnover Cheese-Filled Tomato-Based Sauce—Frozen—Unprepared ☛ Vitamin K = 19.6 mcg; Serving size: 1 serving 4.5 oz, 127 g

Turnover Chicken- Or Turkey- And Vegetable-Filled Reduced Fat—

Frozen ☛ Vitamin K = 17 mcg; Serving size: 1 piece turnover 1 serving, 127 g

Turnover Filled—With Egg Meat And Cheese—Frozen ☛ Vitamin K = 4.8 mcg; Serving size: 1 piece turnover 1 serving, 127 g

Turnover Filled—With Ground Beef And Cabbage ☛ Vitamin K = 56.5 mcg; Serving size: 1 bierock, 215 g

Turnover Meat- And Cheese-Filled Tomato-Based Sauce Reduced Fat —Frozen ☛ Vitamin K = 2.4 mcg; Serving size: 1 piece turnover 1 serving, 127 g

Vada Fried Dumpling ☛ Vitamin K = 4.2 mcg; Serving size: 1 vada, 29 g

Veal Lasagna—Diet—Frozen Meal ☛ Vitamin K = 29.4 mcg; Serving size: 1 meal (10.25 oz), 291 g

Vegetable Combination—With Carrots Broccoli And/or Dark-Green Leafy; Cooked—With Soy-Based Sauce ☛ Vitamin K = 104.2 mcg; Serving size: 1 cup, 185 g

Vegetable Combination—Without Carrots Broccoli And Dark-Green Leafy; Cooked—With Soy-Based Sauce ☛ Vitamin K = 55.9 mcg; Serving size: 1 cup, 185 g

Wonton Fried Filled—With Meat Poultry Or Seafood ☛ Vitamin K = 12.2 mcg; Serving size: 1 wonton, any size, 19 g

Wonton Fried Filled—With Meat Poultry Or Seafood And Vegetable ☛ Vitamin K = 12.2 mcg; Serving size: 1 wonton, any size, 19 g

Wonton Fried Meatless ☛ Vitamin K = 12.2 mcg; Serving size: 1 wonton, any size, 19 g

Yellow Rice—With Seasoning Dry Packet Mix—Unprepared ☛ Vitamin K = 0.3 mcg; Serving size: 1 serving (2 oz), 57 g

Zucchini Lasagna—Diet—Frozen Meal ☛ Vitamin K = 8.7 mcg; Serving size: 1 lean cuisine meal (11 oz), 312 g

25

RESTAURANT FOODS

Applebees—Chicken Tenders From Kids Menu ☞ Vitamin K = 8.8 mcg; Serving size: 1 piece, 35 g

Applebees—Coleslaw ☞ Vitamin K = 49.5 mcg; Serving size: 1 serving, 76 g

Applebees—Double Crunch Shrimp ☞ Vitamin K = 59.9 mcg; Serving size: 1 serving, 206 g

Applebees—French Fries ☞ Vitamin K = 54.8 mcg; Serving size: 1 serving, 164 g

Applebees—Mozzarella Sticks ☞ Vitamin K = 7.1 mcg; Serving size: 1 piece, 32 g

Carrabba's Italian Grill—Spaghetti With Meat Sauce ☞ Vitamin K = 17.7 mcg; Serving size: 1 serving, 537 g

Carrabba's Italian Grill—Spaghetti With Pomodoro Sauce ☞ Vitamin K = 21.5 mcg; Serving size: 1 serving, 489 g

Cracker Barrel—Chicken Tenderloin Platter Fried From Kids Menu ☞ Vitamin K = 34.3 mcg; Serving size: 1 serving, 103 g

Cracker Barrel—Coleslaw ☛ Vitamin K = 147.1 mcg; Serving size: 1 serving, 167 g

Cracker Barrel—Farm Raised Catfish Platter ☛ Vitamin K = 44 mcg; Serving size: 1 serving, 178 g

Cracker Barrel—Grilled Sirloin Steak ☛ Vitamin K = 1.5 mcg; Serving size: 1 steak, 151 g

Cracker Barrel—Macaroni N Cheese Plate From Kids Menu ☛ Vitamin K = 25.4 mcg; Serving size: 1 serving, 257 g

Cracker Barrel—Onion Rings Thick-Cut ☛ Vitamin K = 94.2 mcg; Serving size: 1 serving, 261 g

Cracker Barrel—Steak Fries ☛ Vitamin K = 63.6 mcg; Serving size: 1 serving, 198 g

Denny's—Chicken Nuggets Star Shaped From Kids Menu ☛ Vitamin K = 24.5 mcg; Serving size: 1 serving 4 pieces, 67 g

Denny's—Coleslaw ☛ Vitamin K = 78.4 mcg; Serving size: 1 serving, 91 g

Denny's—French Fries ☛ Vitamin K = 47.5 mcg; Serving size: 1 serving, 165 g

Denny's—Golden Fried Shrimp ☛ Vitamin K = 5.6 mcg; Serving size: 1 piece, 16 g

Denny's—Hash Browns ☛ Vitamin K = 40.4 mcg; Serving size: 1 serving, 124 g

Denny's—Macaroni & Cheese From Kids Menu ☛ Vitamin K = 5.4 mcg; Serving size: 1 serving, 180 g

Denny's—Mozzarella Cheese Sticks ☛ Vitamin K = 57.9 mcg; Serving size: 1 serving, 228 g

Denny's—Onion Rings ☛ Vitamin K = 84 mcg; Serving size: 1 serving, 166 g

Denny's—Top Sirloin Steak ☛ Vitamin K = 1.1 mcg; Serving size: 1 steak, 107 g

French Fries ☛ Vitamin K = 1.6 mcg; Serving size: 10 strip, 69 g

Fried Onion Rings ☛ Vitamin K = 143.9 mcg; Serving size: 1 serving, 350 g

Hash Browns ☛ Vitamin K = 5.8 mcg; Serving size: 1 cup, 156 g

Olive Garden—Lasagna Classico ☛ Vitamin K = 28.7 mcg; Serving size: 1 serving, 422 g

Olive Garden—Spaghetti With Meat Sauce ☛ Vitamin K = 22.6 mcg; Serving size: 1 serving, 525 g

Olive Garden—Spaghetti With Pomodoro Sauce ☛ Vitamin K = 20.1 mcg; Serving size: 1 serving, 478 g

On The Border—Mexican Rice ☛ Vitamin K = 14 mcg; Serving size: 1 cup, 114 g

On The Border—Refried Beans ☛ Vitamin K = 2.8 mcg; Serving size: 1 cup, 135 g

Onion Rings ☛ Vitamin K = 16.4 mcg; Serving size: 1 cup, 48 g

Restaurant Chinese—Beef And Vegetables ☛ Vitamin K = 294.5 mcg; Serving size: 1 order, 574 g

Restaurant Chinese—Chicken And Vegetables ☛ Vitamin K = 379.1 mcg; Serving size: 1 order, 693 g

Restaurant Chinese—Chicken Chow Mein ☛ Vitamin K = 132.9 mcg; Serving size: 1 order, 604 g

Restaurant Chinese—Egg Rolls Assorted ☛ Vitamin K = 52.4 mcg; Serving size: 1 piece, 89 g

Restaurant Chinese—Fried Rice Without Meat ☛ Vitamin K = 3.8 mcg; Serving size: 1 cup, 137 g

Restaurant Chinese—General Tsos Chicken ☞ Vitamin K = 204.4 mcg; Serving size: 1 order, 535 g

Restaurant Chinese—Kung Pao Chicken ☞ Vitamin K = 82.1 mcg; Serving size: 1 order, 604 g

Restaurant Chinese—Lemon Chicken ☞ Vitamin K = 152 mcg; Serving size: 1 order, 623 g

Restaurant Chinese—Orange Chicken ☞ Vitamin K = 158.1 mcg; Serving size: 1 order, 648 g

Restaurant Chinese—Sesame Chicken ☞ Vitamin K = 148.2 mcg; Serving size: 1 order, 547 g

Restaurant Chinese—Shrimp And Vegetables ☞ Vitamin K = 312.5 mcg; Serving size: 1 order, 601 g

Restaurant Chinese—Sweet And Sour Chicken ☞ Vitamin K = 158.9 mcg; Serving size: 1 order, 706 g

Restaurant Chinese—Sweet And Sour Pork ☞ Vitamin K = 169.9 mcg; Serving size: 1 order, 609 g

Restaurant Chinese—Vegetable Chow Mein Without Meat Or Noodles ☞ Vitamin K = 146.9 mcg; Serving size: 1 order, 777 g

Restaurant Chinese—Vegetable Lo Mein Without Meat ☞ Vitamin K = 94.1 mcg; Serving size: 1 order, 741 g

Restaurant Family Style—Chicken Fingers From Kids Menu ☞ Vitamin K = 31.9 mcg; Serving size: 1 serving, 114 g

Restaurant Family Style—Chili With Meat And Beans ☞ Vitamin K = 4.2 mcg; Serving size: 1 cup, 136 g

Restaurant Family Style—Coleslaw ☞ Vitamin K = 85.3 mcg; Serving size: 1 serving, 108 g

Restaurant Family Style—Fish Fillet Battered Or Breaded Fried ☞ Vitamin K = 0.2 mcg; Serving size: 1 serving, 226 g

Restaurant Family Style—French Fries ☞ Vitamin K = 61 mcg; Serving size: 1 serving, 170 g

Restaurant Family Style—Fried Mozzarella Sticks ☞ Vitamin K = 56.1 mcg; Serving size: 1 serving, 245 g

Restaurant Family Style—Hash Browns ☞ Vitamin K = 30.6 mcg; Serving size: 1 cup, 94 g

Restaurant Family Style—Macaroni & Cheese From Kids Menu ☞ Vitamin K = 0.7 mcg; Serving size: 1 cup, 136 g

Restaurant Family Style—Onion Rings ☞ Vitamin K = 110.3 mcg; Serving size: 1 serving, 259 g

Restaurant Family Style—Shrimp Breaded And Fried ☞ Vitamin K = 54.4 mcg; Serving size: 1 serving, 169 g

Restaurant Italian—Lasagna With Meat ☞ Vitamin K = 31.1 mcg; Serving size: 1 serving, 457 g

Restaurant Italian—Spaghetti With Meat Sauce ☞ Vitamin K = 23.3 mcg; Serving size: 1 serving, 554 g

Restaurant Italian—Spaghetti With Pomodoro Sauce (No Meat) ☞ Vitamin K = 20.4 mcg; Serving size: 1 serving, 510 g

Restaurant Latino—Arepa (Unleavened Cornmeal Bread) ☞ Vitamin K = 3.4 mcg; Serving size: 1 piece, 98 g

Restaurant Latino—Arroz Con Frijoles Negros (Rice And Black Beans) ☞ Vitamin K = 47.5 mcg; Serving size: 1 serving, 461 g

Restaurant Latino—Arroz Con Grandules (Rice And Pigeonpeas) ☞ Vitamin K = 82.3 mcg; Serving size: 1 serving, 653 g

Restaurant Latino—Arroz Con Habichuelas Colorados (Rice And Red Beans) ☞ Vitamin K = 46 mcg; Serving size: 1 serving, 590 g

Restaurant Latino—Black Bean Soup ☞ Vitamin K = 14.8 mcg; Serving size: 1 cup, 246 g

Restaurant Latino—Bunuelos (Fried Yeast Bread) ☞ Vitamin K = 18.1 mcg; Serving size: 1 piece, 70 g

Restaurant Latino—Chicken And Rice Entree Prepared ☞ Vitamin K = 5.6 mcg; Serving size: 1 cup, 141 g

Restaurant Latino—Empanadas Beef Prepared ☞ Vitamin K = 5.4 mcg; Serving size: 1 piece, 89 g

Restaurant Latino—Pupusas Con Frijoles (Pupusas Bean) ☞ Vitamin K = 9.3 mcg; Serving size: 1 piece, 126 g

Restaurant Latino—Pupusas Con Queso (Pupusas Cheese) ☞ Vitamin K = 2 mcg; Serving size: 1 piece, 117 g

Restaurant Latino—Pupusas Del Cerdo (Pupusas Pork) ☞ Vitamin K = 1.3 mcg; Serving size: 1 piece, 122 g

Restaurant Latino—Tamale Corn ☞ Vitamin K = 9 mcg; Serving size: 1 piece, 166 g

Restaurant Latino—Tamale Pork ☞ Vitamin K = 7.2 mcg; Serving size: 1 piece, 142 g

Restaurant Latino—Tripe Soup ☞ Vitamin K = 4.6 mcg; Serving size: 1 cup, 200 g

Restaurant Mexican—Refried Beans ☞ Vitamin K = 19.7 mcg; Serving size: 1 cup, 148 g

Restaurant Mexican—Spanish Rice ☞ Vitamin K = 15.1 mcg; Serving size: 1 cup, 116 g

T.G.I. Friday's—Chicken Fingers From Kids Menu ☞ Vitamin K = 10.4 mcg; Serving size: 1 piece, 41 g

T.G.I. Friday's—French Fries ☞ Vitamin K = 79.3 mcg; Serving size: 1 serving, 184 g

26

SNACKS

Bagel Chips Plain ☞ Vitamin K = 1.5 mcg; Serving size: 1 oz, 28.4 g

Banana Chips ☞ Vitamin K = 0.4 mcg; Serving size: 1 oz, 28.4 g

Bean Chips ☞ Vitamin K = 0.1 mcg; Serving size: 1 chip, 3 g

Beef Jerky Chopped And Formed ☞ Vitamin K = 0.7 mcg; Serving size: 1 oz, 28.4 g

Breadsticks Hard Reduced Sodium ☞ Vitamin K = 0.1 mcg; Serving size: 1 snack size stick, 2 g

Breadsticks Hard Whole Wheat ☞ Vitamin K = 0.1 mcg; Serving size: 1 snack size stick, 2 g

Breakfast Bar—Cereal Crust—With Fruit Filling Reduced Fat ☞ Vitamin K = 5.1 mcg; Serving size: 1 bar, 37 g

Breakfast Bar—Corn Flake Crust—With Fruit ☞ Vitamin K = 3.9 mcg; Serving size: 1 oz, 28.4 g

Breakfast Bar—Nfs ☞ Vitamin K = 5.9 mcg; Serving size: 1 bar, 43 g

Brown Rice Chips ☞ Vitamin K = 0.6 mcg; Serving size: 1 cake, 9 g

Candy Bits Yogurt Covered—With Vitamin C ☞ Vitamin K = 2.7 mcg; Serving size: 1 package, 20 g

Corn Cakes ☞ Vitamin K = 0 mcg; Serving size: 1 cake, 9 g

Corn Chips—Flavored ☞ Vitamin K = 0.1 mcg; Serving size: 1 chip, 1 g

Corn Chips—Plain ☞ Vitamin K = 0.1 mcg; Serving size: 1 chip, 1 g

Corn Chips—Reduced Sodium ☞ Vitamin K = 0.1 mcg; Serving size: 1 chip, 1 g

Crackers—Breakfast Biscuit ☞ Vitamin K = 2 mcg; Serving size: 1 biscuit, 15 g

Crackers—Flatbread ☞ Vitamin K = 0.4 mcg; Serving size: 1 flatbread, 10 g

Crackers—Rice And Nuts ☞ Vitamin K = 0.1 mcg; Serving size: 1 cracker, 3 g

Crackers—Saltine Reduced Sodium ☞ Vitamin K = 0.5 mcg; Serving size: 1 cracker, 3 g

Crackers—Wheat ☞ Vitamin K = 0.6 mcg; Serving size: 1 cracker, 3 g

Crackers—Woven Wheat ☞ Vitamin K = 1 mcg; Serving size: 1 cracker, 5 g

Granola Bar—Chewy Reduced Sugar All Flavors ☞ Vitamin K = 0.6 mcg; Serving size: 1 bar, 24 g

Granola Bar—General Mills Nature Valley Chewy Trail Mix ☞ Vitamin K = 2.6 mcg; Serving size: 1 bar, 35 g

Granola Bar—General Mills Nature Valley Sweet&salty Nut Peanut ☞ Vitamin K = 4.1 mcg; Serving size: 1 bar, 35 g

Granola Bar—General Mills Nature Valley—With Yogurt Coating ☞ Vitamin K = 2.4 mcg; Serving size: 1 bar, 35 g

Granola Bar—Hard Plain ☛ Vitamin K = 3.1 mcg; Serving size: 1 bar, 21 g

Granola Bar—Kashi Golean Chewy Mixed Flavors ☛ Vitamin K = 2.8 mcg; Serving size: 1 bar, 78 g

Granola Bar—Kashi Golean Crunchy Mixed Flavors ☛ Vitamin K = 0.8 mcg; Serving size: 1 bar, 47 g

Granola Bar—Kashi Tlc Bar Chewy Mixed Flavors ☛ Vitamin K = 0.9 mcg; Serving size: 1 bar, 35 g

Granola Bar—Kashi Tlc Bar Crunchy Mixed Flavors ☛ Vitamin K = 3.9 mcg; Serving size: 2 bar, 40 g

Granola Bar—Quaker Chewy 90 Calorie Bar ☛ Vitamin K = 0.7 mcg; Serving size: 1 bar, 24 g

Granola Bar—Quaker Dipps All Flavors ☛ Vitamin K = 0.6 mcg; Serving size: 1 bar, 31 g

Granola Bar—Quaker Oatmeal To Go All Flavors ☛ Vitamin K = 4.1 mcg; Serving size: 1 bar, 60 g

Granola Bar—Soft Almond Confectioners Coating ☛ Vitamin K = 0.5 mcg; Serving size: 1 bar, 35 g

Granola Bar—Soft Coated Milk Chocolate Coating Peanut Butter ☛ Vitamin K = 3.7 mcg; Serving size: 1 oz, 28.4 g

Granola Bar—Soft Milk Chocolate Coated Peanut Butter ☛ Vitamin K = 1.6 mcg; Serving size: 1 oz, 28.4 g

Granola Bar—Soft Uncoated Chocolate Chip ☛ Vitamin K = 7.1 mcg; Serving size: 1 bar (1.5 oz), 43 g

Granola Bar—With Coconut Chocolate Coated ☛ Vitamin K = 0.4 mcg; Serving size: 1 oz, 28.4 g

Granola Bites Mixed Flavors ☛ Vitamin K = 1.8 mcg; Serving size: 1 package, 20 g

M&M'S—Mars Combos Cheddar Cheese Pretzel ☛ Vitamin K = 0.9 mcg; Serving size: 1 oz, 28.4 g

Nutrition Bar Or Meal Replacement Bar ☛ Vitamin K = 0.5 mcg; Serving size: 1 bar, 34 g

Oriental Mix Rice-Based ☛ Vitamin K = 0.7 mcg; Serving size: 1 oz, 28.4 g

Pita Chips—Salted ☛ Vitamin K = 0.3 mcg; Serving size: 1 oz, 28.4 g

Plantain Chips—Salted ☛ Vitamin K = 8.1 mcg; Serving size: 1 oz, 28.4 g

Popcorn—Air-Popped ☛ Vitamin K = 0.1 mcg; Serving size: 1 cup, 8 g

Popcorn—Air-Popped Unbuttered ☛ Vitamin K = 0.1 mcg; Serving size: 1 cup, popped, 8 g

Popcorn—Air-Popped—With Added Butter Or Margarine ☛ Vitamin K = 0.9 mcg; Serving size: 1 cup, popped, 11 g

Popcorn—Cakes ☛ Vitamin K = 0.1 mcg; Serving size: 1 cake, 10 g

Popcorn—Caramel Coated ☛ Vitamin K = 4.3 mcg; Serving size: 1 cup, 35 g

Popcorn—Caramel Coated—With Nuts ☛ Vitamin K = 1.6 mcg; Serving size: 1 cup, 42 g

Popcorn—Caramel-Coated—With Peanuts ☛ Vitamin K = 1.1 mcg; Serving size: 1 oz, 28.4 g

Popcorn—Caramel-Coated—Without Peanuts ☛ Vitamin K = 3.6 mcg; Serving size: 1 oz, 28.4 g

Popcorn—Cheese-Flavor ☛ Vitamin K = 0.9 mcg; Serving size: 1 cup, 11 g

Popcorn—Chips—Other Flavors ☛ Vitamin K = 0.2 mcg; Serving size: 1 chip, 1 g

Popcorn—Chips—Plain ☞ Vitamin K = 0.2 mcg; Serving size: 1 chip, 1 g

Popcorn—Chips—Sweet Flavors ☞ Vitamin K = 0.2 mcg; Serving size: 1 chip, 1 g

Popcorn—Home-Prepared Oil-Popped—Unsalted ☞ Vitamin K = 0.3 mcg; Serving size: 1 cup, 8 g

Popcorn—Microwave Butter Flavored ☞ Vitamin K = 3.6 mcg; Serving size: 1 regular microwave bag, 85 g

Popcorn—Movie Theater Unbuttered ☞ Vitamin K = 2 mcg; Serving size: 1 kids size order, 66 g

Popcorn—Movie Theater—With Added Butter ☞ Vitamin K = 3.5 mcg; Serving size: 1 kids size order, 84 g

Popcorn—Oil-Popped Microwave Regular Flavor No Trans Fat ☞ Vitamin K = 0.5 mcg; Serving size: 1 cup, 11 g

Popcorn—Popped In Oil Unbuttered ☞ Vitamin K = 0.5 mcg; Serving size: 1 cup, popped, 11 g

Potato Chips—Baked Flavored ☞ Vitamin K = 0.1 mcg; Serving size: 1 chip, 2 g

Potato Chips—Barbecue-Flavor ☞ Vitamin K = 4.6 mcg; Serving size: 1 oz, 28.4 g

Potato Chips—Fat-Free ☞ Vitamin K = 0.1 mcg; Serving size: 1 chip, 1 g

Potato Chips—Fat-Free—Salted ☞ Vitamin K = 2.6 mcg; Serving size: 1 oz, 28.4 g

Potato Chips—Fat-Free Made—With Olestra ☞ Vitamin K = 0 mcg; Serving size: 1 oz, 28.4 g

Potato Chips—Lightly—Salted ☞ Vitamin K = 6.2 mcg; Serving size: pieces, 28 g

Potato Chips—Lightly—Salted ☛ Vitamin K = 0.4 mcg; Serving size: 1 chip, 2 g

Potato Chips—Made From Dried Potatoes Fat-Free Made—With Olestra ☛ Vitamin K = 93.3 mcg; Serving size: 1 oz, 28.4 g

Potato Chips—Plain—Salted ☛ Vitamin K = 6.2 mcg; Serving size: 1 oz, 28 g

Potato Chips—Plain—Unsalted ☛ Vitamin K = 6.3 mcg; Serving size: 1 oz, 28.4 g

Potato Chips—Popped Flavored ☛ Vitamin K = 0.1 mcg; Serving size: 1 chip, 1 g

Potato Chips—Reduced Fat ☛ Vitamin K = 3.8 mcg; Serving size: 1 oz, 28.4 g

Potato Chips—Reduced Fat ☛ Vitamin K = 0.3 mcg; Serving size: 1 chip, 2 g

Potato Chips—Restructured Flavored ☛ Vitamin K = 0.1 mcg; Serving size: 1 chip, 2 g

Potato Chips—Restructured Lightly—Salted ☛ Vitamin K = 0.4 mcg; Serving size: 1 chip, 2 g

Potato Chips—Restructured Plain ☛ Vitamin K = 0.1 mcg; Serving size: 1 chip, 2 g

Potato Chips—Unsalted ☛ Vitamin K = 0.2 mcg; Serving size: 1 chip, 2 g

Potato Chips—White Restructured Baked ☛ Vitamin K = 2.4 mcg; Serving size: 1 cup, 34 g

Potato Chips—Without Salt Reduced Fat ☛ Vitamin K = 3.8 mcg; Serving size: 1 oz, 28.4 g

Potato Sticks ☛ Vitamin K = 6.3 mcg; Serving size: 1 oz, 28.4 g

Potato Sticks—Flavored ☛ Vitamin K = 0.7 mcg; Serving size: 10

sticks, 3 g

Potato Sticks—Fry Shaped ☞ Vitamin K = 0.7 mcg; Serving size: 10 sticks, 3 g

Pretzel Chips—Hard Flavored ☞ Vitamin K = 0.1 mcg; Serving size: 1 pretzel chip/crisp/thin, 3 g

Pretzel Chips—Hard Gluten-Free ☞ Vitamin K = 0 mcg; Serving size: 1 pretzel chip/crisp/thin, 3 g

Pretzel Chips—Hard Plain ☞ Vitamin K = 0.1 mcg; Serving size: 1 pretzel chip/crisp/thin, 3 g

Pretzels—Hard Coated Gluten-Free ☞ Vitamin K = 0.2 mcg; Serving size: 1 miniature/bite size, 4 g

Pretzels—Hard Confectioners Coating Chocolate-Flavor ☞ Vitamin K = 3.2 mcg; Serving size: 1 oz, 28.4 g

Pretzels—Hard Flavored ☞ Vitamin K = 0.1 mcg; Serving size: 1 miniature/bite size, 2 g

Pretzels—Hard Flavored Gluten-Free ☞ Vitamin K = 0 mcg; Serving size: 1 pretzel stick, 1 g

Pretzels—Hard Multigrain ☞ Vitamin K = 0.1 mcg; Serving size: 1 miniature/bite size, 2 g

Pretzels—Hard Peanut Butter Filled ☞ Vitamin K = 0.1 mcg; Serving size: 1 miniature/bite size, 3 g

Pretzels—Hard Plain Lightly—Salted ☞ Vitamin K = 0 mcg; Serving size: 1 miniature/bite size, 2 g

Pretzels—Soft Multigrain ☞ Vitamin K = 1.7 mcg; Serving size: 1 small, 62 g

Rice Cake—Brown Rice Plain—Unsalted ☞ Vitamin K = 0.2 mcg; Serving size: 1 cake, 9 g

Rice Cracker—Brown Rice Plain ☞ Vitamin K = 0.2 mcg; Serving size: 1 cake, 9 g

Rice Paper ☛ Vitamin K = 0 mcg; Serving size: 1 small paper (6-3/8" dia), 5 g

Sesame Sticks—Wheat-Based—Salted ☛ Vitamin K = 2.3 mcg; Serving size: 1 oz, 28.4 g

Soychips ☛ Vitamin K = 3.4 mcg; Serving size: 1 oz, 28.4 g

Sweet Potato Chips ☛ Vitamin K = 0.5 mcg; Serving size: 1 chip, 2 g

Sweet Potato Chips—Unsalted ☛ Vitamin K = 7 mcg; Serving size: 1 oz, 28.4 g

Taro Chips ☛ Vitamin K = 5.1 mcg; Serving size: 1 oz, 28.4 g

Tortilla Chips—Nacho Cheese ☛ Vitamin K = 0.4 mcg; Serving size: 1 oz, 28.4 g

Tortilla Chips—Reduced Fat Baked—Without Fat ☛ Vitamin K = 0.1 mcg; Serving size: 1 oz, 28.4 g

Tortilla Chips—Reduced Fat Made—With Olestra Nacho Cheese ☛ Vitamin K = 54.5 mcg; Serving size: 1 oz, 28.4 g

Tortilla Chips—Reduced Fat—Unsalted ☛ Vitamin K = 5.9 mcg; Serving size: 1 oz, 28.4 g

Tortilla Chips—Yellow Plain—Salted ☛ Vitamin K = 0.2 mcg; Serving size: 1 oz, 28.4 g

Trail Mix ☛ Vitamin K = 9.5 mcg; Serving size: 1 cup, 146 g

Vegetable Chips ☛ Vitamin K = 0.6 mcg; Serving size: 1 chip, 2 g

Vegetable Chips—Hain Celestial Group Terra Chips ☛ Vitamin K = 12.6 mcg; Serving size: 1 oz, 28.4 g

Vegetable Chips—Made From Garden Vegetables ☛ Vitamin K = 5 mcg; Serving size: 1 oz, 28.4 g

Yucca Chips—Salted ☛ Vitamin K = 1.5 mcg; Serving size: 1 oz, 28.4 g

27

SPICES AND HERBS

Apple Cider Vinegar ☞ Vitamin K = 0 mcg; Serving size: 1 tbsp, 14.9 g

Basil ☞ Vitamin K = 10.4 mcg; Serving size: 5 leaves, 2.5 g

Black Pepper ☞ Vitamin K = 3.8 mcg; Serving size: 1 tsp, ground, 2.3 g

Capers ☞ Vitamin K = 2.1 mcg; Serving size: 1 tbsp, drained, 8.6 g

Caraway Seed ☞ Vitamin K = 0 mcg; Serving size: 1 tsp, 2.1 g

Cayenne Pepper ☞ Vitamin K = 1.4 mcg; Serving size: 1 tsp, 1.8 g

Celery Seed ☞ Vitamin K = 0 mcg; Serving size: 1 tsp, 2 g

Chili Powder ☞ Vitamin K = 2.9 mcg; Serving size: 1 tsp, 2.7 g

Cinnamon ☞ Vitamin K = 0.8 mcg; Serving size: 1 tsp, 2.6 g

Cumin Seed ☞ Vitamin K = 0.1 mcg; Serving size: 1 tsp, whole, 2.1 g

Curry Powder ☞ Vitamin K = 2 mcg; Serving size: 1 tsp, 2 g

Distilled Vinegar ☞ Vitamin K = 0 mcg; Serving size: 1 tbsp, 14.9 g

Dried Basil ☞ Vitamin K = 12 mcg; Serving size: 1 tsp, leaves, 0.7 g

Dried Coriander ☛ Vitamin K = 8.2 mcg; Serving size: 1 tsp, 0.6 g

Dried Marjoram ☛ Vitamin K = 3.7 mcg; Serving size: 1 tsp, 0.6 g

Dried Oregano ☛ Vitamin K = 6.2 mcg; Serving size: 1 tsp, leaves, 1 g

Dried Parsley ☛ Vitamin K = 6.8 mcg; Serving size: 1 tsp, 0.5 g

Garlic Powder ☛ Vitamin K = 0 mcg; Serving size: 1 tsp, 3.1 g

Ground Cloves ☛ Vitamin K = 3 mcg; Serving size: 1 tsp, 2.1 g

Ground Ginger ☛ Vitamin K = 0 mcg; Serving size: 1 tsp, 1.8 g

Ground Mustard Seed ☛ Vitamin K = 0.1 mcg; Serving size: 1 tsp, 2 g

Ground Nutmeg ☛ Vitamin K = 0 mcg; Serving size: 1 tsp, 2.2 g

Ground Sage ☛ Vitamin K = 12 mcg; Serving size: 1 tsp, 0.7 g

Ground Turmeric ☛ Vitamin K = 0.4 mcg; Serving size: 1 tsp, 3 g

Horseradish ☛ Vitamin K = 0.1 mcg; Serving size: 1 tsp, 5 g

Onion Powder ☛ Vitamin K = 0.1 mcg; Serving size: 1 tsp, 2.4 g

Paprika ☛ Vitamin K = 1.8 mcg; Serving size: 1 tsp, 2.3 g

Poppy Seeds ☛ Vitamin K = 0 mcg; Serving size: 1 tsp, 2.8 g

Poultry Seasoning ☛ Vitamin K = 12.1 mcg; Serving size: 1 tsp, 1.5 g

Pumpkin Pie Spice ☛ Vitamin K = 0.5 mcg; Serving size: 1 tsp, 1.7 g

Spices Thyme Dried ☛ Vitamin K = 17.1 mcg; Serving size: 1 tsp, leaves, 1 g

Table Salt ☛ Vitamin K = 0 mcg; Serving size: 1 tsp, 6 g

Vanilla Extract ☛ Vitamin K = 0 mcg; Serving size: 1 tsp, 4.2 g

Yellow Mustard ☛ Vitamin K = 0.1 mcg; Serving size: 1 tsp or 1 packet, 5 g

28

VEGETABLES AND VEGETABLES PRODUCTS

Alfalfa Sprouts ☛ Vitamin K = 10.1 mcg; Serving size: 1 cup, 33 g

Amaranth Leaves—Raw ☛ Vitamin K = 319.2 mcg; Serving size: 1 cup, 28 g

Artichoke Salad In Oil ☛ Vitamin K = 24.1 mcg; Serving size: 1 cup, 130 g

Artichoke—Cooked—From Canned—Cooked—Without Fat ☛ Vitamin K = 12.5 mcg; Serving size: 1 small globe, 100 g

Artichoke—Cooked—From Fresh—Cooked—Without Fat ☛ Vitamin K = 14.7 mcg; Serving size: 1 small globe, 100 g

Artichoke—Cooked—From Frozen—Cooked—Without Fat ☛ Vitamin K = 21 mcg; Serving size: 1 cup, hearts, 168 g

Artichokes (Globe Or French) ☛ Vitamin K = 18.9 mcg; Serving size: 1 artichoke, medium, 128 g

Artichokes (Globe Or French)—Cooked Boiled—Drained—With Salt ☛ Vitamin K = 17.8 mcg; Serving size: 1 artichoke, medium, 120 g

Artichokes (Globe Or French)—Cooked Boiled—Drained—Without Salt ☞ Vitamin K = 17.8 mcg; Serving size: 1 artichoke, medium, 120 g

Artichokes (Globe Or French)—Frozen—Cooked Boiled—Drained—With Salt ☞ Vitamin K = 21.2 mcg; Serving size: 1 cup, 168 g

Artichokes Stuffed ☞ Vitamin K = 74 mcg; Serving size: 1 stuffed globe, 251 g

Arugula ☞ Vitamin K = 2.2 mcg; Serving size: 1 leaf, 2 g

Asparagus ☞ Vitamin K = 55.7 mcg; Serving size: 1 cup, 134 g

Asparagus—Canned—No Salt Added—Solids And Liquids ☞ Vitamin K = 47.6 mcg; Serving size: 1/2 cup, 122 g

Asparagus—Cooked Boiled—Drained—With Salt ☞ Vitamin K = 45.5 mcg; Serving size: 1/2 cup, 90 g

Asparagus—Cooked—From Canned—Cooked—Without Fat ☞ Vitamin K = 99.5 mcg; Serving size: 1 cup, 242 g

Asparagus—Cooked—From Fresh—Cooked—Without Fat ☞ Vitamin K = 1.5 mcg; Serving size: 1 piece, 3 g

Asparagus—Cooked—From Frozen—Cooked—Without Fat ☞ Vitamin K = 2.4 mcg; Serving size: 1 piece, 3 g

Asparagus—From Canned—Creamed Or With Cheese Sauce ☞ Vitamin K = 72.9 mcg; Serving size: 1 cup, 235 g

Asparagus—From Fresh—Creamed Or With Cheese Sauce ☞ Vitamin K = 82.3 mcg; Serving size: 1 cup, 235 g

Asparagus—From Frozen—Creamed Or With Cheese Sauce ☞ Vitamin K = 129.5 mcg; Serving size: 1 cup, 235 g

Asparagus—Frozen—Cooked Boiled—Drained—With Salt ☞ Vitamin K = 144 mcg; Serving size: 1 cup, 180 g

Asparagus—Frozen—Cooked Boiled—Drained—Without Salt ☞ Vitamin K = 144 mcg; Serving size: 1 cup, 180 g

Baby Carrots ☛ Vitamin K = 1.4 mcg; Serving size: 1 large, 15 g

Bamboo Shoots ☛ Vitamin K = 0 mcg; Serving size: 1 cup (1/2 inch slices), 151 g

Bamboo Shoots—Canned ☛ Vitamin K = 0 mcg; Serving size: 1 cup (1/8 inch slices), 131 g

Bamboo Shoots—Cooked—Cooked With Fat ☛ Vitamin K = 7.5 mcg; Serving size: 1 cup, 156 g

Bamboo Shoots—Cooked—Cooked—Without Fat ☛ Vitamin K = 0 mcg; Serving size: 1 cup, slices, 120 g

Banana Peppers ☛ Vitamin K = 11.8 mcg; Serving size: 1 cup, 124 g

Bean Salad— Yellow And/or Green String Beans ☛ Vitamin K = 41 mcg; Serving size: 1 cup, 150 g

Bean Sprouts—Cooked—From Fresh—Cooked With Fat ☛ Vitamin K = 59.2 mcg; Serving size: 1 cup, 129 g

Beet Greens—Cooked Boiled—Drained—With Salt ☛ Vitamin K = 697 mcg; Serving size: 1 cup (1 inch pieces), 144 g

Beet Greens—Cooked—Cooked—Without Fat ☛ Vitamin K = 692.2 mcg; Serving size: 1 cup, 144 g

Beet Greens—Raw ☛ Vitamin K = 152 mcg; Serving size: 1 cup, 38 g

Beets—Canned Low Sodium—Cooked—Without Fat ☛ Vitamin K = 0.3 mcg; Serving size: 1 cup, 170 g

Beets—Canned Regular Pack—Solids And Liquids ☛ Vitamin K = 0.5 mcg; Serving size: 1 cup, 246 g

Beets—Canned—Drained Solids ☛ Vitamin K = 0.3 mcg; Serving size: 1 cup, diced, 157 g

Beets—Canned—No Salt Added—Solids And Liquids ☛ Vitamin K = 0.2 mcg; Serving size: 1 cup, 246 g

Beets—Cooked Boiled.—Drained—With Salt ☛ Vitamin K = 0.2 mcg; Serving size: 1/2 cup slices, 85 g

Beets—Cooked—From Canned—Cooked—Without Fat ☛ Vitamin K = 0.3 mcg; Serving size: 1 cup, whole, 163 g

Beets—Cooked—From Fresh—Cooked—Without Fat ☛ Vitamin K = 0.3 mcg; Serving size: 1 cup, whole, 163 g

Beets—Cooked—From Frozen—Cooked—Without Fat ☛ Vitamin K = 0.3 mcg; Serving size: 1 cup, whole, 163 g

Beets—Raw ☛ Vitamin K = 0.3 mcg; Serving size: 1 cup, 136 g

Bitter Melon—Cooked—Cooked With Fat ☛ Vitamin K = 11.2 mcg; Serving size: 1 cup, 129 g

Bitter Melon—Cooked—Cooked—Without Fat ☛ Vitamin K = 6 mcg; Serving size: 1 cup, 124 g

Boiled Potatoes ☛ Vitamin K = 1.7 mcg; Serving size: 1/2 cup, 78 g

Boiled Sweet Potatoes ☛ Vitamin K = 6.9 mcg; Serving size: 1 cup, mashed, 328 g

Bok Choy ☛ Vitamin K = 31.9 mcg; Serving size: 1 cup, shredded, 70 g

Breadfruit Fried ☛ Vitamin K = 8.7 mcg; Serving size: 1 cup, 170 g

Breadfruit—Cooked—Cooked With Fat ☛ Vitamin K = 5.1 mcg; Serving size: 1 cup, 257 g

Breadfruit—Cooked—Cooked—Without Fat ☛ Vitamin K = 1.5 mcg; Serving size: 1 cup, 252 g

Broccoflower—Cooked—Cooked—Without Fat ☛ Vitamin K = 17 mcg; Serving size: 1 cup, fresh, 82 g

Broccoli ☛ Vitamin K = 92.5 mcg; Serving size: 1 cup chopped, 91 g

Broccoli—Batter-Dipped And Fried ☛ Vitamin K = 71.5 mcg; Serving size: 1 cup, 85 g

Broccoli—Casserole With Noodles ☛ Vitamin K = 105.3 mcg; Serving size: 1 cup, 228 g

Broccoli—Casserole With Rice ☛ Vitamin K = 105.3 mcg; Serving size: 1 cup, 228 g

Broccoli—Chinese—Cooked—From Fresh—Cooked—Without Fat ☛ Vitamin K = 73.7 mcg; Serving size: 1 cup, 88 g

Broccoli—Chinese—Cooked—From Frozen—Cooked—Without Fat ☛ Vitamin K = 73.7 mcg; Serving size: 1 cup, 88 g

Broccoli—Cooked Boiled—Drained—With Salt ☛ Vitamin K = 110.1 mcg; Serving size: 1/2 cup, chopped, 78 g

Broccoli—Cooked—From Fresh With Cheese Sauce ☛ Vitamin K = 212 mcg; Serving size: 1 cup, 228 g

Broccoli—Cooked—From Fresh With Mushroom Sauce ☛ Vitamin K = 199.3 mcg; Serving size: 1 cup, 228 g

Broccoli—Cooked—From Fresh—Cooked—Without Fat ☛ Vitamin K = 218.7 mcg; Serving size: 1 cup, fresh, cut stalks, 156 g

Broccoli—Cooked—From Fresh—With Cream Sauce ☛ Vitamin K = 179.2 mcg; Serving size: 1 cup, 228 g

Broccoli—Cooked—From Frozen With Cheese Sauce ☛ Vitamin K = 140 mcg; Serving size: 1 cup, 228 g

Broccoli—Cooked—From Frozen With Mushroom Sauce ☛ Vitamin K = 136.3 mcg; Serving size: 1 cup, 228 g

Broccoli—Cooked—From Frozen—Cooked—Without Fat ☛ Vitamin K = 8.8 mcg; Serving size: 1 piece, 10 g

Broccoli—Cooked—From Frozen—With Cream Sauce ☛ Vitamin K = 120.4 mcg; Serving size: 1 cup, 228 g

Broccoli—Frozen Chopped—Cooked Boiled—Drained—With Salt ☛ Vitamin K = 162.1 mcg; Serving size: 1 cup, 184 g

Broccoli—Frozen Chopped—Cooked Boiled—Drained—Without Salt ☞ Vitamin K = 162.1 mcg; Serving size: 1 cup, 184 g

Broccoli—Frozen Chopped—Unprepared ☞ Vitamin K = 126.5 mcg; Serving size: 1 cup, 156 g

Broccoli—Frozen Spears—Cooked Boiled—Drained—With Salt ☞ Vitamin K = 91.5 mcg; Serving size: 1/2 cup, 92 g

Broccoli—Frozen Spears—Cooked Boiled—Drained—Without Salt ☞ Vitamin K = 81.1 mcg; Serving size: 1/2 cup, 92 g

Broccoli—Frozen Spears—Unprepared ☞ Vitamin K = 96.3 mcg; Serving size: 1/3 package (10 oz), 95 g

Broccoli—Raab ☞ Vitamin K = 89.6 mcg; Serving size: 1 cup chopped, 40 g

Broccoli—Raab—Cooked—Cooked—Without Fat ☞ Vitamin K = 432.7 mcg; Serving size: 1 cup, 170 g

Broccoli—Salad With Cauliflower—Cheese Bacon Bits And Dressing ☞ Vitamin K = 92.6 mcg; Serving size: 1 cup, 154 g

Broccoli—Slaw Salad ☞ Vitamin K = 150.3 mcg; Serving size: 1 cup, 186 g

Brussels Sprouts—Cooked Boiled—Drained—With Salt ☞ Vitamin K = 29.5 mcg; Serving size: 1 sprout, 21 g

Brussels Sprouts—Cooked—From Fresh—Cooked—Without Fat ☞ Vitamin K = 216.1 mcg; Serving size: 1 cup, 155 g

Brussels Sprouts—Cooked—From Frozen—Cooked—Without Fat ☞ Vitamin K = 298.1 mcg; Serving size: 1 cup, 155 g

Brussels Sprouts—From Fresh—Creamed ☞ Vitamin K = 178.3 mcg; Serving size: 1 cup, 228 g

Brussels Sprouts—From Frozen—Creamed ☞ Vitamin K = 244.9 mcg; Serving size: 1 cup, 228 g

Brussels Sprouts—Frozen—Cooked Boiled—Drained—With Salt ☛ Vitamin K = 299.9 mcg; Serving size: 1 cup, 155 g

Brussels Sprouts—Frozen—Cooked Boiled—Drained—Without Salt ☛ Vitamin K = 299.9 mcg; Serving size: 1 cup, 155 g

Brussels Sprouts—Frozen—Unprepared ☛ Vitamin K = 179.3 mcg; Serving size: 1/3 package (10 oz), 95 g

Brussels Sprouts—Raw ☛ Vitamin K = 155.8 mcg; Serving size: 1 cup, 88 g

Burdock Root—Cooked Boiled—Drained—With Salt ☛ Vitamin K = 2.5 mcg; Serving size: 1 cup (1 inch pieces), 125 g

Burdock Root—Raw ☛ Vitamin K = 1.9 mcg; Serving size: 1 cup (1 inch pieces), 118 g

Burdock—Cooked—Cooked With Fat ☛ Vitamin K = 7.8 mcg; Serving size: 1 cup, 130 g

Burdock—Cooked—Cooked—Without Fat ☛ Vitamin K = 2.5 mcg; Serving size: 1 cup, 125 g

Cabbage ☛ Vitamin K = 67.6 mcg; Serving size: 1 cup, chopped, 89 g

Cabbage Chinese (Pak-Choi)—Cooked Boiled—Drained—With Salt ☛ Vitamin K = 57.8 mcg; Serving size: 1 cup, shredded, 170 g

Cabbage Chinese (Pe-Tsai)—Raw ☛ Vitamin K = 32.6 mcg; Serving size: 1 cup, shredded, 76 g

Cabbage Chinese Salad With Dressing ☛ Vitamin K = 23.1 mcg; Serving size: 1 cup, 76 g

Cabbage Chinese—Cooked—Cooked—Without Fat ☛ Vitamin K = 57.5 mcg; Serving size: 1 cup, 170 g

Cabbage Common—Cooked Boiled—Drained—With Salt ☛ Vitamin K = 81.5 mcg; Serving size: 1/2 cup, shredded, 75 g

Cabbage Green—Cooked—Cooked—Without Fat ☞ Vitamin K = 162 mcg; Serving size: 1 cup, 150 g

Cabbage Japanese—Style Fresh Pickled ☞ Vitamin K = 188.9 mcg; Serving size: 1 cup, 150 g

Cabbage Mustard—Salted ☞ Vitamin K = 148 mcg; Serving size: 1 cup, 128 g

Cabbage Red—Cooked Boiled—Drained—With Salt ☞ Vitamin K = 10.5 mcg; Serving size: 1 leaf, 22 g

Cabbage Red—Cooked—Cooked—Without Fat ☞ Vitamin K = 71 mcg; Serving size: 1 cup, 150 g

Cabbage Salad Or Coleslaw—Made With Any Type Of Fat-free Dressing ☞ Vitamin K = 121.5 mcg; Serving size: 1 cup, 219 g

Cabbage Salad Or Coleslaw—Made With Coleslaw Dressing ☞ Vitamin K = 141 mcg; Serving size: 1 cup, 219 g

Cabbage Salad Or Coleslaw—Made With Italian Dressing ☞ Vitamin K = 137.5 mcg; Serving size: 1 cup, 219 g

Cabbage Salad Or Coleslaw—Made With Light Coleslaw Dressing ☞ Vitamin K = 128.6 mcg; Serving size: 1 cup, 219 g

Cabbage Salad Or Coleslaw—Made With Light Creamy Dressing ☞ Vitamin K = 109.5 mcg; Serving size: 1 cup, 219 g

Cabbage Salad Or Coleslaw—Made With Light Italian Dressing ☞ Vitamin K = 116.5 mcg; Serving size: 1 cup, 219 g

Cabbage Salad Or Coleslaw—Made—With Creamy Dressing ☞ Vitamin K = 175 mcg; Serving size: 1 cup, 219 g

Cabbage Salad Or Coleslaw—With Apples And/or Raisins With Dressing ☞ Vitamin K = 112.8 mcg; Serving size: 1 cup, 219 g

Cabbage Salad Or Coleslaw—With Pineapple With Dressing ☞ Vitamin K = 121.8 mcg; Serving size: 1 cup, 219 g

Cabbage Savoy—Cooked—Cooked—Without Fat ☛ Vitamin K = 103.2 mcg; Serving size: 1 cup, 145 g

Cabbage—Creamed ☛ Vitamin K = 119.2 mcg; Serving size: 1 cup, 200 g

Cactus—Cooked—Cooked—Without Fat ☛ Vitamin K = 7.6 mcg; Serving size: 1 cup, 149 g

Caesar Salad With Romaine—No Dressing ☛ Vitamin K = 70.4 mcg; Serving size: 1 cup, 79 g

Calabaza—Cooked ☛ Vitamin K = 27.4 mcg; Serving size: 1 cup, cubes, 166 g

Candied Ripe Plantain—Puerto Rican Style ☛ Vitamin K = 12.3 mcg; Serving size: 1 serving (1/2 plantain with syrup), 140 g

Carrot Dehydrated ☛ Vitamin K = 79.9 mcg; Serving size: 1 cup, 74 g

Carrot Juice—Canned ☛ Vitamin K = 36.6 mcg; Serving size: 1 cup, 236 g

Carrots ☛ Vitamin K = 16.9 mcg; Serving size: 1 cup chopped, 128 g

Carrots—Canned Regular Pack—Drained Solids ☛ Vitamin K = 14.3 mcg; Serving size: 1 cup, sliced, 146 g

Carrots—Canned Regular Pack—Solids And Liquids ☛ Vitamin K = 12.1 mcg; Serving size: 1/2 cup slices, 123 g

Carrots—Canned—No Salt Added—Drained Solids ☛ Vitamin K = 14.3 mcg; Serving size: 1 cup, sliced, 146 g

Carrots—Canned—No Salt Added—Solids And Liquids ☛ Vitamin K = 12.1 mcg; Serving size: 1/2 cup slices, 123 g

Carrots—Cooked Boiled—Drained—With Salt ☛ Vitamin K = 1.3 mcg; Serving size: 1 tbsp, 9.7 g

Carrots—Cooked—From Canned Glazed ☛ Vitamin K = 14.2 mcg; Serving size: 1 cup, 161 g

Carrots—Cooked—From Canned With Cheese Sauce ☛ Vitamin K = 15 mcg; Serving size: 1 cup, 228 g

Carrots—Cooked—From Canned—Cooked—Without Fat ☛ Vitamin K = 0.2 mcg; Serving size: 1 baby carrot, 2 g

Carrots—Cooked—From Canned—Creamed ☛ Vitamin K = 13 mcg; Serving size: 1 cup, 228 g

Carrots—Cooked—From Fresh Glazed ☛ Vitamin K = 1.2 mcg; Serving size: 1 baby carrot, 10 g

Carrots—Cooked—From Fresh With Cheese Sauce ☛ Vitamin K = 21.2 mcg; Serving size: 1 cup, 228 g

Carrots—Cooked—From Fresh—Cooked—Without Fat ☛ Vitamin K = 1.2 mcg; Serving size: 1 baby carrot, 9 g

Carrots—Cooked—From Fresh—Creamed ☛ Vitamin K = 18.2 mcg; Serving size: 1 cup, 228 g

Carrots—Cooked—From Frozen Glazed ☛ Vitamin K = 19.6 mcg; Serving size: 1 cup, 161 g

Carrots—Cooked—From Frozen With Cheese Sauce ☛ Vitamin K = 20.7 mcg; Serving size: 1 cup, 228 g

Carrots—Cooked—From Frozen—Cooked—Without Fat ☛ Vitamin K = 0.7 mcg; Serving size: 1 baby carrot, 5 g

Carrots—Cooked—From Frozen—Creamed ☛ Vitamin K = 17.6 mcg; Serving size: 1 cup, 228 g

Carrots—Frozen—Cooked Boiled—Drained—With Salt ☛ Vitamin K = 19.9 mcg; Serving size: 1 cup slices, 146 g

Carrots—Frozen—Cooked Boiled—Drained—Without Salt ☛ Vitamin K = 19.9 mcg; Serving size: 1 cup, sliced, 146 g

Carrots—Frozen—Unprepared ☛ Vitamin K = 11.3 mcg; Serving size: 1/2 cup slices, 64 g

Carrots—In Tomato Sauce ☞ Vitamin K = 17.2 mcg; Serving size: 1 cup, 176 g

Carrots—Raw Salad ☞ Vitamin K = 74.2 mcg; Serving size: 1 cup, 175 g

Carrots—Raw Salad With Apples ☞ Vitamin K = 73.5 mcg; Serving size: 1 cup, 171 g

Cassava ☞ Vitamin K = 3.9 mcg; Serving size: 1 cup, 206 g

Cassava With Creole Sauce—Puerto Rican Style ☞ Vitamin K = 9 mcg; Serving size: 1 serving (2 pieces with sauce), 230 g

Cassava—Cooked—Cooked—Without Fat ☞ Vitamin K = 0.4 mcg; Serving size: 1 piece, 20 g

Cauliflower ☞ Vitamin K = 16.6 mcg; Serving size: 1 cup chopped (1/2 inch pieces), 107 g

Cauliflower—Batter-Dipped Fried ☞ Vitamin K = 4.1 mcg; Serving size: 1 floweret, 26 g

Cauliflower—Cooked Boiled—Drained—With Salt ☞ Vitamin K = 8.6 mcg; Serving size: 1/2 cup (1 inch pieces), 62 g

Cauliflower—Cooked—From Canned—Cooked—Without Fat ☞ Vitamin K = 21.2 mcg; Serving size: 1 cup, 180 g

Cauliflower—Cooked—From Fresh—Cooked—Without Fat ☞ Vitamin K = 3 mcg; Serving size: 1 piece, 22 g

Cauliflower—Cooked—From Frozen—Cooked—Without Fat ☞ Vitamin K = 21.2 mcg; Serving size: 1 cup, 180 g

Cauliflower—From Canned—Creamed ☞ Vitamin K = 16.9 mcg; Serving size: 1 cup, 228 g

Cauliflower—From Fresh—Creamed ☞ Vitamin K = 16.6 mcg; Serving size: 1 cup, 228 g

Cauliflower—From Frozen—Creamed ☞ Vitamin K = 16.9 mcg; Serving size: 1 cup, 228 g

Cauliflower—Frozen—Cooked Boiled—Drained—With Salt ☛ Vitamin K = 21.4 mcg; Serving size: 1 cup (1 inch pieces), 180 g

Cauliflower—Frozen—Cooked Boiled—Drained—Without Salt ☛ Vitamin K = 21.4 mcg; Serving size: 1 cup (1 inch pieces), 180 g

Cauliflower—Frozen—Unprepared ☛ Vitamin K = 9.8 mcg; Serving size: 1/2 cup (1 inch pieces), 66 g

Celeriac ☛ Vitamin K = 64 mcg; Serving size: 1 cup, 156 g

Celeriac—Cooked ☛ Vitamin K = 66.5 mcg; Serving size: 1 cup, pieces, 155 g

Celery ☛ Vitamin K = 29.6 mcg; Serving size: 1 cup chopped, 101 g

Celery—Cooked Boiled—Drained—With Salt ☛ Vitamin K = 56.7 mcg; Serving size: 1 cup, diced, 150 g

Celery—Cooked—Cooked—Without Fat ☛ Vitamin K = 56.4 mcg; Serving size: 1 cup, diced, 150 g

Celery—Creamed ☛ Vitamin K = 47.9 mcg; Serving size: 1 cup, 228 g

Celery—Stuffed With Cheese ☛ Vitamin K = 6.7 mcg; Serving size: 1 small stalk (5" long), 32 g

Chamnamul—Cooked—Cooked With Fat ☛ Vitamin K = 583.2 mcg; Serving size: 1 cup, 151 g

Chamnamul—Cooked—Cooked—Without Fat ☛ Vitamin K = 591.2 mcg; Serving size: 1 cup, 146 g

Channa Saag ☛ Vitamin K = 776.9 mcg; Serving size: 1 cup, 245 g

Chard Swiss—Cooked Boiled—Drained—With Salt ☛ Vitamin K = 572.8 mcg; Serving size: 1 cup, chopped, 175 g

Chard—Cooked—Cooked—Without Fat ☛ Vitamin K = 471.8 mcg; Serving size: 1 cup, stalk and leaves, 145 g

Chayote Fruit—Cooked Boiled—Drained—With Salt ☛ Vitamin K = 7.5 mcg; Serving size: 1 cup (1 inch pieces), 160 g

Chayote Fruit—Raw ☛ Vitamin K = 5.4 mcg; Serving size: 1 cup (1 inch pieces), 132 g

Chicory Greens ☛ Vitamin K = 86.3 mcg; Serving size: 1 cup, chopped, 29 g

Chives ☛ Vitamin K = 6.4 mcg; Serving size: 1 tbsp chopped, 3 g

Christophine—Cooked—Cooked With Fat ☛ Vitamin K = 9.6 mcg; Serving size: 1 cup, 165 g

Christophine—Cooked—Cooked—Without Fat ☛ Vitamin K = 7.5 mcg; Serving size: 1 cup, 160 g

Chrysanthemum ☛ Vitamin K = 87.5 mcg; Serving size: 1 cup (1 inch pieces), 25 g

Chrysanthemum Garland—Cooked Boiled—Drained—With Salt ☛ Vitamin K = 142.7 mcg; Serving size: 1 cup (1 inch pieces), 100 g

Cilantro ☛ Vitamin K = 12.4 mcg; Serving size: 1/4 cup, 4 g

Cobb Salad—No Dressing ☛ Vitamin K = 35.4 mcg; Serving size: 1 cup, 105 g

Collards ☛ Vitamin K = 157.4 mcg; Serving size: 1 cup, chopped, 36 g

Collards—Cooked Boiled—Drained—With Salt ☛ Vitamin K = 772.5 mcg; Serving size: 1 cup, chopped, 190 g

Collards—Cooked—From Canned—Cooked—Without Fat ☛ Vitamin K = 650.4 mcg; Serving size: 1 cup, canned, 162 g

Collards—Cooked—From Fresh—Cooked—Without Fat ☛ Vitamin K = 517.8 mcg; Serving size: 1 cup, fresh, 128 g

Collards—Cooked—From Frozen—Cooked—Without Fat ☛ Vitamin K = 1053.3 mcg; Serving size: 1 cup, frozen, 170 g

Collards—Frozen Chopped—Cooked Boiled—Drained—With Salt ☛ Vitamin K = 1059.4 mcg; Serving size: 1 cup, chopped, 170 g

Collards—Frozen Chopped—Cooked Boiled—Drained—Without Salt ☛ Vitamin K = 1059.4 mcg; Serving size: 1 cup, chopped, 170 g

Corn Dried—Cooked ☛ Vitamin K = 2 mcg; Serving size: 1 oz, 28 g

Corn Fritter ☛ Vitamin K = 11.8 mcg; Serving size: 1 cup, 107 g

Corn Pudding—Home Made ☛ Vitamin K = 1.3 mcg; Serving size: 1 cup, 250 g

Corn Scalloped Or Pudding ☛ Vitamin K = 6.8 mcg; Serving size: 1 cup, 214 g

Corn Sweet White—Canned Whole Kernel—Drained Solids ☛ Vitamin K = 0 mcg; Serving size: 1 cup, 164 g

Corn Sweet White—Canned—Cream Style Regular Pack ☛ Vitamin K = 0 mcg; Serving size: 1 cup, 256 g

Corn Sweet White—Canned—Cream Style—No Salt Added ☛ Vitamin K = 0.8 mcg; Serving size: 1 cup, 256 g

Corn Sweet White—Cooked Boiled—Drained—With Salt ☛ Vitamin K = 0.4 mcg; Serving size: 1 ear, small (5-1/2 inch to 6-1/2 inch long), 89 g

Corn Sweet White—Frozen Kernels Cut Off Cob Boiled—Drained—With Salt ☛ Vitamin K = 0.5 mcg; Serving size: 1 cup, 165 g

Corn Sweet White—Frozen Kernels Cut Off Cob Boiled—Drained—Without Salt ☛ Vitamin K = 0.5 mcg; Serving size: 1 cup, 165 g

Corn Sweet White—Frozen Kernels Cut Off Cob—Unprepared ☛ Vitamin K = 0.5 mcg; Serving size: 1 cup, 165 g

Corn Sweet Yellow—Canned Brine Pack Regular Pack—Solids And Liquids ☛ Vitamin K = 0 mcg; Serving size: 1 cup, 256 g

Corn Sweet Yellow—Canned Whole Kernel—Drained Solids ☞ Vitamin K = 0 mcg; Serving size: 1 cup, 164 g

Corn Sweet Yellow—Canned—Cream Style Regular Pack ☞ Vitamin K = 0 mcg; Serving size: 1 cup, 256 g

Corn Sweet Yellow—Canned—Cream Style—No Salt Added ☞ Vitamin K = 0 mcg; Serving size: 1 cup, 256 g

Corn Sweet Yellow—Canned—No Salt Added—Solids And Liquids ☞ Vitamin K = 0 mcg; Serving size: 1 cup, 256 g

Corn Sweet Yellow—Canned—Vacuum Pack—No Salt Added ☞ Vitamin K = 0 mcg; Serving size: 1 cup, 210 g

Corn Sweet Yellow—Canned—Vacuum Pack—Regular Pack ☞ Vitamin K = 0 mcg; Serving size: 1 cup, 210 g

Corn Sweet Yellow—Cooked Boiled—Drained—With Salt ☞ Vitamin K = 0.4 mcg; Serving size: 1 ear small (5-1/2 inch to 6-1/2 inch long), 89 g

Corn Sweet Yellow—Frozen Kernels Cut Off Cob Boiled—Drained— With Salt ☞ Vitamin K = 0.5 mcg; Serving size: 1 cup, 165 g

Corn Sweet Yellow—Frozen Kernels Cut Off Cob Boiled—Drained— Without Salt ☞ Vitamin K = 0.5 mcg; Serving size: 1 cup, 165 g

Corn Sweet Yellow—Frozen Kernels Cut Off Cob—Unprepared ☞ Vitamin K = 0.4 mcg; Serving size: 1 cup, 136 g

Corn Sweet Yellow—Frozen Kernels On Cob—Cooked Boiled— Drained—With Salt ☞ Vitamin K = 0.7 mcg; Serving size: 1 cup kernels, 165 g

Corn Sweet Yellow—Frozen Kernels On Cob—Cooked Boiled— Drained—Without Salt ☞ Vitamin K = 0.7 mcg; Serving size: 1 cup kernels, 165 g

Corn Sweet Yellow—Frozen Kernels On Cob—Unprepared ☞ Vitamin K = 0.7 mcg; Serving size: 1 cup kernels, 165 g

Corn White—Cooked—From Canned—Cooked—Without Fat ☛ Vitamin K = 0 mcg; Serving size: 1 cup, 164 g

Corn White—From Canned—Cream Style ☛ Vitamin K = 0 mcg; Serving size: 1 cup, 256 g

Corn Yellow And White—Cooked—From Canned—Cooked—Without Fat ☛ Vitamin K = 0 mcg; Serving size: 1 cup, 164 g

Corn Yellow Whole Kernel—Frozen—Microwaved ☛ Vitamin K = 0.6 mcg; Serving size: 1 cup, 141 g

Corn Yellow—Cooked—From Canned—Cooked—Without Fat ☛ Vitamin K = 0 mcg; Serving size: 1 cup, 164 g

Corn Yellow—From Canned—Cream Style ☛ Vitamin K = 0 mcg; Serving size: 1 cup, 256 g

Corn Yellow—From Canned—Cream Style—Cooked With Fat ☛ Vitamin K = 2.1 mcg; Serving size: 1 cup, 261 g

Corn—Cooked—From Canned—With Cream Sauce Made With Milk ☛ Vitamin K = 1 mcg; Serving size: 1 cup, 256 g

Corn—Cooked—From Fresh—With Cream Sauce Made With Milk ☛ Vitamin K = 1.5 mcg; Serving size: 1 cup, 256 g

Corn—Cooked—From Frozen—With Cream Sauce Made With Milk ☛ Vitamin K = 1.5 mcg; Serving size: 1 cup, 256 g

Cowpeas (Blackeyes)—Immature Seeds—Frozen—Cooked Boiled—Drained—With Salt ☛ Vitamin K = 62.6 mcg; Serving size: 1 cup, 170 g

Cowpeas (Blackeyes)—Immature Seeds—Frozen—Cooked Boiled—Drained—Without Salt ☛ Vitamin K = 62.6 mcg; Serving size: 1 cup, 170 g

Cowpeas With Snap Beans—Cooked—Cooked With Fat ☛ Vitamin K = 44.5 mcg; Serving size: 1 cup, 143 g

Cowpeas With Snap Beans—Cooked—Cooked—Without Fat ☛ Vitamin K = 42.4 mcg; Serving size: 1 cup, 138 g

Cowpeas Young Pods With Seeds—Raw ☛ Vitamin K = 29.6 mcg; Serving size: 1 cup, 94 g

Creamed Christophine—Puerto Rican Style ☛ Vitamin K = 7 mcg; Serving size: 1 serving (1/2 chayote, 4-1/2" x 3-1/2" x 1-1/2") (without shell), 107 g

Cremini Mushrooms ☛ Vitamin K = 0 mcg; Serving size: 1 cup whole, 87 g

Cress Garden—Cooked Boiled—Drained—With Salt ☛ Vitamin K = 517.6 mcg; Serving size: 1 cup, 135 g

Cress—Cooked—From Canned—Cooked—Without Fat ☛ Vitamin K = 513.8 mcg; Serving size: 1 cup, 135 g

Cress—Cooked—From Fresh—Cooked—Without Fat ☛ Vitamin K = 513.8 mcg; Serving size: 1 cup, 135 g

Crookneck Summer Squash ☛ Vitamin K = 4.1 mcg; Serving size: 1 cup sliced, 127 g

Cucumber ☛ Vitamin K = 8.5 mcg; Serving size: 1/2 cup slices, 52 g

Cucumber— Peeled—Raw ☛ Vitamin K = 9.6 mcg; Serving size: 1 cup, pared, chopped, 133 g

Cucumber— Salad Made With Cucumber— And Vinegar ☛ Vitamin K = 15.9 mcg; Serving size: 1 cup, 159 g

Cucumber— Salad Made With Italian Dressing ☛ Vitamin K = 32 mcg; Serving size: 1 cup, 159 g

Cucumber— Salad Made With Sour Cream Dressing ☛ Vitamin K = 7.3 mcg; Serving size: 1 cup, 133 g

Cucumber——Raw ☛ Vitamin K = 0.5 mcg; Serving size: 1 piece, 7 g

Cucumber—Cooked—Cooked—Without Fat ☞ Vitamin K = 36.2 mcg; Serving size: 1 cup, 180 g

Dandelion Greens ☞ Vitamin K = 428.1 mcg; Serving size: 1 cup, chopped, 55 g

Dandelion Greens—Cooked Boiled—Drained—With Salt ☞ Vitamin K = 376.8 mcg; Serving size: 1 cup, chopped, 105 g

Dandelion Greens—Cooked—Cooked—Without Fat ☞ Vitamin K = 573.5 mcg; Serving size: 1 cup, chopped, 105 g

Dasheen Boiled ☞ Vitamin K = 1.7 mcg; Serving size: 1 cup, pieces, 142 g

Dasheen Fried ☞ Vitamin K = 7.5 mcg; Serving size: 1 cup, pieces, 123 g

Dill Pickles ☞ Vitamin K = 6.1 mcg; Serving size: 1 spear, small, 35 g

Drumstick Leaves—Cooked Boiled—Drained—With Salt ☞ Vitamin K = 45.4 mcg; Serving size: 1 cup, chopped, 42 g

Drumstick Leaves—Cooked Boiled—Drained—Without Salt ☞ Vitamin K = 45.4 mcg; Serving size: 1 cup, chopped, 42 g

Edamame—Frozen—Unprepared ☞ Vitamin K = 37.1 mcg; Serving size: 1 cup, 118 g

Egg Curry ☞ Vitamin K = 118.7 mcg; Serving size: 1 cup, 236 g

Eggplant ☞ Vitamin K = 2.9 mcg; Serving size: 1 cup, cubes, 82 g

Eggplant—Batter-Dipped Fried ☞ Vitamin K = 18.3 mcg; Serving size: 1 cup, 220 g

Eggplant—Cooked Boiled—Drained—With Salt ☞ Vitamin K = 2.9 mcg; Serving size: 1 cup (1 inch cubes), 99 g

Eggplant—Cooked—Cooked—Without Fat ☞ Vitamin K = 15.6 mcg; Serving size: 1 eggplant, 538 g

Eggplant—In Tomato Sauce—Cooked—Cooked—Without Fat ☛ Vitamin K = 6.5 mcg; Serving size: 1 cup, 231 g

Eggplant—Parmesan Casserole Regular ☛ Vitamin K = 17.2 mcg; Serving size: 1 cup, 198 g

Eggplant—Pickled ☛ Vitamin K = 5 mcg; Serving size: 1 cup, 136 g

Eggplant—With Cheese And Tomato Sauce ☛ Vitamin K = 5.3 mcg; Serving size: 1 cup, 198 g

Endive ☛ Vitamin K = 57.8 mcg; Serving size: 1/2 cup, chopped, 25 g

Enoki Mushrooms ☛ Vitamin K = 0 mcg; Serving size: 1 large, 5 g

Escarole—Cooked—Cooked—Without Fat ☛ Vitamin K = 273.4 mcg; Serving size: 1 cup, 130 g

Escarole—Creamed ☛ Vitamin K = 220.6 mcg; Serving size: 1 cup, 200 g

Fennel ☛ Vitamin K = 54.6 mcg; Serving size: 1 cup, sliced, 87 g

Fennel Bulb—Cooked—Cooked—Without Fat ☛ Vitamin K = 209.1 mcg; Serving size: 1 fennel bulb, 211 g

Garden Cress ☛ Vitamin K = 271 mcg; Serving size: 1 cup, 50 g

Garlic ☛ Vitamin K = 2.3 mcg; Serving size: 1 cup, 136 g

Ginger ☛ Vitamin K = 0 mcg; Serving size: 1 tsp, 2 g

Ginger Root Pickled—Canned With Artificial Sweetener ☛ Vitamin K = 0.6 mcg; Serving size: 2 tablespoon, 25 g

Gourd Dishcloth—Cooked Boiled—Drained—With Salt ☛ Vitamin K = 3 mcg; Serving size: 1 cup (1 inch pieces), 178 g

Gourd Dishcloth—Cooked Boiled—Drained—Without Salt ☛ Vitamin K = 3 mcg; Serving size: 1 cup (1 inch pieces), 178 g

Gourd Dishcloth—Raw ☛ Vitamin K = 0.7 mcg; Serving size: 1 cup (1 inch pieces), 95 g

Grape Leaves—Canned ☛ Vitamin K = 3.9 mcg; Serving size: 1 leaf, 4 g

Grape Leaves—Raw ☛ Vitamin K = 15.2 mcg; Serving size: 1 cup, 14 g

Greek Salad—No Dressing ☛ Vitamin K = 67.7 mcg; Serving size: 1 cup, 105 g

Green Banana Fried ☛ Vitamin K = 1.8 mcg; Serving size: 1 slice, 23 g

Green Banana—Cooked In Salt Water ☛ Vitamin K = 0.3 mcg; Serving size: 1 small, 54 g

Green Bell Peppers ☛ Vitamin K = 11 mcg; Serving size: 1 cup, chopped, 149 g

Green Cauliflower ☛ Vitamin K = 12.9 mcg; Serving size: 1 cup, 64 g

Green Leaf Lettuce ☛ Vitamin K = 45.5 mcg; Serving size: 1 cup shredded, 36 g

Green Peppers And Onions—Cooked—Cooked—Without Fat ☛ Vitamin K = 5.7 mcg; Serving size: 1 cup, 139 g

Green Plantain With Cracklings—Puerto Rican Style ☛ Vitamin K = 9 mcg; Serving size: 1 ball (3" dia), 64 g

Green Plantains Boiled ☛ Vitamin K = 0.2 mcg; Serving size: 1 slice, 27 g

Green Snap Beans—Raw ☛ Vitamin K = 43 mcg; Serving size: 1 cup 1/2 inch pieces, 100 g

Green Tomatoes ☛ Vitamin K = 18.2 mcg; Serving size: 1 cup, 180 g

Greens With Ham Or Pork ☛ Vitamin K = 716.8 mcg; Serving size: 1 cup, 144 g

Greens—Cooked—From Canned—Cooked—Without Fat ☛ Vitamin K = 860.5 mcg; Serving size: 1 cup, 170 g

Greens—Cooked—From Fresh—Cooked—Without Fat 🖛 Vitamin K = 739.1 mcg; Serving size: 1 cup, 146 g

Greens—Cooked—From Frozen—Cooked—Without Fat 🖛 Vitamin K = 1053.9 mcg; Serving size: 1 cup, 161 g

Hot Green Chili Peppers 🖛 Vitamin K = 6.4 mcg; Serving size: 1 pepper, 45 g

Hubbard Squash 🖛 Vitamin K = 1.5 mcg; Serving size: 1 cup, cubes, 116 g

Hungarian Peppers 🖛 Vitamin K = 2.7 mcg; Serving size: 1 pepper, 27 g

Hyacinth-Beans—Immature Seeds—Raw 🖛 Vitamin K = 14.5 mcg; Serving size: 1 cup, 80 g

Iceberg Lettuce 🖛 Vitamin K = 17.4 mcg; Serving size: 1 cup shredded, 72 g

Irishmoss Seaweed 🖛 Vitamin K = 0.5 mcg; Serving size: 2 tbsp (1/8 cup), 10 g

Jalapeno Peppers 🖛 Vitamin K = 16.7 mcg; Serving size: 1 cup, sliced, 90 g

Jerusalem-Artichokes—Raw 🖛 Vitamin K = 0.2 mcg; Serving size: 1 cup slices, 150 g

Jute Potherb—Cooked Boiled—Drained—With Salt 🖛 Vitamin K = 94 mcg; Serving size: 1 cup, 87 g

Kale 🖛 Vitamin K = 62.3 mcg; Serving size: 1 cup 1 inch pieces, loosely packed, 16 g

Kale—Cooked Boiled—Drained—With Salt 🖛 Vitamin K = 544.1 mcg; Serving size: 1 cup, chopped, 130 g

Kale—Cooked—From Canned—Cooked—Without Fat 🖛 Vitamin K = 1321.6 mcg; Serving size: 1 cup, canned, 163 g

Kale—Cooked—From Fresh—Cooked—Without Fat ☞ Vitamin K = 1054 mcg; Serving size: 1 cup, fresh, 130 g

Kale—Cooked—From Frozen—Cooked—Without Fat ☞ Vitamin K = 1137.9 mcg; Serving size: 1 cup, frozen, 130 g

Kale—Frozen—Cooked Boiled—Drained—With Salt ☞ Vitamin K = 544.1 mcg; Serving size: 1 cup, chopped, 130 g

Kale—Frozen—Cooked Boiled—Drained—Without Salt ☞ Vitamin K = 544.1 mcg; Serving size: 1 cup, chopped, 130 g

Kale—Frozen—Unprepared ☞ Vitamin K = 313.6 mcg; Serving size: 1/3 package (10 oz), 94 g

Kelp Seaweed ☞ Vitamin K = 6.6 mcg; Serving size: 2 tbsp (1/8 cup), 10 g

Ketchup ☞ Vitamin K = 0.5 mcg; Serving size: 1 tbsp, 17 g

Kimchi ☞ Vitamin K = 65.4 mcg; Serving size: 1 cup, 150 g

Kohlrabi ☞ Vitamin K = 0.1 mcg; Serving size: 1 cup, 135 g

Kohlrabi—Cooked Boiled—Drained—With Salt ☞ Vitamin K = 0.2 mcg; Serving size: 1 cup slices, 165 g

Kohlrabi—Cooked—Cooked With Fat ☞ Vitamin K = 2.2 mcg; Serving size: 1 cup, 170 g

Kohlrabi—Cooked—Cooked—Without Fat ☞ Vitamin K = 0.2 mcg; Serving size: 1 cup, 165 g

Kohlrabi—Creamed ☞ Vitamin K = 0.7 mcg; Serving size: 1 cup, 187 g

Lambsquarter—Cooked—Cooked—Without Fat ☞ Vitamin K = 884.7 mcg; Serving size: 1 cup, 180 g

Lambsquarters—Cooked Boiled—Drained—With Salt ☞ Vitamin K = 889.6 mcg; Serving size: 1 cup, chopped, 180 g

Lambsquarters—Cooked   Boiled—Drained—Without   Salt   ☛ Vitamin K = 889.6 mcg; Serving size: 1 cup, chopped, 180 g

Laver Seaweed ☛ Vitamin K = 1 mcg; Serving size: 10 sheets, 26 g

Leeks ☛ Vitamin K = 41.8 mcg; Serving size: 1 cup, 89 g

Leeks (Bulb And Lower Leaf-Portion)—Cooked Boiled—Drained— With Salt ☛ Vitamin K = 31.5 mcg; Serving size: 1 leek, 124 g

Lettuce Salad—With Assorted Vegetables Excluding Tomatoes And Carrots—No Dressing ☛ Vitamin K = 87.1 mcg; Serving size: 1 cup, 74 g

Lettuce Salad—With Assorted Vegetables Including Tomatoes And/or Carrots—No Dressing ☛ Vitamin K = 78.2 mcg; Serving size: 1 cup, 73 g

Lettuce Salad—With Avocado Tomato And/or Carrots—With Or Without Other Vegetables—No Dressing ☛ Vitamin K = 79.2 mcg; Serving size: 1 cup, 87 g

Lettuce Salad—With Cheese Tomato And/or Carrots—With Or Without Other Vegetables—No Dressing ☛ Vitamin K = 68.5 mcg; Serving size: 1 cup, 77 g

Lettuce Salad—With Egg Cheese Tomato And/or Carrots—With Or Without Other Vegetables—No Dressing ☛ Vitamin K = 175.1 mcg; Serving size: 1 garden salad, 236 g

Lettuce Salad—With Egg Tomato And/or Carrots—With Or Without Other Vegetables—No Dressing ☛ Vitamin K = 75.2 mcg; Serving size: 1 cup, 88 g

Lettuce Wilted With Bacon Dressing ☛ Vitamin K = 125.4 mcg; Serving size: 1 cup, 125 g

Lettuce—Cooked—Cooked With Fat ☛ Vitamin K = 31.6 mcg; Serving size: 1 cup, 86 g

Lettuce—Cooked—Cooked—Without Fat ☞ Vitamin K = 19.4 mcg; Serving size: 1 cup, 81 g

Lima Beans And Corn—Cooked—Cooked—Without Fat ☞ Vitamin K = 5.2 mcg; Serving size: 1 cup, 192 g

Lima Beans Immature—Cooked—From Canned With Mushroom Sauce ☞ Vitamin K = 20.1 mcg; Serving size: 1 cup, 228 g

Lima Beans Immature—Cooked—From Canned—Cooked—Without Fat ☞ Vitamin K = 8.9 mcg; Serving size: 1 cup, 174 g

Lima Beans Immature—Cooked—From Fresh With Mushroom Sauce ☞ Vitamin K = 21.7 mcg; Serving size: 1 cup, 228 g

Lima Beans Immature—Cooked—From Fresh—Cooked—Without Fat ☞ Vitamin K = 10.5 mcg; Serving size: 1 cup, 170 g

Lima Beans Immature—Cooked—From Frozen With Mushroom Sauce ☞ Vitamin K = 20.1 mcg; Serving size: 1 cup, 228 g

Lima Beans Immature—Cooked—From Frozen—Cooked—Without Fat ☞ Vitamin K = 9.2 mcg; Serving size: 1 cup, 180 g

Lima Beans Immature—From Canned—Creamed Or With Cheese Sauce ☞ Vitamin K = 8.4 mcg; Serving size: 1 cup, 228 g

Lima Beans Immature—From Fresh—Creamed Or With Cheese Sauce ☞ Vitamin K = 10.3 mcg; Serving size: 1 cup, 228 g

Lima Beans Immature—From Frozen—Creamed Or With Cheese Sauce ☞ Vitamin K = 8.4 mcg; Serving size: 1 cup, 228 g

Lima Beans—Immature Seeds—Cooked Boiled—Drained—With Salt ☞ Vitamin K = 10.5 mcg; Serving size: 1 cup, 170 g

Lima Beans—Immature Seeds—Frozen Baby—Cooked Boiled—Drained—With Salt ☞ Vitamin K = 9.4 mcg; Serving size: 1 cup, 180 g

Lima Beans—Immature Seeds—Frozen Baby—Cooked Boiled—

Drained—Without Salt ☞ Vitamin K = 9.4 mcg; Serving size: 1 cup, 180 g

Lima Beans—Immature Seeds—Frozen Fordhook—Cooked Boiled —Drained—Without Salt ☞ Vitamin K = 8.7 mcg; Serving size: 1 cup, 170 g

Lima Beans—Immature Seeds—Frozen Fordhook—Unprepared ☞ Vitamin K = 8.5 mcg; Serving size: 1 cup, 160 g

Lima Beans—Immature Seeds—Raw ☞ Vitamin K = 8.7 mcg; Serving size: 1 cup, 156 g

Lotus Root—Cooked—Cooked With Fat ☞ Vitamin K = 10.4 mcg; Serving size: 1 cup, 125 g

Lotus Root—Cooked—Cooked—Without Fat ☞ Vitamin K = 0.1 mcg; Serving size: 1 cup, 120 g

Low Sodium Ketchup ☞ Vitamin K = 0.5 mcg; Serving size: 1 tbsp, 17 g

Low Sodium Sour Pickles ☞ Vitamin K = 67.2 mcg; Serving size: 1 cup, chopped or diced, 143 g

Low Sodium Sweet Pickles ☞ Vitamin K = 4.6 mcg; Serving size: 1 slice, 6 g

Luffa—Cooked—Cooked With Fat ☞ Vitamin K = 76.7 mcg; Serving size: 1 cup, 183 g

Luffa—Cooked—Cooked—Without Fat ☞ Vitamin K = 70.8 mcg; Serving size: 1 cup, 178 g

Maitake Mushrooms ☞ Vitamin K = 0 mcg; Serving size: 1 cup diced, 70 g

Mashed Sweet Potatoes ☞ Vitamin K = 6.1 mcg; Serving size: 1 cup, 255 g

Mixed Vegetables—Cooked—From Canned—Cooked –Without Fat ☞ Vitamin K = 33.1 mcg; Serving size: 1 cup, 182 g

Mixed Vegetables—Cooked—From Frozen—Cooked—Without Fat ☛ Vitamin K = 42.6 mcg; Serving size: 1 cup, 182 g

Mountain Yam Hawaii—Raw ☛ Vitamin K = 1 mcg; Serving size: 1/2 cup, cubes, 68 g

Mung Bean Sprouts ☛ Vitamin K = 34.3 mcg; Serving size: 1 cup, 104 g

Mung Beans—Mature Seeds Sprouted—Cooked Boiled—Drained—With Salt ☛ Vitamin K = 28.1 mcg; Serving size: 1 cup, 124 g

Mung Beans—Mature Seeds Sprouted—Cooked Boiled—Drained—Without Salt ☛ Vitamin K = 28.1 mcg; Serving size: 1 cup, 124 g

Mushroom Asian—Cooked From Dried ☛ Vitamin K = 0 mcg; Serving size: 1 cup, 145 g

Mushrooms Batter-Dipped Fried ☛ Vitamin K = 0.2 mcg; Serving size: 1 small, 8 g

Mushrooms Portobellos Grilled ☛ Vitamin K = 0 mcg; Serving size: 1 cup sliced, 121 g

Mushrooms Shiitake—Cooked—With Salt ☛ Vitamin K = 0 mcg; Serving size: 1 cup pieces, 145 g

Mushrooms Shiitake—Stir-Fried ☛ Vitamin K = 0 mcg; Serving size: 1 cup whole, 89 g

Mushrooms Stuffed ☛ Vitamin K = 3.3 mcg; Serving size: 1 stuffed cap, 24 g

Mushrooms White—Cooked Boiled—Drained—With Salt ☛ Vitamin K = 0 mcg; Serving size: 1 cup pieces, 156 g

Mushrooms—Cooked—From Canned—Cooked—Without Fat ☛ Vitamin K = 0 mcg; Serving size: 1 piece, 4 g

Mushrooms—Cooked—From Fresh—Cooked—Without Fat ☛ Vitamin K = 0 mcg; Serving size: 1 piece, 4 g

Mushrooms—Cooked—From Frozen—Cooked—Without Fat ☞ Vitamin K = 0 mcg; Serving size: 1 piece, 4 g

Mushrooms—From Canned—Creamed ☞ Vitamin K = 0.9 mcg; Serving size: 1 cup, 217 g

Mushrooms—From Fresh—Creamed ☞ Vitamin K = 0.9 mcg; Serving size: 1 cup, 217 g

Mushrooms—From Frozen—Creamed ☞ Vitamin K = 0.9 mcg; Serving size: 1 cup, 217 g

Mustard Cabbage—Cooked—Cooked With Fat ☞ Vitamin K = 59.7 mcg; Serving size: 1 cup, 175 g

Mustard Cabbage—Cooked—Cooked—Without Fat ☞ Vitamin K = 57.5 mcg; Serving size: 1 cup, 170 g

Mustard Greens ☞ Vitamin K = 144.2 mcg; Serving size: 1 cup, chopped, 56 g

Mustard Greens—Cooked Boiled—Drained—With Salt ☞ Vitamin K = 829.8 mcg; Serving size: 1 cup, chopped, 140 g

Mustard Greens—Cooked—From Canned—Cooked—Without Fat ☞ Vitamin K = 900.4 mcg; Serving size: 1 cup, canned, 153 g

Mustard Greens—Cooked—From Fresh—Cooked—Without Fat ☞ Vitamin K = 823.9 mcg; Serving size: 1 cup, fresh, 140 g

Mustard Greens—Cooked—From Frozen—Cooked—Without Fat ☞ Vitamin K = 499.4 mcg; Serving size: 1 cup, frozen, 150 g

Mustard Greens—Frozen—Cooked Boiled—Drained—With Salt ☞ Vitamin K = 502.7 mcg; Serving size: 1 cup, chopped or diced, 150 g

Mustard Greens—Frozen—Cooked Boiled—Drained—Without Salt ☞ Vitamin K = 502.7 mcg; Serving size: 1 cup, chopped, 150 g

New Zealand Spinach ☞ Vitamin K = 188.7 mcg; Serving size: 1 cup, chopped, 56 g

New Zealand Spinach—Cooked Boiled—Drained—With Salt ☞ Vitamin K = 525.6 mcg; Serving size: 1 cup, chopped, 180 g

Nopales ☞ Vitamin K = 4.6 mcg; Serving size: 1 cup, sliced, 86 g

Okra ☞ Vitamin K = 31.3 mcg; Serving size: 1 cup, 100 g

Okra—Batter-Dipped Fried ☞ Vitamin K = 19.7 mcg; Serving size: 1 cup, 92 g

Okra—Cooked Boiled—Drained—With Salt ☞ Vitamin K = 32 mcg; Serving size: 1/2 cup slices, 80 g

Okra—Cooked—From Canned—Cooked—Without Fat ☞ Vitamin K = 66.5 mcg; Serving size: 1 cup, 167 g

Okra—Cooked—From Fresh—Cooked—Without Fat ☞ Vitamin K = 63.7 mcg; Serving size: 1 cup, 160 g

Okra—Cooked—From Frozen—Cooked—Without Fat ☞ Vitamin K = 87.4 mcg; Serving size: 1 cup, 184 g

Okra—Frozen—Cooked Boiled—Drained—With Salt ☞ Vitamin K = 44 mcg; Serving size: 1/2 cup slices, 92 g

Okra—Frozen—Unprepared ☞ Vitamin K = 46.9 mcg; Serving size: 1/3 package (10 oz), 95 g

Onion Rings—From Fresh Batter-Dipped Baked Or Fried ☞ Vitamin K = 10.4 mcg; Serving size: 10 small rings (1" - 2" dia), 48 g

Onions ☞ Vitamin K = 0.6 mcg; Serving size: 1 cup, chopped, 160 g

Onions Dehydrated Flakes ☞ Vitamin K = 0.2 mcg; Serving size: 1 tbsp, 5 g

Onions Green—Cooked—From Fresh—Cooked With Fat ☞ Vitamin K = 477.6 mcg; Serving size: 1 cup, 224 g

Onions Green—Cooked—From Fresh—Cooked—Without Fat ☞ Vitamin K = 472.4 mcg; Serving size: 1 cup, 219 g

Onions Pearl—Cooked—From Canned ☛ Vitamin K = 0.9 mcg; Serving size: 1 cup, 185 g

Onions Pearl—Cooked—From Fresh ☛ Vitamin K = 0.9 mcg; Serving size: 1 cup, 185 g

Onions Pearl—Cooked—From Frozen ☛ Vitamin K = 0.6 mcg; Serving size: 1 cup, 185 g

Onions Young Green Tops Only ☛ Vitamin K = 9.4 mcg; Serving size: 1 tbsp, 6 g

Onions—Canned—Solids And Liquids ☛ Vitamin K = 0.1 mcg; Serving size: 1 onion, 63 g

Onions—Cooked Boiled—Drained—With Salt ☛ Vitamin K = 1.1 mcg; Serving size: 1 cup, 210 g

Onions—Cooked—From Fresh—Cooked—Without Fat ☛ Vitamin K = 1.1 mcg; Serving size: 1 cup, 210 g

Onions—Cooked—From Frozen—Cooked—Without Fat ☛ Vitamin K = 0.6 mcg; Serving size: 1 cup, 210 g

Onions—From Fresh—Creamed ☛ Vitamin K = 1.4 mcg; Serving size: 1 cup, 228 g

Onions—Frozen Chopped—Cooked Boiled—Drained—With Salt ☛ Vitamin K = 0 mcg; Serving size: 1 tbsp chopped, 15 g

Onions—Frozen Chopped—Cooked Boiled—Drained—Without Salt ☛ Vitamin K = 0 mcg; Serving size: 1 tbsp chopped, 15 g

Onions—Frozen Whole—Cooked Boiled—Drained—With Salt ☛ Vitamin K = 0.6 mcg; Serving size: 1 cup, 210 g

Onions—Frozen Whole—Cooked Boiled—Drained—Without Salt ☛ Vitamin K = 0.6 mcg; Serving size: 1 cup, 210 g

Onions—Frozen Whole—Unprepared ☛ Vitamin K = 0.4 mcg; Serving size: 1/3 package (10 oz), 95 g

Oriental Radishes ☛ Vitamin K = 0.3 mcg; Serving size: 1 cup slices, 116 g

Oyster Mushrooms ☛ Vitamin K = 0 mcg; Serving size: 1 large, 148 g

Palak Paneer ☛ Vitamin K = 356.2 mcg; Serving size: 1 cup, 200 g

Palm Hearts—Cooked Assume—Cooked—Without Fat ☛ Vitamin K = 0 mcg; Serving size: 1 cup, 146 g

Parsley ☛ Vitamin K = 984 mcg; Serving size: 1 cup chopped, 60 g

Parsnips ☛ Vitamin K = 29.9 mcg; Serving size: 1 cup slices, 133 g

Parsnips—Cooked Boiled—Drained—With Salt ☛ Vitamin K = 0.8 mcg; Serving size: 1/2 cup slices, 78 g

Parsnips—Cooked—Cooked—Without Fat ☛ Vitamin K = 1.6 mcg; Serving size: 1 cup, pieces, 156 g

Parsnips—Creamed ☛ Vitamin K = 2.3 mcg; Serving size: 1 cup, 228 g

Pea Salad ☛ Vitamin K = 115.6 mcg; Serving size: 1 cup, 214 g

Pea Salad With Cheese ☛ Vitamin K = 104.4 mcg; Serving size: 1 cup, 214 g

Peas ☛ Vitamin K = 36 mcg; Serving size: 1 cup, 145 g

Peas And Carrots—Canned—No Salt Added—Solids And Liquids ☛ Vitamin K = 33.4 mcg; Serving size: 1 cup, 255 g

Peas And Carrots—Cooked—From Canned—Cooked—Without Fat ☛ Vitamin K = 38.9 mcg; Serving size: 1 cup, 160 g

Peas And Carrots—Cooked—From Fresh—Cooked—Without Fat ☛ Vitamin K = 31.7 mcg; Serving size: 1 cup, 160 g

Peas And Carrots—Cooked—From Frozen—Cooked—Without Fat ☛ Vitamin K = 29.9 mcg; Serving size: 1 cup, 160 g

Peas And Carrots—From Canned—Creamed ☛ Vitamin K = 34.2 mcg; Serving size: 1 cup, 244 g

Peas And Carrots—From Fresh—Creamed ☛ Vitamin K = 28.1 mcg; Serving size: 1 cup, 244 g

Peas And Carrots—From Frozen—Creamed ☛ Vitamin K = 26.6 mcg; Serving size: 1 cup, 244 g

Peas And Carrots—Frozen—Cooked Boiled—Drained—With Salt ☛ Vitamin K = 15 mcg; Serving size: 1/2 cup, 80 g

Peas And Carrots—Frozen—Cooked Boiled—Drained—Without Salt ☛ Vitamin K = 52.3 mcg; Serving size: 1 package (10 oz) yields, 278 g

Peas And Corn—Cooked—Cooked—Without Fat ☛ Vitamin K = 20.9 mcg; Serving size: 1 cup, 162 g

Peas And Mushrooms—Cooked—Cooked—Without Fat ☛ Vitamin K = 28.6 mcg; Serving size: 1 cup, 159 g

Peas And Onions—Cooked—Cooked—Without Fat ☛ Vitamin K = 21.6 mcg; Serving size: 1 cup, 180 g

Peas And Onions—Frozen—Cooked Boiled—Drained—With Salt ☛ Vitamin K = 21.8 mcg; Serving size: 1 cup, 180 g

Peas And Onions—Frozen—Cooked Boiled—Drained—Without Salt ☛ Vitamin K = 21.8 mcg; Serving size: 1 cup, 180 g

Peas And Potatoes—Cooked—Cooked—Without Fat ☛ Vitamin K = 22.3 mcg; Serving size: 1 cup, 158 g

Peas Cowpeas Field Peas Or Blackeye Peas Not Dried—Cooked—From Canned—Cooked Without Fat ☛ Vitamin K = 65.5 mcg; Serving size: 1 cup, 180 g

Peas Cowpeas Field Peas Or Blackeye Peas Not Dried—Cooked—From Fresh—Cooked—Without Fat ☛ Vitamin K = 43.6 mcg; Serving size: 1 cup, 165 g

Peas Cowpeas Field Peas Or Blackeye Peas Not Dried—Cooked—

From Frozen—Cooked—Without Fat ☛ Vitamin K = 62.2 mcg; Serving size: 1 cup, 170 g

Peas Edible-Podded—Cooked Boiled—Drained—With Salt ☛ Vitamin K = 40 mcg; Serving size: 1 cup, 160 g

Peas Edible-Podded—Frozen—Cooked Boiled—Drained—With Salt ☛ Vitamin K = 48.3 mcg; Serving size: 1 cup, 160 g

Peas Green (Includes Baby And Lesuer Types)—Canned—Drained Solids—Unprepared ☛ Vitamin K = 64.4 mcg; Serving size: 1 cup, 175 g

Peas Green—Canned Low Sodium—Cooked—Without Fat ☛ Vitamin K = 43.9 mcg; Serving size: 1 cup, 170 g

Peas Green—Canned Regular Pack—Solids And Liquids ☛ Vitamin K = 25.7 mcg; Serving size: 1/2 cup, 124 g

Peas Green—Canned—No Salt Added—Drained Solids ☛ Vitamin K = 18.2 mcg; Serving size: 1/2 cup, 85 g

Peas Green—Canned—No Salt Added—Solids And Liquids ☛ Vitamin K = 20.5 mcg; Serving size: 1/2 cup, 124 g

Peas Green—Cooked—From Canned—Cooked—Without Fat ☛ Vitamin K = 62.4 mcg; Serving size: 1 cup, 170 g

Peas Green—Cooked—From Fresh—Cooked—Without Fat ☛ Vitamin K = 41.1 mcg; Serving size: 1 cup, 160 g

Peas Green—Cooked—From Frozen—Cooked—Without Fat ☛ Vitamin K = 38.2 mcg; Serving size: 1 cup, 160 g

Peas Green—Frozen—Cooked Boiled—Drained—With Salt ☛ Vitamin K = 19.2 mcg; Serving size: 1/2 cup, 80 g

Peas Green—Frozen—Cooked Boiled—Drained—Without Salt ☛ Vitamin K = 19.2 mcg; Serving size: 1/2 cup, 80 g

Peas Green—Frozen—Unprepared ☞ Vitamin K = 37.4 mcg; Serving size: 1 cup, 134 g

Peas—Cooked—From Canned With Mushroom Sauce ☞ Vitamin K = 67.8 mcg; Serving size: 1 cup, 244 g

Peas—Cooked—From Canned With Tomato Sauce ☞ Vitamin K = 62 mcg; Serving size: 1 cup, 244 g

Peas—Cooked—From Fresh With Mushroom Sauce ☞ Vitamin K = 51.5 mcg; Serving size: 1 cup, 244 g

Peas—Cooked—From Fresh With Tomato Sauce ☞ Vitamin K = 43.4 mcg; Serving size: 1 cup, 244 g

Peas—Cooked—From Frozen With Mushroom Sauce ☞ Vitamin K = 48.8 mcg; Serving size: 1 cup, 244 g

Peas—Cooked—From Frozen With Tomato Sauce ☞ Vitamin K = 40.5 mcg; Serving size: 1 cup, 244 g

Peas—From Canned—Creamed ☞ Vitamin K = 52.7 mcg; Serving size: 1 cup, 244 g

Peas—From Fresh—Creamed ☞ Vitamin K = 36.4 mcg; Serving size: 1 cup, 244 g

Peas—From Frozen—Creamed ☞ Vitamin K = 33.7 mcg; Serving size: 1 cup, 244 g

Pepper Sweet Red—Raw ☞ Vitamin K = 0.5 mcg; Serving size: 1 piece, 10 g

Peppers Green—Cooked—Cooked—Without Fat ☞ Vitamin K = 13.2 mcg; Serving size: 1 cup, 136 g

Peppers Hot Chili Green—Canned Pods Excluding Seeds—Solids And Liquids ☞ Vitamin K = 6.4 mcg; Serving size: 1 pepper, 73 g

Peppers Hot Chili Red—Canned Excluding Seeds—Solids And Liquids ☞ Vitamin K = 6.4 mcg; Serving size: 1 pepper, 73 g

Peppers Hot Pickled—Canned ☛ Vitamin K = 7.4 mcg; Serving size: 1/4 cup drained, 34 g

Peppers Jalapeno—Canned—Solids And Liquids ☛ Vitamin K = 17.5 mcg; Serving size: 1 cup, chopped, 136 g

Peppers Red—Cooked—Cooked—Without Fat ☛ Vitamin K = 6.9 mcg; Serving size: 1 cup, 136 g

Peppers Sweet Green—Cooked Boiled—Drained—With Salt ☛ Vitamin K = 1.1 mcg; Serving size: 1 tbsp, 11.6 g

Peppers Sweet Red Freeze-Dried ☛ Vitamin K = 0.5 mcg; Serving size: 1 tbsp, 0.4 g

Peppers Sweet Red—Cooked Boiled—Drained—With Salt ☛ Vitamin K = 0.6 mcg; Serving size: 1 tbsp, 12 g

Peppers Sweet Red—Frozen Chopped Boiled—Drained—With Salt ☛ Vitamin K = 4.6 mcg; Serving size: 1 cup, chopped or strips, 135 g

Peppers Sweet Red—Frozen Chopped Boiled—Drained—Without Salt ☛ Vitamin K = 4.6 mcg; Serving size: 1 cup, chopped or strips, 135 g

Peppers Sweet Red—Frozen Chopped—Unprepared ☛ Vitamin K = 3.6 mcg; Serving size: 1/3 package (10 oz), 95 g

Pickled Beets ☛ Vitamin K = 0.7 mcg; Serving size: 1 cup slices, 227 g

Pickles Chowchow With Cauliflower—Onion Mustard Sweet ☛ Vitamin K = 150.9 mcg; Serving size: 1 cup, 245 g

Pigeon Peas—Cooked—From Canned—Cooked With Fat ☛ Vitamin K = 32.2 mcg; Serving size: 1 cup, 158 g

Pigeon Peas—Cooked—From Canned—Cooked—Without Fat ☛ Vitamin K = 30.1 mcg; Serving size: 1 cup, 153 g

Pigeon Peas—Cooked—From Fresh—Cooked With Fat ☛ Vitamin K = 32.2 mcg; Serving size: 1 cup, 158 g

Pigeon Peas—Cooked—From Fresh—Cooked—Without Fat ☛ Vitamin K = 30.1 mcg; Serving size: 1 cup, 153 g

Pigeonpeas—Immature Seeds—Cooked Boiled—Drained—With Salt ☛ Vitamin K = 30.3 mcg; Serving size: 1 cup, 153 g

Pigeonpeas—Immature Seeds—Cooked Boiled—Drained—Without Salt ☛ Vitamin K = 30.3 mcg; Serving size: 1 cup, 153 g

Pigeonpeas—Immature Seeds—Raw ☛ Vitamin K = 37 mcg; Serving size: 1 cup, 154 g

Pinacbet ☛ Vitamin K = 13.5 mcg; Serving size: 1 cup, 214 g

Plantain Ripe Rolled In Flour Fried ☛ Vitamin K = 6.4 mcg; Serving size: 1 piece (2-1/2" long), 45 g

Poi ☛ Vitamin K = 2.4 mcg; Serving size: 1 cup, 240 g

Poke Greens—Cooked—Cooked—Without Fat ☛ Vitamin K = 166.3 mcg; Serving size: 1 cup, 155 g

Pokeberry Shoots (Poke)—Cooked Boiled—Drained—With Salt ☛ Vitamin K = 178.2 mcg; Serving size: 1 cup, 165 g

Pokeberry Shoots (Poke)—Cooked Boiled—Drained—Without Salt ☛ Vitamin K = 178.2 mcg; Serving size: 1 cup, 165 g

Portobellos (Exposed To Sunlight Or Uv) ☛ Vitamin K = 0 mcg; Serving size: 1 cup sliced, 121 g

Portobellos Mushrooms ☛ Vitamin K = 0 mcg; Serving size: 1 cup diced, 86 g

Potato Baked—Peel Eaten ☛ Vitamin K = 4.6 mcg; Serving size: 1 small, 230 g

Potato Baked—Peel Eaten With Meat ☛ Vitamin K = 5.5 mcg; Serving size: 1 small, 260 g

Potato Baked—Peel Eaten With Vegetables ☛ Vitamin K = 18.7 mcg; Serving size: 1 small, 260 g

Potato Baked—Peel Not Eaten ☛ Vitamin K = 0.7 mcg; Serving size: 1 small, 230 g

Potato Baked—Peel Not Eaten With Cheese ☛ Vitamin K = 2.1 mcg; Serving size: 1 small, 260 g

Potato Baked—Peel Not Eaten With Chili ☛ Vitamin K = 3.6 mcg; Serving size: 1 small, 260 g

Potato Baked—Peel Not Eaten With Meat ☛ Vitamin K = 2.1 mcg; Serving size: 1 small, 260 g

Potato Baked—Peel Not Eaten With Sour Cream ☛ Vitamin K = 1.8 mcg; Serving size: 1 small, 260 g

Potato Baked—Peel Not Eaten With Vegetables ☛ Vitamin K = 15.1 mcg; Serving size: 1 small, 260 g

Potato Boiled—From Fresh Peel Eaten—Cooked—Without Fat ☛ Vitamin K = 1.2 mcg; Serving size: 1 baby potato, 60 g

Potato Boiled—From Fresh Peel Not Eaten—Cooked—Without Fat ☛ Vitamin K = 0.2 mcg; Serving size: 1 baby potato, 60 g

Potato Boiled—Ready-To-Heat ☛ Vitamin K = 2.5 mcg; Serving size: 1 baby potato, 60 g

Potato Flour ☛ Vitamin K = 0 mcg; Serving size: 1 cup, 160 g

Potato Only From Puerto Rican Mixed Dishes Gravy And Other Components Reported Separately ☛ Vitamin K = 2.1 mcg; Serving size: 1 small, 97 g

Potato Pancakes ☛ Vitamin K = 0.6 mcg; Serving size: 1 small 2-3/4 in. dia., 5/8 in. thick., 22 g

Potato Puffs—Frozen Oven-Heated ☛ Vitamin K = 2.9 mcg; Serving size: 10 puffs, 79 g

Potato Puffs—Frozen—Unprepared ☛ Vitamin K = 3 mcg; Serving size: 1 cup, 120 g

Potato Roasted—From Fresh Peel Eaten—Cooked—Without Fat ☞ Vitamin K = 1.2 mcg; Serving size: 1 baby potato, 60 g

Potato Roasted—From Fresh Peel Not Eaten—Cooked—Without Fat ☞ Vitamin K = 0.2 mcg; Serving size: 1 baby potato, 60 g

Potato Roasted—Ready-To-Heat ☞ Vitamin K = 2.5 mcg; Serving size: 1 baby potato, 60 g

Potato—Canned—Cooked—Without Fat ☞ Vitamin K = 0.5 mcg; Serving size: 1 whole, canned, 35 g

Potatoes Baked—Flesh And Skin—With Salt ☞ Vitamin K = 1.2 mcg; Serving size: 1/2 cup, 61 g

Potatoes Baked—Flesh—With Salt ☞ Vitamin K = 0.2 mcg; Serving size: 1/2 cup, 61 g

Potatoes Baked—Skin Only—With Salt ☞ Vitamin K = 1 mcg; Serving size: 1 skin, 58 g

Potatoes Baked—Skin—Without Salt ☞ Vitamin K = 1 mcg; Serving size: 1 skin, 58 g

Potatoes Boiled—Cooked In Skin Flesh—With Salt ☞ Vitamin K = 1.7 mcg; Serving size: 1/2 cup, 78 g

Potatoes Boiled—Cooked Without Skin Flesh—With Salt ☞ Vitamin K = 1.7 mcg; Serving size: 1/2 cup, 78 g

Potatoes Boiled—Cooked Without Skin Flesh—Without Salt ☞ Vitamin K = 1.7 mcg; Serving size: 1/2 cup, 78 g

Potatoes Flesh And Skin—Raw ☞ Vitamin K = 1.5 mcg; Serving size: 1/2 cup, diced, 75 g

Potatoes French Fried—All Types Salt Added In Processing—Frozen —Home-Made Oven Heated ☞ Vitamin K = 5.6 mcg; Serving size: 10 fries, 76 g

Potatoes French Fried—All Types Salt Added In Processing—Frozen —Unprepared ☛ Vitamin K = 2 mcg; Serving size: 10 strip, 89 g

Potatoes French Fried—All Types Salt Not Added In Processing— Frozen As Purchased ☛ Vitamin K = 1.4 mcg; Serving size: 10 strips, 65 g

Potatoes French Fried—All Types Salt Not Added In Processing— Frozen Oven-Heated ☛ Vitamin K = 1.9 mcg; Serving size: 10 strip, 74 g

Potatoes French Fried—Crinkle Or Regular Cut Salt Added In Processing—Frozen As Purchased ☛ Vitamin K = 1.7 mcg; Serving size: 10 strip, 82 g

Potatoes French Fried—Shoestring Salt Added In Processing— Frozen As Purchased ☛ Vitamin K = 0.8 mcg; Serving size: 10 strip, 30 g

Potatoes French Fried—Shoestring Salt Added In Processing— Frozen Oven-Heated ☛ Vitamin K = 0.6 mcg; Serving size: 10 strip, 21 g

Potatoes French Fried—Steak Fries Salt Added In Processing— Frozen As Purchased ☛ Vitamin K = 2.8 mcg; Serving size: 10 strip, 153 g

Potatoes French Fried—Steak Fries Salt Added In Processing— Frozen Oven-Heated ☛ Vitamin K = 3.1 mcg; Serving size: 10 strip, 133 g

Potatoes Hash Brown—Refrigerated Made Pan-Fried In Canola Oil ☛ Vitamin K = 25.5 mcg; Serving size: 1 cup prepared, 130 g

Potatoes Hash Brown—Refrigerated—Unprepared ☛ Vitamin K = 0.6 mcg; Serving size: 1 cup unprepared, 159 g

Potatoes Hash Brown—Frozen Plain Made Pan Fried In Canola Oil ☛ Vitamin K = 27.2 mcg; Serving size: 1 cup prepared, 150 g

Potatoes Mashed—Dehydrated Flakes—Without Milk—Dry Form ☞ Vitamin K = 5.2 mcg; Serving size: 1 cup, 60 g

Potatoes Mashed—Dehydrated Granules With Milk Dry Form ☞ Vitamin K = 17.4 mcg; Serving size: 1 cup, 200 g

Potatoes Mashed—Dehydrated Granules—Without Milk—Dry Form ☞ Vitamin K = 18 mcg; Serving size: 1 cup, 200 g

Potatoes Mashed—Ready-To-Eat ☞ Vitamin K = 5.5 mcg; Serving size: 1 cup, 229 g

Potatoes Mashed—Home-Made Whole Milk Added ☞ Vitamin K = 3.8 mcg; Serving size: 1 cup, 210 g

Potatoes—Red Flesh And Skin—Raw ☞ Vitamin K = 2.2 mcg; Serving size: 1/2 cup, diced, 75 g

Potatoes—Russet Flesh And Skin—Raw ☞ Vitamin K = 1.4 mcg; Serving size: 1/2 cup, diced, 75 g

Potatoes—White Flesh And Skin—Raw ☞ Vitamin K = 1.2 mcg; Serving size: 1/2 cup, diced, 75 g

Potatoes—Canned—Drained Solids—No Salt Added ☞ Vitamin K = 2.7 mcg; Serving size: 1 cup, 180 g

Pumpkin Flowers—Cooked Boiled—Drained—With Salt ☞ Vitamin K = 0 mcg; Serving size: 1 cup, 134 g

Pumpkin Fritters—Puerto Rican Style ☞ Vitamin K = 0.3 mcg; Serving size: 1 fritter (2" dia), 35 g

Pumpkin Leaves—Cooked Boiled—Drained—With Salt ☞ Vitamin K = 76.7 mcg; Serving size: 1 cup, 71 g

Pumpkin—Canned—With Salt ☞ Vitamin K = 39.2 mcg; Serving size: 1 cup, 245 g

Pumpkin—Cooked Boiled—Drained—With Salt ☞ Vitamin K = 2 mcg; Serving size: 1 cup, mashed, 245 g

Pumpkin—Cooked—From Canned—Cooked—Without Fat ☛ Vitamin K = 39 mcg; Serving size: 1 cup, 245 g

Pumpkin—Cooked—From Fresh—Cooked—Without Fat ☛ Vitamin K = 2 mcg; Serving size: 1 cup, 245 g

Pumpkin—Cooked—From Frozen—Cooked—Without Fat ☛ Vitamin K = 2 mcg; Serving size: 1 cup, 245 g

Pumpkin—Raw ☛ Vitamin K = 1.3 mcg; Serving size: 1 cup (1 inch cubes), 116 g

Radicchio ☛ Vitamin K = 102.1 mcg; Serving size: 1 cup, shredded, 40 g

Radish Daikon—Cooked—Cooked With Fat ☛ Vitamin K = 5.8 mcg; Serving size: 1 cup, 153 g

Radish Daikon—Cooked—Cooked—Without Fat ☛ Vitamin K = 0.4 mcg; Serving size: 1 cup, 147 g

Radishes ☛ Vitamin K = 1.5 mcg; Serving size: 1 cup slices, 116 g

Radishes Hawaiian Style Pickled ☛ Vitamin K = 0.8 mcg; Serving size: 1 cup, 150 g

Radishes Oriental Dried ☛ Vitamin K = 5.2 mcg; Serving size: 1 cup, 116 g

Radishes Oriental—Cooked Boiled—Drained—With Salt ☛ Vitamin K = 0.4 mcg; Serving size: 1 cup slices, 147 g

Ratatouille ☛ Vitamin K = 13.5 mcg; Serving size: 1 cup, 214 g

Red Cabbage ☛ Vitamin K = 34 mcg; Serving size: 1 cup, chopped, 89 g

Red Chili Peppers ☛ Vitamin K = 6.3 mcg; Serving size: 1 pepper, 45 g

Red Leaf Lettuce ☛ Vitamin K = 39.3 mcg; Serving size: 1 cup shredded, 28 g

Reduced Sodium Dill Pickles ☛ Vitamin K = 6.1 mcg; Serving size: 1 spear, small, 35 g

Ripe Plantain Fritters—Puerto Rican Style ☛ Vitamin K = 14.6 mcg; Serving size: 1 pionono (2"x 2-1/2" x 3/4"), 58 g

Romaine Lettuce ☛ Vitamin K = 48.2 mcg; Serving size: 1 cup shredded, 47 g

Rutabaga—Cooked—Cooked—Without Fat ☛ Vitamin K = 0.3 mcg; Serving size: 1 cup, pieces, 170 g

Rutabagas (Neeps Swedes) ☛ Vitamin K = 0.4 mcg; Serving size: 1 cup, cubes, 140 g

Rutabagas—Cooked Boiled—Drained—With Salt ☛ Vitamin K = 0.2 mcg; Serving size: 1/2 cup, mashed, 120 g

Salsify—Cooked Boiled—Drained—With Salt ☛ Vitamin K = 0.4 mcg; Serving size: 1 cup slices, 135 g

Salsify—Cooked Boiled—Drained—Without Salt ☛ Vitamin K = 0.4 mcg; Serving size: 1 cup, sliced, 135 g

Salsify—Cooked—Cooked With Fat ☛ Vitamin K = 2.5 mcg; Serving size: 1 cup, 140 g

Salsify—Cooked—Cooked—Without Fat ☛ Vitamin K = 0.4 mcg; Serving size: 1 cup, 135 g

Sambar Vegetable Stew ☛ Vitamin K = 17.9 mcg; Serving size: 1 cup, 248 g

Sauerkraut ☛ Vitamin K = 18.5 mcg; Serving size: 1 cup, 142 g

Sauteed Green Bell Peppers ☛ Vitamin K = 24.5 mcg; Serving size: 1 cup chopped, 115 g

Savoy Cabbage ☛ Vitamin K – 48.2 mcg; Serving size: 1 cup, shredded, 70 g

Scallop Squash ☛ Vitamin K = 4.3 mcg; Serving size: 1 cup slices,

130 g

Seaweed Agar—Raw ☛ Vitamin K = 0.2 mcg; Serving size: 2 tbsp (1/8 cup), 10 g

Seaweed—Raw ☛ Vitamin K = 15.4 mcg; Serving size: 1 cup, 80 g

Serrano Peppers ☛ Vitamin K = 12.4 mcg; Serving size: 1 cup, chopped, 105 g

Seven-Layer Salad Lettuce Salad—Made With A Combination Of Onion Celery—Green Pepper Peas Mayonnaise Cheese Eggs And/or Bacon ☛ Vitamin K = 58.7 mcg; Serving size: 1 cup, 119 g

Shallots ☛ Vitamin K = 0.1 mcg; Serving size: 1 tbsp chopped, 10 g

Shallots Freeze-Dried ☛ Vitamin K = 0 mcg; Serving size: 1 tbsp, 0.9 g

Shellie Beans—Canned—Solids And Liquids ☛ Vitamin K = 19.6 mcg; Serving size: 1 cup, 245 g

Snap Beans (Green)—Canned Regular Pack—Drained Solids ☛ Vitamin K = 52.5 mcg; Serving size: 1 cup, 135 g

Snap Beans (Green)—Canned—No Salt Added—Drained Solids ☛ Vitamin K = 59.5 mcg; Serving size: 1 cup, 153 g

Snap Beans (Green)—Cooked Boiled—Drained—With Salt ☛ Vitamin K = 59.9 mcg; Serving size: 1 cup, 125 g

Snap Beans (Green)—Frozen All Styles—Microwaved ☛ Vitamin K = 64 mcg; Serving size: 1 cup, 111 g

Snap Beans (Green)—Frozen All Styles—Unprepared ☛ Vitamin K = 54.2 mcg; Serving size: 1 cup, 121 g

Snap Beans (Green)—Frozen—Cooked Boiled—Drained—With Salt ☛ Vitamin K = 51.4 mcg; Serving size: 1 cup, 135 g

Snap Beans (Yellow)—Canned Regular Pack—Drained Solids ☛ Vitamin K = 60.1 mcg; Serving size: 1 cup, 153 g

Snap Beans (Yellow)—Canned Regular Pack—Solids And Liquids 🖝 Vitamin K = 37.4 mcg; Serving size: 1/2 cup, 120 g

Snap Beans (Yellow)—Canned—No Salt Added—Drained Solids 🖝 Vitamin K = 59.5 mcg; Serving size: 1 cup, 153 g

Snap Beans (Yellow)—Canned—No Salt Added—Solids And Liquids 🖝 Vitamin K = 37.4 mcg; Serving size: 1/2 cup, 120 g

Snap Beans (Yellow)—Cooked Boiled—Drained—With Salt 🖝 Vitamin K = 59.9 mcg; Serving size: 1 cup, 125 g

Snap Beans (Yellow)—Frozen All Styles—Unprepared 🖝 Vitamin K = 54.5 mcg; Serving size: 1 cup, 121 g

Snap Beans (Yellow)—Frozen—Cooked Boiled—Drained—With Salt 🖝 Vitamin K = 51.4 mcg; Serving size: 1 cup, 135 g

Snap Beans (Yellow)—Frozen—Cooked Boiled—Drained—Without Salt 🖝 Vitamin K = 51.4 mcg; Serving size: 1 cup, 135 g

Snow Peas 🖝 Vitamin K = 24.5 mcg; Serving size: 1 cup, chopped, 98 g

Snowpea—Cooked—From Fresh—Cooked—Without Fat 🖝 Vitamin K = 39.7 mcg; Serving size: 1 cup, 160 g

Snowpea—Cooked—From Frozen—Cooked—Without Fat 🖝 Vitamin K = 48 mcg; Serving size: 1 cup, 160 g

Sour Pickled Cucumber 🖝 Vitamin K = 72.9 mcg; Serving size: 1 cup, 155 g

Soybeans—Mature Seeds Sprouted—Cooked Steamed—With Salt 🖝 Vitamin K = 31 mcg; Serving size: 1 cup, 94 g

Spaghetti Squash 🖝 Vitamin K = 0.9 mcg; Serving size: 1 cup, cubes, 101 g

Spinach 🖝 Vitamin K = 144.9 mcg; Serving size: 1 cup, 30 g

Spinach And Cheese Casserole 🖝 Vitamin K = 489.2 mcg; Serving size: 1 cup, 200 g

Spinach Salad—No Dressing ☞ Vitamin K = 257.4 mcg; Serving size: 1 cup, 74 g

Spinach Souffle ☞ Vitamin K = 172 mcg; Serving size: 1 cup, 136 g

Spinach—Canned Regular Pack—Drained Solids ☞ Vitamin K = 987.8 mcg; Serving size: 1 cup, 214 g

Spinach—Canned Regular Pack—Solids And Liquids ☞ Vitamin K = 891.1 mcg; Serving size: 1 cup, 234 g

Spinach—Canned—No Salt Added—Solids And Liquids ☞ Vitamin K = 891.1 mcg; Serving size: 1 cup, 234 g

Spinach—Cooked Boiled—Drained—With Salt ☞ Vitamin K = 888.5 mcg; Serving size: 1 cup, 180 g

Spinach—Cooked—From Canned With Cheese Sauce ☞ Vitamin K = 664 mcg; Serving size: 1 cup, 200 g

Spinach—Cooked—From Canned—Cooked—Without Fat ☞ Vitamin K = 985.9 mcg; Serving size: 1 cup, canned, 214 g

Spinach—Cooked—From Fresh With Cheese Sauce ☞ Vitamin K = 680.4 mcg; Serving size: 1 cup, 200 g

Spinach—Cooked—From Fresh—Cooked—Without Fat ☞ Vitamin K = 883.6 mcg; Serving size: 1 cup, fresh, 180 g

Spinach—Cooked—From Frozen With Cheese Sauce ☞ Vitamin K = 757.6 mcg; Serving size: 1 cup, 200 g

Spinach—Cooked—From Frozen—Cooked—Without Fat ☞ Vitamin K = 1022 mcg; Serving size: 1 cup, frozen, leaf, 190 g

Spinach—From Canned—Creamed ☞ Vitamin K = 583.4 mcg; Serving size: 1 cup, 200 g

Spinach—From Fresh—Creamed ☞ Vitamin K = 582.6 mcg; Serving size: 1 cup, 200 g

Spinach—From Frozen—Creamed ☛ Vitamin K = 652.2 mcg; Serving size: 1 cup, 200 g

Spinach—Frozen Chopped Or Leaf—Cooked Boiled—Drained— With Salt ☛ Vitamin K = 513.7 mcg; Serving size: 1/2 cup, 95 g

Spinach—Frozen Chopped Or Leaf—Cooked Boiled—Drained— Without Salt ☛ Vitamin K = 513.7 mcg; Serving size: 1/2 cup, 95 g

Spinach—Frozen Chopped Or Leaf—Unprepared ☛ Vitamin K = 580.3 mcg; Serving size: 1 cup, 156 g

Spring Onions ☛ Vitamin K = 207 mcg; Serving size: 1 cup, chopped, 100 g

Squash Fritter Or Cake ☛ Vitamin K = 3.1 mcg; Serving size: 1 fritter, 24 g

Squash Spaghetti—Cooked—Cooked—Without Fat ☛ Vitamin K = 1.2 mcg; Serving size: 1 cup, cooked, 155 g

Squash Summer—All Varieties—Cooked Boiled—Drained—With Salt ☛ Vitamin K = 6.3 mcg; Serving size: 1 cup slices, 180 g

Squash Summer Casserole—With Cheese Sauce ☛ Vitamin K = 7.4 mcg; Serving size: 1 cup, 217 g

Squash Summer Casserole—With Rice And Tomato Sauce ☛ Vitamin K = 6.1 mcg; Serving size: 1 cup, 233 g

Squash Summer Casserole—With Tomato And Cheese ☛ Vitamin K = 7.8 mcg; Serving size: 1 cup, 217 g

Squash Summer Crookneck—And Straightneck—Canned—Drained Solid—Without Salt ☛ Vitamin K = 5.9 mcg; Serving size: 1 cup, diced, 210 g

Squash Summer Crookneck—And Straightneck—Cooked Boiled— Drained—With Salt ☛ Vitamin K = 7.9 mcg; Serving size: 1 cup slices, 180 g

Squash Summer Crookneck—And Straightneck—Frozen—Cooked Boiled—Drained—With Salt ☛ Vitamin K = 10.4 mcg; Serving size: 1 cup slices, 192 g

Squash Summer Crookneck—And Straightneck—Frozen—Cooked Boiled—Drained—Without Salt ☛ Vitamin K = 10.4 mcg; Serving size: 1 cup slices, 192 g

Squash Summer Scallop—Cooked Boiled—Drained—With Salt ☛ Vitamin K = 3.2 mcg; Serving size: 1/2 cup slices, 90 g

Squash Summer—Yellow Or Green And Onions—Cooked—Cooked With Fat ☛ Vitamin K = 7 mcg; Serving size: 1 cup, 190 g

Squash Summer—Yellow Or Green And Onions—Cooked—Cooked —Without Fat ☛ Vitamin K = 4.8 mcg; Serving size: 1 cup, 185 g

Squash Summer—Yellow Or Green—Breaded Or Battered Baked ☛ Vitamin K = 5.1 mcg; Serving size: 1 cup, 220 g

Squash Summer—Yellow Or Green—Breaded Or Battered Fried ☛ Vitamin K = 37.4 mcg; Serving size: 1 cup, 220 g

Squash Summer—Yellow Or Green With Tomato Sauce—Cooked— Cooked With Fat ☛ Vitamin K = 9.5 mcg; Serving size: 1 cup, 238 g

Squash Summer—Yellow Or Green With Tomato Sauce—Cooked— Cooked—Without Fat ☛ Vitamin K = 7.7 mcg; Serving size: 1 cup, 233 g

Squash Summer—Yellow Or Green—Cooked—From Canned— Cooked—Without Fat ☛ Vitamin K = 6 mcg; Serving size: 1 cup, 216 g

Squash Summer—Yellow Or Green—Cooked—From Fresh— Cooked—Without Fat ☛ Vitamin K = 6.3 mcg; Serving size: 1 cup, 180 g

Squash Summer—Yellow Or Green—Cooked—From Frozen— Cooked—Without Fat ☛ Vitamin K = 8.5 mcg; Serving size: 1 cup, 180 g

Squash Summer—Zucchini Includes Skin—Cooked Boiled—Drained—With Salt ☛ Vitamin K = 3.8 mcg; Serving size: 1/2 cup slices, 90 g

Squash Summer—Zucchini Includes Skin—Frozen—Cooked Boiled—Drained—With Salt ☛ Vitamin K = 9.4 mcg; Serving size: 1 cup, 223 g

Squash Summer—Zucchini Includes Skin—Frozen—Cooked Boiled—Drained—Without Salt ☛ Vitamin K = 9.4 mcg; Serving size: 1 cup, 223 g

Squash Summer—Zucchini Includes Skin—Frozen—Unprepared ☛ Vitamin K = 4 mcg; Serving size: 1/3 package (10 oz), 95 g

Squash Summer—From Canned—Creamed ☛ Vitamin K = 4.6 mcg; Serving size: 1 cup, 217 g

Squash Summer—From Fresh—Creamed ☛ Vitamin K = 5.2 mcg; Serving size: 1 cup, 217 g

Squash Summer—From Frozen—Creamed ☛ Vitamin K = 7.2 mcg; Serving size: 1 cup, 217 g

Squash Winter All Varieties—Cooked Baked—With Salt ☛ Vitamin K = 9 mcg; Serving size: 1 cup, cubes, 205 g

Squash Winter Baked With Cheese ☛ Vitamin K = 17.2 mcg; Serving size: 1 cup, 224 g

Squash Winter Hubbard Baked—With Salt ☛ Vitamin K = 3.3 mcg; Serving size: 1 cup, cubes, 205 g

Squash Winter Hubbard –Cooked Boiled Mashed—With Salt ☛ Vitamin K = 2.4 mcg; Serving size: 1 cup, mashed, 236 g

Squash Winter Hubbard—Cooked Boiled Mashed—Without Salt ☛ Vitamin K = 2.4 mcg; Serving size: 1 cup, mashed, 236 g

Squash Winter Spaghetti—Cooked Boiled—Drained Or Baked—With Salt ☛ Vitamin K = 1.2 mcg; Serving size: 1 cup, 155 g

Squash Winter Type Baked Fat And Sugar Added In Cooking ☞ Vitamin K = 10.7 mcg; Serving size: 1 cup, cubes, all varieties, 214 g

Squash Winter Type Baked No Fat Or Sugar Added In Cooking ☞ Vitamin K = 9 mcg; Serving size: 1 cup, cubes, all varieties, 205 g

Squash Winter Type Baked No—Cooked With Fat Sugar Added In Cooking ☞ Vitamin K = 8.6 mcg; Serving size: 1 cup, cubes, all varieties, 209 g

Squash Winter Type Mashed Fat And Sugar Added In Cooking ☞ Vitamin K = 12.9 mcg; Serving size: 1 cup, ns as to variety, 257 g

Squash Winter Type Mashed No Fat Or Sugar Added In Cooking ☞ Vitamin K = 10.6 mcg; Serving size: 1 cup, ns as to variety, 240 g

Squash Winter Type Mashed—Cooked With Fat No Sugar Added In Cooking ☞ Vitamin K = 13 mcg; Serving size: 1 cup, ns as to variety, 245 g

Starchy Vegetables Including Tannier White Sweet Potato And Yam No Plantain—Puerto Rican Style ☞ Vitamin K = 3.4 mcg; Serving size: 1 cup, 190 g

Starchy Vegetables Including Tannier White Sweet Potato And Yam With Green Or Ripe Plantains—Puerto Rican Style ☞ Vitamin K = 2.9 mcg; Serving size: 1 cup, 195 g

String Beans (Green) And Potatoes—Cooked—Cooked—Without Fat ☞ Vitamin K = 30.9 mcg; Serving size: 1 cup, 138 g

String Beans (Green) With Almonds—Cooked—Cooked—Without Fat ☞ Vitamin K = 52.3 mcg; Serving size: 1 cup, 122 g

String Beans (Green) With Chickpeas—Cooked—Cooked With Fat ☞ Vitamin K = 48.1 mcg; Serving size: 1 cup, 139 g

String Beans (Green) With Chickpeas—Cooked—Cooked—Without Fat ☞ Vitamin K = 46 mcg; Serving size: 1 cup, 134 g

String Beans (Green) With Onions—Cooked—Cooked—Without Fat ☞ Vitamin K = 44.8 mcg; Serving size: 1 cup, 146 g

String Beans (Green) With Pinto Beans—Cooked—Cooked With Fat ☞ Vitamin K = 48.1 mcg; Serving size: 1 cup, 141 g

String Beans (Green) With Pinto Beans—Cooked—Cooked— Without Fat ☞ Vitamin K = 45.8 mcg; Serving size: 1 cup, 136 g

String Beans (Green) With Spaetzel—Cooked—Cooked With Fat ☞ Vitamin K = 51.2 mcg; Serving size: 1 cup, 152 g

String Beans (Green) With Spaetzel—Cooked—Cooked—Without Fat ☞ Vitamin K = 49 mcg; Serving size: 1 cup, 147 g

String Beans (Green) With Tomatoes—Cooked—Cooked With Fat ☞ Vitamin K = 45.6 mcg; Serving size: 1 cup, 153 g

String Beans (Green) With Tomatoes—Cooked—Cooked—Without Fat ☞ Vitamin K = 43.7 mcg; Serving size: 1 cup, 148 g

String Beans (Green)—Cooked—From Canned With Mushroom Sauce ☞ Vitamin K = 64.8 mcg; Serving size: 1 cup, 228 g

String Beans (Green)—Cooked—From Canned—Cooked—Without Fat ☞ Vitamin K = 59.4 mcg; Serving size: 1 cup, canned, 153 g

String Beans (Green)—Cooked—From Fresh With Mushroom Sauce ☞ Vitamin K = 72.7 mcg; Serving size: 1 cup, 228 g

String Beans (Green)—Cooked—From Fresh—Cooked—Without Fat ☞ Vitamin K = 59.4 mcg; Serving size: 1 cup, fresh, 125 g

String Beans (Green)—Cooked—From Frozen With Mushroom Sauce ☞ Vitamin K = 62 mcg; Serving size: 1 cup, 228 g

String Beans (Green)—Cooked—From Frozen—Cooked—Without Fat ☞ Vitamin K = 51 mcg; Serving size: 1 cup, frozen, 135 g

String Beans (Green)—From Canned—Creamed Or With Cheese Sauce ☞ Vitamin K = 58.4 mcg; Serving size: 1 cup, 228 g

String Beans (Green)—From Fresh—Creamed Or With Cheese Sauce ☞ Vitamin K = 66.6 mcg; Serving size: 1 cup, 228 g

String Beans (Green)—From Frozen—Creamed Or With Cheese Sauce ☞ Vitamin K = 54.7 mcg; Serving size: 1 cup, 228 g

String Beans (Yellow)—Cooked—From Canned—Cooked—Without Fat ☞ Vitamin K = 60 mcg; Serving size: 1 cup, 153 g

String Beans (Yellow)—Cooked—From Fresh—Cooked—Without Fat ☞ Vitamin K = 59.4 mcg; Serving size: 1 cup, 125 g

String Beans (Yellow)—Cooked—From Frozen—Cooked—Without Fat ☞ Vitamin K = 51 mcg; Serving size: 1 cup, 135 g

String Beans (Yellow)—From Canned—Creamed Or With Cheese Sauce ☞ Vitamin K = 58.8 mcg; Serving size: 1 cup, 228 g

String Beans (Yellow)—From Fresh—Creamed Or With Cheese Sauce ☞ Vitamin K = 66.6 mcg; Serving size: 1 cup, 228 g

String Beans (Yellow)—From Frozen—Creamed Or With Cheese Sauce ☞ Vitamin K = 54.7 mcg; Serving size: 1 cup, 228 g

Stuffed Green Pepper—Frozen Meal ☞ Vitamin K = 103.2 mcg; Serving size: 1 meal (14 oz), 397 g

Stuffed Pepper With Meat ☞ Vitamin K = 23.5 mcg; Serving size: 1/2 pepper with filling, 149 g

Stuffed Pepper With Rice And Meat ☞ Vitamin K = 16.4 mcg; Serving size: 1/2 pepper with filling, 149 g

Stuffed Pepper With Rice Meatless ☞ Vitamin K = 21.6 mcg; Serving size: 1/2 pepper with filling, 149 g

Stuffed Tomato With Rice And Meat ☞ Vitamin K = 12.1 mcg; Serving size: 1 tomato with filling, 149 g

Stuffed Tomato With Rice Meatless ☞ Vitamin K = 11.5 mcg; Serving size: 1 tomato with filling, 149 g

Succotash (Corn And Limas)—Frozen—Cooked Boiled—Drained—
With Salt ☞ Vitamin K = 4.6 mcg; Serving size: 1 cup, 170 g

Succotash (Corn And Limas)—Frozen—Cooked Boiled—Drained—
Without Salt ☞ Vitamin K = 4.6 mcg; Serving size: 1 cup, 170 g

Summer Squash ☞ Vitamin K = 3.4 mcg; Serving size: 1 cup, sliced,
113 g

Sun-Dried Hot Chile Peppers ☞ Vitamin K = 40 mcg; Serving size: 1
cup, 37 g

Sun-Dried Tomatoes ☞ Vitamin K = 23.2 mcg; Serving size: 1 cup, 54 g

Sweet Onions ☞ Vitamin K = 0.4 mcg; Serving size: 1 nlea serving,
148 g

Sweet Pickled Cucumbers ☞ Vitamin K = 75.4 mcg; Serving size: 1
cup, chopped, 160 g

Sweet Pickled Relish ☞ Vitamin K = 12.6 mcg; Serving size: 1 tbsp, 15 g

Sweet Potato And Pumpkin Casserole—Puerto Rican Style ☞
Vitamin K = 12.5 mcg; Serving size: 1 cup, 266 g

Sweet Potato Baked—Peel Eaten—Cooked—Without Fat ☞ Vitamin
K = 1.8 mcg; Serving size: 1 small, 80 g

Sweet Potato Baked—Peel Not Eaten—Cooked—Without Fat ☞
Vitamin K = 1.8 mcg; Serving size: 1 small, 80 g

Sweet Potato Boiled—Cooked—Without Fat ☞ Vitamin K = 1.7 mcg;
Serving size: 1 small, 80 g

Sweet Potato Candied ☞ Vitamin K = 2 mcg; Serving size: 1 piece, 45 g

Sweet Potato Casserole Or Mashed ☞ Vitamin K = 4.8 mcg; Serving
size: 1 cup, 250 g

Sweet Potato Fries—From Fresh Baked ☞ Vitamin K = 6.4 mcg;
Serving size: 1 fry, any cut, 50 g

Sweet Potato Fries—From Fresh Fried ☞ Vitamin K = 8.7 mcg; Serving size: 1 fry, any cut, 50 g

Sweet Potato Leaves Squash Leaves Pumpkin Leaves Chrysanthemum Leaves Bean Leaves Or Swamp Cabbage—Cooked—Cooked With Fat ☞ Vitamin K = 70.9 mcg; Serving size: 1 cup, sweet potato leaves, 69 g

Sweet Potato Leaves—Cooked Steamed—With Salt ☞ Vitamin K = 69.5 mcg; Serving size: 1 cup, 64 g

Sweet Potato Leaves—Cooked Steamed—Without Salt ☞ Vitamin K = 69.5 mcg; Serving size: 1 cup, 64 g

Sweet Potato Leaves—Raw ☞ Vitamin K = 105.8 mcg; Serving size: 1 cup, chopped, 35 g

Sweet Potato Yellow Puerto Rican—Cooked ☞ Vitamin K = 2.9 mcg; Serving size: 1 cup, 140 g

Sweet Potato—Canned Syrup Pack—Drained Solids ☞ Vitamin K = 5.1 mcg; Serving size: 1 cup, 196 g

Sweet Potato—Canned Syrup Pack—Solids And Liquids ☞ Vitamin K = 4.8 mcg; Serving size: 1 cup, 228 g

Sweet Potato—Canned Vacuum Pack ☞ Vitamin K = 5.6 mcg; Serving size: 1 cup, mashed, 255 g

Sweet Potato—Canned—Cooked With Fat ☞ Vitamin K = 14.8 mcg; Serving size: 1 cup, pieces, 250 g

Sweet Potato—Canned—Cooked—Without Fat ☞ Vitamin K = 5.5 mcg; Serving size: 1 cup, pieces, 250 g

Sweet Potato—Cooked Baked In Skin Flesh—With Salt ☞ Vitamin K = 2.6 mcg; Serving size: 1 medium (2 inch dia, 5 inch long, raw), 114 g

Sweet Potato—Cooked Boiled Without Skin—With Salt ☞ Vitamin K = 6.9 mcg; Serving size: 1 cup, mashed, 328 g

Sweet Potato—Cooked Candied—Home-Made ☛ Vitamin K = 2.2 mcg; Serving size: 1 piece (2-1/2 inch x 2 inch dia), 105 g

Sweet Potato—Frozen—Cooked Baked—Without Salt ☛ Vitamin K = 4.4 mcg; Serving size: 1 cup, cubes, 176 g

Sweet Potatoes ☛ Vitamin K = 2.4 mcg; Serving size: 1 cup, cubes, 133 g

Sweet Potatoes—French Fried—Frozen As Packaged Salt Added In Processing ☛ Vitamin K = 2.3 mcg; Serving size: 12 fries, 51 g

Sweet Red Bell Peppers ☛ Vitamin K = 7.3 mcg; Serving size: 1 cup, chopped, 149 g

Sweet White Corn ☛ Vitamin K = 0.2 mcg; Serving size: 1 ear, small (5-1/2 inch to 6-1/2 inch long), 73 g

Swiss Chard ☛ Vitamin K = 298.8 mcg; Serving size: 1 cup, 36 g

Tannier Fritters—Puerto Rican Style ☛ Vitamin K = 1.8 mcg; Serving size: 1 fritter (2-1/2" x 1-1/2"x 1/2"), 20 g

Tannier—Cooked ☛ Vitamin K = 2.7 mcg; Serving size: 1 cup, 190 g

Taro ☛ Vitamin K = 1 mcg; Serving size: 1 cup, sliced, 104 g

Taro Baked ☛ Vitamin K = 1.7 mcg; Serving size: 1 cup, 132 g

Taro Leaves—Raw ☛ Vitamin K = 30.4 mcg; Serving size: 1 cup, 28 g

Taro—Cooked—With Salt ☛ Vitamin K = 1.6 mcg; Serving size: 1 cup slices, 132 g

Thistle Leaves—Cooked—Cooked With Fat ☛ Vitamin K = 683.2 mcg; Serving size: 1 cup, 185 g

Thistle Leaves—Cooked—Cooked—Without Fat ☛ Vitamin K = 685.1 mcg; Serving size: 1 cup, 180 g

Tomatillos ☛ Vitamin K = 3.4 mcg; Serving size: 1 medium, 34 g

Tomato And Celery—Cooked—Cooked With Fat ☞ Vitamin K = 23.9 mcg; Serving size: 1 cup, 249 g

Tomato And Celery—Cooked—Cooked—Without Fat ☞ Vitamin K = 21.5 mcg; Serving size: 1 cup, 244 g

Tomato And Corn—Cooked—Cooked With Fat ☞ Vitamin K = 6.2 mcg; Serving size: 1 cup, 247 g

Tomato And Corn—Cooked—Cooked—Without Fat ☞ Vitamin K = 3.6 mcg; Serving size: 1 cup, 242 g

Tomato And Cucumber— Salad Made With Tomato Cucumber— Oil And Vinegar ☞ Vitamin K = 28.9 mcg; Serving size: 1 cup, 159 g

Tomato And Okra—Cooked—Cooked—Without Fat ☞ Vitamin K = 38 mcg; Serving size: 1 cup, 217 g

Tomato And Onion—Cooked—Cooked—Without Fat ☞ Vitamin K = 5.5 mcg; Serving size: 1 cup, 237 g

Tomato And Vegetable Juice—Low Sodium ☞ Vitamin K = 12.8 mcg; Serving size: 1 cup, 242 g

Tomato Aspic ☞ Vitamin K = 4.1 mcg; Serving size: 1 cup, 227 g

Tomato Juice—Canned—With Salt Added ☞ Vitamin K = 5.6 mcg; Serving size: 1 cup, 243 g

Tomato Juice—Canned—Without Salt Added ☞ Vitamin K = 5.6 mcg; Serving size: 1 cup, 243 g

Tomato Products—Canned Puree—With Salt Added ☞ Vitamin K = 8.5 mcg; Serving size: 1 cup, 250 g

Tomato Products—Canned Sauce ☞ Vitamin K = 6.9 mcg; Serving size: 1 cup, 245 g

Tomato Products—Canned Sauce With Mushrooms ☞ Vitamin K = 9.3 mcg; Serving size: 1 cup, 245 g

Tomato Products—Canned Sauce With Onions Green Peppers And Celery ☛ Vitamin K = 9.3 mcg; Serving size: 1 cup, 250 g

Tomato Sauce—Canned—No Salt Added ☛ Vitamin K = 6.9 mcg; Serving size: 1 cup, 245 g

Tomato With Corn And Okra—Cooked—Cooked—Without Fat ☛ Vitamin K = 26.3 mcg; Serving size: 1 cup, 212 g

Tomatoes ☛ Vitamin K = 11.8 mcg; Serving size: 1 cup cherry tomatoes, 149 g

Tomatoes Crushed—Canned ☛ Vitamin K = 6.4 mcg; Serving size: 1/2 cup, 121 g

Tomatoes Green—Cooked—From Fresh ☛ Vitamin K = 17.8 mcg; Serving size: 1 small, 75 g

Tomatoes Red Ripe—Canned Packed In Tomato Juice ☛ Vitamin K = 6.2 mcg; Serving size: 1 cup, 240 g

Tomatoes Red Ripe—Canned Packed In Tomato Juice—No Salt Added ☛ Vitamin K = 7 mcg; Serving size: 1 cup, 240 g

Tomatoes Red Ripe—Canned Stewed ☛ Vitamin K = 6.1 mcg; Serving size: 1 cup, 255 g

Tomatoes Red Ripe—Cooked—With Salt ☛ Vitamin K = 6.7 mcg; Serving size: 1 cup, 240 g

Tomatoes Red—From Fresh Fried ☛ Vitamin K = 15 mcg; Serving size: 1 small, 75 g

Tomatoes—From Fresh Broiled ☛ Vitamin K = 1.4 mcg; Serving size: 1 cherry, 14 g

Tomatoes—From Fresh Scalloped ☛ Vitamin K = 21.9 mcg; Serving size: 1 cup, 235 g

Tomatoes—From Fresh Stewed ☛ Vitamin K = 7.1 mcg; Serving size: 1 tomato, 114 g

Turnip Greens ☛ Vitamin K = 138.1 mcg; Serving size: 1 cup, chopped, 55 g

Turnip Greens And Turnips—Frozen—Cooked Boiled—Drained—With Salt ☛ Vitamin K = 676.6 mcg; Serving size: 1 cup, 163 g

Turnip Greens And Turnips—Frozen—Cooked Boiled—Drained—Without Salt ☛ Vitamin K = 676.6 mcg; Serving size: 1 cup, 163 g

Turnip Greens With Roots—Cooked—From Canned—Cooked With Fat ☛ Vitamin K = 225.3 mcg; Serving size: 1 cup, 168 g

Turnip Greens With Roots—Cooked—From Canned—Cooked—Without Fat ☛ Vitamin K = 223.1 mcg; Serving size: 1 cup, 163 g

Turnip Greens With Roots—Cooked—From Fresh—Cooked With Fat ☛ Vitamin K = 288 mcg; Serving size: 1 cup, 168 g

Turnip Greens With Roots—Cooked—From Fresh—Cooked—Without Fat ☛ Vitamin K = 285.7 mcg; Serving size: 1 cup, 163 g

Turnip Greens With Roots—Cooked—From Frozen—Cooked With Fat ☛ Vitamin K = 676.9 mcg; Serving size: 1 cup, 168 g

Turnip Greens With Roots—Cooked—From Frozen—Cooked—Without Fat ☛ Vitamin K = 672.7 mcg; Serving size: 1 cup, 163 g

Turnip Greens—Canned Reduced Sodium—Cooked—Cooked With Fat Made With Any Type Of Fat ☛ Vitamin K = 458.1 mcg; Serving size: 1 cup, 164 g

Turnip Greens—Canned—No Salt Added ☛ Vitamin K = 413.3 mcg; Serving size: 1 cup, 144 g

Turnip Greens—Cooked Boiled—Drained—With Salt ☛ Vitamin K = 529.3 mcg; Serving size: 1 cup, chopped, 144 g

Turnip Greens—Cooked—From Canned—Cooked—Without Fat ☛ Vitamin K = 453.2 mcg; Serving size: 1 cup, canned, 159 g

Turnip Greens—Cooked—From Fresh—Cooked—Without Fat ☞ Vitamin K = 525.7 mcg; Serving size: 1 cup, fresh, 144 g

Turnip Greens—Cooked—From Frozen—Cooked—Without Fat ☞ Vitamin K = 851.1 mcg; Serving size: 1 cup, frozen, 165 g

Turnip Greens—Frozen—Cooked Boiled—Drained—With Salt ☞ Vitamin K = 425.5 mcg; Serving size: 1/2 cup, 82 g

Turnip Greens—Frozen—Cooked Boiled—Drained—Without Salt ☞ Vitamin K = 851 mcg; Serving size: 1 cup, 164 g

Turnip—Cooked—From Canned—Cooked—Without Fat ☞ Vitamin K = 0.2 mcg; Serving size: 1 cup, pieces, 155 g

Turnip—Cooked—From Fresh—Cooked—Without Fat ☞ Vitamin K = 0.2 mcg; Serving size: 1 cup, pieces, 155 g

Turnip—Cooked—From Frozen—Cooked—Without Fat ☞ Vitamin K = 0.2 mcg; Serving size: 1 cup, pieces, 155 g

Turnips ☞ Vitamin K = 0.1 mcg; Serving size: 1 cup, cubes, 130 g

Turnips—Cooked Boiled—Drained—With Salt ☞ Vitamin K = 0.2 mcg; Serving size: 1 cup, cubes, 156 g

Turnips—From Canned—Creamed ☞ Vitamin K = 1.1 mcg; Serving size: 1 cup, 226 g

Turnips—From Fresh—Creamed ☞ Vitamin K = 1.1 mcg; Serving size: 1 cup, 226 g

Turnips—From Frozen—Creamed ☞ Vitamin K = 1.1 mcg; Serving size: 1 cup, 226 g

Turnips—Frozen—Cooked Boiled—Drained—With Salt ☞ Vitamin K = 0.2 mcg; Serving size: 1 cup, 156 g

Turnips—Frozen—Cooked Boiled—Drained—Without Salt ☞ Vitamin K = 0.2 mcg; Serving size: 1 cup, 156 g

Vegetable And Pasta Combinations—With Cream Or Cheese Sauce

Broccoli—Pasta Carrots—Corn Zucchini Peppers Cauliflower Peas—Cooked ☞ Vitamin K = 42.4 mcg; Serving size: 1 cup, 162 g

Vegetable Combinations—Excluding Carrots—Broccoli—And Dark-Green Leafy;—Cooked—With Cream Sauce ☞ Vitamin K = 23.7 mcg; Serving size: 1 cup, 228 g

Vegetable Combinations—Including Carrots—Broccoli—And/or Dark-Green Leafy;—Cooked—With Cream Sauce ☞ Vitamin K = 68.4 mcg; Serving size: 1 cup, 228 g

Vegetable Combinations—Excluding Carrots—Broccoli—And Dark-Green Leafy;—Cooked With Cheese Sauce ☞ Vitamin K = 23.9 mcg; Serving size: 1 cup, 228 g

Vegetable Combinations—Excluding Carrots—Broccoli—And Dark-Green Leafy;—Cooked With Pasta ☞ Vitamin K = 17.3 mcg; Serving size: 1 cup, 137 g

Vegetable Combinations—Excluding Carrots—Broccoli—And Dark-Green Leafy;—Cooked With Tomato Sauce ☞ Vitamin K = 25.1 mcg; Serving size: 1 cup, 228 g

Vegetable Combinations—Including Carrots—Broccoli—And/or Dark-Green Leafy;—Cooked With Cheese Sauce ☞ Vitamin K = 69.1 mcg; Serving size: 1 cup, 228 g

Vegetable Combinations—Including Carrots—Broccoli—And/or Dark-Green Leafy;—Cooked With Pasta ☞ Vitamin K = 48.6 mcg; Serving size: 1 cup, 137 g

Vegetable Combinations—Including Carrots—Broccoli—And/or Dark-Green Leafy;—Cooked With Tomato Sauce ☞ Vitamin K = 69.3 mcg; Serving size: 1 cup, 228 g

Vegetable Curry ☞ Vitamin K = 123.9 mcg; Serving size: 1 cup, 236 g

Vegetable Juice—Bolthouse Farms Daily Greens ☞ Vitamin K = 284.1 mcg; Serving size: 1 cup, 269 g

Vegetable Juice—Cocktail Low Sodium—Canned ☛ Vitamin K = 15.5 mcg; Serving size: 1 cup, 254 g

Vegetable Juice—Cocktail—Canned ☛ Vitamin K = 15.4 mcg; Serving size: 1 cup, 253 g

Vegetable Stew Without Meat ☛ Vitamin K = 10.8 mcg; Serving size: 1 cup, 239 g

Vegetable Tempura ☛ Vitamin K = 18.1 mcg; Serving size: 1 cup, 63 g

Vegetables Mixed—Corn Lima Beans Peas Green Beans Carrots—Canned—No Salt Added ☛ Vitamin K = 33.1 mcg; Serving size: 1 cup, 182 g

Vegetables Mixed—Canned—Drained Solids ☛ Vitamin K = 29.7 mcg; Serving size: 1 cup, 163 g

Vegetables Mixed—Frozen—Cooked Boiled—Drained—With Salt ☛ Vitamin K = 21.4 mcg; Serving size: 1/2 cup, 91 g

Vegetables Mixed—Frozen—Cooked Boiled—Drained—Without Salt ☛ Vitamin K = 21.4 mcg; Serving size: 1/2 cup, 91 g

Vegetables Stew Type—Cooked—Cooked—Without Fat ☛ Vitamin K = 16.2 mcg; Serving size: 1 cup, 160 g

Wakame ☛ Vitamin K = 0.5 mcg; Serving size: 2 tbsp (1/8 cup), 10 g

Water Chestnut ☛ Vitamin K = 0.5 mcg; Serving size: 1 cup, 158 g

Waterchestnuts Chinese (Matai)—Raw ☛ Vitamin K = 0.2 mcg; Serving size: 1/2 cup slices, 62 g

Waterchestnuts Chinese—Canned—Solids And Liquids ☛ Vitamin K = 0.1 mcg; Serving size: 1/2 cup slices, 70 g

Watercress ☛ Vitamin K = 85 mcg; Serving size: 1 cup, chopped, 34 g

Watercress—Cooked—Cooked With Fat ☛ Vitamin K = 334.3 mcg; Serving size: 1 cup, 142 g

Watercress—Cooked—Cooked—Without Fat ☞ Vitamin K = 340.4 mcg; Serving size: 1 cup, 137 g

Waxgourd—Cooked Boiled—Drained—With Salt ☞ Vitamin K = 4.9 mcg; Serving size: 1 cup, cubes, 175 g

Waxgourd—Cooked Boiled—Drained—Without Salt ☞ Vitamin K = 4.9 mcg; Serving size: 1 cup, cubes, 175 g

White Button Mushrooms ☞ Vitamin K = 0 mcg; Serving size: 1 cup, pieces or slices, 70 g

White Button Mushrooms (Stir-Fried) ☞ Vitamin K = 0 mcg; Serving size: 1 cup sliced, 108 g

Winter Melon—Cooked ☞ Vitamin K = 4.9 mcg; Serving size: 1 cup, 175 g

Winter Squash ☞ Vitamin K = 1.3 mcg; Serving size: 1 cup, cubes, 116 g

Yam ☞ Vitamin K = 3.5 mcg; Serving size: 1 cup, cubes, 150 g

Yam—Cooked Boiled—Drained Or Baked—With Salt ☞ Vitamin K = 3.1 mcg; Serving size: 1 cup, cubes, 136 g

Yam—Cooked Puerto Rican ☞ Vitamin K = 3.2 mcg; Serving size: 1 cup, 140 g

Yambean (Jicama)—Raw ☞ Vitamin K = 0.4 mcg; Serving size: 1 cup slices, 120 g

Yellow Onions ☞ Vitamin K = 18.8 mcg; Serving size: 1 cup chopped, 87 g

Yellow Snap Beans ☞ Vitamin K = 43.2 mcg; Serving size: 1 cup 1/2 inch pieces, 100 g

Yellow Sweet Corn ☞ Vitamin K = 0.4 mcg; Serving size: 1 cup, 145 g

Yuca Fries ☞ Vitamin K = 25.1 mcg; Serving size: 1 cup, 140 g

Zucchini ☞ Vitamin K = 5.3 mcg; Serving size: 1 cup, chopped, 124 g

ABOUT THE AUTHOR

"Dr. H. Maher" is a joint pen name under which Dr. Y. Naitlho, PharmD, and H. Naitlho, MS/MBA, co-write books.

Dr. Y. Naitlho PharmD has over 25 years of pharmacy practice, applied nutrition research, and writing. He is currently a pharmacist and health and nutrition writer. He is the author of several books in the field of food science and human nutrition, and applied nutrition.

Dr. Y. Naitlho received his Doctor of Pharmacy from Perm State Pharmaceutical Academy. As a pharmacist and nutrition professional, He ensures that book design meets readers' dynamic learning needs and that content meets reliability and integrity standards.

H. Naitlho has over 30 years of engineering practice and science and engineering Research. He is the author of several books in the field of business management and coauthor of numerous books in food science and human nutrition, food engineering, and applied nutrition.

H. Naitlho holds an Engineering degree from the École Supérieure d'Aéronautique et de l'Espace (Sup'Aéro), an Engineering degree from the École de l'Air (Salon de Provence) and has an MBA from Laureate International Universities, a post-graduate degree in Automatics from Paul Sabatier University, and a further post-graduate degree in Mechanics from Aix Marseille University.

H. Naitlho brings the engineering mindset and scientific rigor. He consistently refines ideas, analyzes data, and carries consistency and a great sense of detail to their work.